QUALITY OF LIFE AFTER OPEN HEART SURGERY

Developments in Cardiovascular Medicine

VOLUME 132

The titles published in this series are listed at the end of this volume.

Quality of Life after Open Heart Surgery

edited by

PAUL J. WALTER
University School of Medicine Antwerp,
Antwerp, Belgium

With a foreword by

NANETTE K. WENGER
Emory University School of Medicine,
Atlanta, Georgia, USA

Springer Science+Business Media, B.V.

Library of Congress Cataloging-in-Publication Data

Quality of life after open heart surgery / edited by Paul J. Walter ;
  with a foreword by Nanette K. Wenger.
      p.   cm. -- (Developments in cardiovascular medicine ; v. 132)
    Includes bibliographical references and index.
    ISBN 978-0-7923-1580-3   ISBN 978-94-011-2640-3 (eBook)
    DOI 10.1007/978-94-011-2640-3
    1. Heart--Surgery--Patients--Rehabilitation--Congresses.
  2. Health status indicators--Congresses.   I. Walter, P. J. (Paul
  J.), 1935-   . II. Series.
    [DNLM: 1. Heart Surgery--congresses. 2. Postoperative Period-
  -congresses. 3. Quality of Life--congresses.   W1 DE99VME v.132 /
  WG 169 Q108]
  RD598.Q35 1992
  617.4'1203--dc20
  DNLM/DLC
  for Library of Congress   91-46511

ISBN 978-0-7923-1580-3

Cover illustration by E. Winkel. Reproduced with permission.

Table of contents

Preface by Paul J. Walter   xi

Foreword by Nanette K. Wenger   xv

List of contributors   xix

1. Quality of life: Why the burgeoning interest in the clinical and research
   cardiology communities?   1
   by Nanette K. Wenger

Part One: Quality of life after heart valve replacement

A. *Physiological state*

2. Results after biological heart valve replacement   9
   by Donald N. Ross
3. Quality of life after mitral valve repair   13
   by John Y. M. Relland
4. Quality of life and prognosis following heart valve replacement   19
   by Dieter Horstkotte, Hagen D. Schulte, Wolfgang. Bircks and Bodo E. Strauer

B. *Intellectual functioning*

5. Cognitive function before and after cardiac surgery: A comparison of cardiac
   valvular replacement and coronary artery bypass surgery   39
   by Allen E. Willner
6. Neuropsychologic outcome after heart valve replacement   47
   by Kyösti A. Sotaniemi

C. *Emotional state*

7. Psychosocial state of patients after heart valve surgery   63
   by C. David Jenkins

8. Emotional state of patients one year after heart valve replacement; clinical, functional and psychological correlates   71
   by M. Bullinger and D. Naber

D. *General satisfaction*

9. Aspects of quality of life in patients with mechanical heart valves   91
   by Lars. I. Thulin

E. *Concluding remarks*

Quality of life after heart valve replacement   101
by D. Horstkotte

Part Two: Quality of life after coronary bypass surgery

A. *Physiological state*

10. Morbidity and mortality after myocardial revascularization in patients with ischemic
    heart disease   107
    by W. J. Keon and S. C. Menzies
11. Long-term results of patients after coronary artery bypass surgery   115
    by Charles J. Mullany and Bernard J. Gersh
12. Comprehensive cardiac care and quality of life in patients after surgical revasculariz-
    ation   133
    by Jan J. Kellermann

B. *Intellectual functioning*

13. The intellectual function of patients after coronary bypass surgery   141
    by Pamela J. Shaw
14. Perceived and assessed cognitive function following coronary artery bypass surgery
    – mechanisms and intervention   155
    by Stanton Newman

C. *Emotional state*

15. Psychological status of patients before and after coronary bypass surgery   169
    by H. Boudrez, J. Denollet, B. J. Amsel, G. de Backer, P. J. Walter,
    J. De Beule and R. Mohan
16. The emotional state of patients after coronary bypass surgery   177
    by Elizabeth Lorna Cay and Aine O'Rourke

17. Clinical significance of research on quality of life after coronary artery surgery 185
    by Richard Mayou
18. Psychological reactions to open heart surgery: results of a quantitative and qualitative analysis of the recovery process 193
    by W. Langosch and H-P. Schmoll-Flockerzie

D. *Performance of social roles*

19. Is employment after coronary bypass surgery a measure of the patient's quality of life? 203
    by Paul J. Walter and B. J. Amsel
20. The relationship between medical and occupational rehabilitation in two cohorts of coronary artery bypass patients ten years apart 215
    by Uta Gerhardt
21. Factors influencing quality of life in CABG: a prospective study 227
    by Vadim P. Zaitsev, Tatyana A. Aivazyan, Nataliya I. Gracheva and Dimitry S. Dekin
22. Changes of coronary risk factors in women after elective coronary bypass surgery 235
    by Frank Loskot, Bernd Hartmann, Petrus Novotny and Nikolas Mouselimis

E. *Summary*

Quality of life after coronary bypass surgery 245
by Bernard J. Gersh

Part Three: Quality of life after surgical correction of congenital heart disease

A. *Physiological state*

23. Quality of life 30 to 36 years after closure of isolated ventricular septal defects in 341 patients 253
    by C. Walton Lillehei, Ceeya Patton and James H. Moller
24. Long-term results after atrial correction of transposition of the great vessels 267
    by Marko Turina, Miralem Pasic, Monika Fry and Ludwig von Segesser
25. Congenital heart disease: an analytic approach to functional outcome after open heart surgery 277
    by Catherine A. Neill and Edward B. Clark
26. Quality of life of patients after 'corrective' open heart surgery for congenital heart defects 293
    by F. J. Meijboom and J. Hess
27. Lung function in children after heart surgery 303
    by Milan Šamánek, A. Zapletal, J. Šulc and B. Hučín

B. *Intellectual functioning*

28. Psychointellectual performance after correction of complex congenital heart defects   315
by H. C. Kallfelz, H. Kaemmerer, I. Luhmer, H. Lacher, M. Anacker and
P. Wietzke

C. *Emotional state*

29. Psychosocial aspects of congenital heart disease in children, adolescents and adults   325
by Elisabeth M. W. J. Utens

D. *Performance of social roles*

30. Psychosocial development during school period of children operated for
transposition of the great arteries   335
by E. Stucki, F. P. Stocker, H. Hämmerli, V. Rüfenacht, M. Stucki, J. W. Weber
and P. Schüpbach

E. *General satisfaction*

31. Quality of life after surgical correction of congenital heart disease: the parents'
point of view   347
by M. Dhont, E. De Wit, H. Verhaaren and D. Matthys
32. The role of a parents' organization   355
by R. P. Kamphuis
33. Pediatric heart transplantation: the recipient's perspective   363
by Kathy S. Lawrence, F. Jay Fricker and Susan Cardillo
34. Quality of life of children having undergone heart transplantation   371
by J. Kachaner, J. Le Bidois, D. Sidi, J. F. Piéchaud and P. Vouhé

F. *Summary*

Quality of life after surgical correction of congenital heart disease   383
by Franco P. Stocker

Part Four: Quality of life after heart transplantation

A. *Physiological state*

35. Long-term results: morbidity and mortality of patients after heart transplantation   389
by C. Cabrol, I. Gandjbakhch, A. Pavie, V. Bors, Ph. Leger, E. Vassier,
J. P. Levaseur, M. Desruennes and A. Cabrol

36. Quality of life of patients on LVAD support   397
    by Nancy L. Abow-Awdi and O. H. Frazier
37. Physiological and psychological benefits of exercise rehabilitation after cardiac
    transplantation   403
    by Terence Kavanagh

B. *Intellectual functioning*

38. Neuropsychological function before and after cardiac transplantation   419
    by R. A. Bornstein, R. C. Starling and P. D. Myerowitz

C. *Emotional state*

39. Long-term follow-up of the emotional adjustment of patients after heart trans-
    plantation   427
    by Brett Jones, Frances Taylor, K. Downs and P. Spratt
40. The emotional state of the individual after heart transplantation   439
    by Francois M. Mai and F. Neil McKenzie
41. Psychological well-being of heart transplant patients – cross-sectional and longitudi-
    nal results   445
    by M. Bullinger, C. E. Angermann and B. M. Kemkes
42. Psychosocial outcome after heart transplantation   457
    by G. Magni and G. Borgherini

D. *Performance of social roles*

43. Psychosocial aspects of heart transplantation: a comparative analysis   469
    by Roger W. Evans
44. Changes in partnership after cardiac transplantation   483
    by A. Grundböck, B. Bunzel and M. T. Schubert
45. Quality of life before and after heart transplantation   491
    by N. Caine, L. Sharples and J. Wallwork

E. *General satisfaction*

46. Quality of life and satisfaction after heart transplantation   501
    by B. Bunzel, A. Grundböck and G. Wollenek
47. Quality of life after open heart surgery: strategies to improve quality of life after
    heart transplantation   507
    by Peter A. Shapiro

F. *Summary*

Quality of life after heart transplantation   519
by Peter A. Shapiro

Index   523

Preface

In the early fifties, the outlook for a heart patient, whether young or old, was dismal. Medical treatment was often unable to reduce symptoms or prevent impending death, and the risks of surgery clearly appeared prohibitive. Tribute must be given to the ingenuity and daring of surgeons who then pioneered the advent of cardiopulmonary bypass and hypothermia to facilitate open heart surgery. With further phenomenal advances in all spheres of this challenging field, it has since saved millions of lives and the current state of the art practice is associated with routine success. However, of late, success has begun to mean more than mere operative survival or even long-term survival. The question in the nineties is what kind of life will be possible for the patient after one or the other mode of treatment? Is there a continuation of physical complaints, or a curb on intended activities such as going out to work or to play? Does the sickness interfere with personal relationships and leaves the patient dependent and depressed? Has the operation been a satisfying experience? Considering the increasing need for cost-effective allocation of health care resources, and because open heart surgery is expensive, although common, its real outcome must be judged on the lasting overall benefit it leaves for the patient.

This book comprises the 51 papers presented at the international symposium 'Quality of Life after Open Heart Surgery' which was held at Antwerp, Belgium, from 16 to 18 May 1991. Cardiologists, cardiac surgeons, psychologists, occupational physicians, and general practitioners from several countries participated in a team commitment to explore the quality of life of patients who have undergone open heart surgery.

Although a better quality of life had been the colloquial slogan of every socio-political system since ancient times, the inclusion of 'Quality of Life' as a scientific entity in medical literature occurred only 15 years ago. Awareness spread by the World Health Organisation that health is not just absence of disease but soundness of body and mind, alerted clinicians to the personal and social effects of treatment, as these were often more crucial to the ultimate prognosis than the treatment itself. Recent recognition that the

Paul J. Walter (ed.): Quality of Life after Open Heart Surgery, xi–xiv.
© 1992 Kluwer Academic Publishers.

primary goal of all forms of therapy is not just prolonging life, but improving the quality of life, has forced analysis of what constitutes quality of life, a concept whose structure pervades all walks of life and eludes definition. Global well being, happiness, morale, vitality, fullness of social life, and satisfaction must be integrated and assessed for the effects of the disease and the therapy, in the context of specific personality traits, attitudes to life, family situation, and socio-economic and political freedom. A growing interest in research on this subject has led to a clearer understanding of the components which come to determine quality of a patient's life, and how they can be measured in a reproducible manner so that valid comparisons can be made.

Keeping these recommendations of analysing quality of life within the context of patients who have undergone open heart surgery, it seemed appropriate to me to separate the influence of various forms of open heart surgery into five aspects of life which can comprehensively reflect the quality of life outcome of the operation. These five 'components' are (1) *Physiological state*, which summarises the traditionally reported incidence of operative mortality and morbidity, objectively and subjectively measured physical capacity, and the residual symptoms, treatment and long-term survival. (2) *Intellectual functioning* relates to the psychoneurolgocial deficit in memory, reasoning or judgement because of cerebral microembolism and hypo-perfusion during cardiopulmonary bypass. (3) *Emotional state* pertains to affective well-being, psychological distress measured particularly in scales of depression and anxiety, and spontaneous feeling of happiness. (4) *Performance of social roles* is assessed by the closeness of ties with the spouse and the family, visits to friends or relatives, going to work, and participation in community organisations. Determinants of this component are the patient's own physical, cognitive, and psychological well-being, as well as the chance to perform these roles provided or denied by family members or society. Further, this component influences the emotional state of the patient. (5) *General satisfaction* involves judgement by the patients about their physical and mental health, and the success they have had in the fulfillment of their everyday needs and long-term inner goals.

In the four parts of this book, these components of quality of life are separately analysed after four different kinds of open heart operations, i.e., after heart valve replacement, after coronary artery bypass surgery, after surgery for congenital heart disease, and after heart transplantation.

This book thus offers a holistic scope of quality of life, with an integration of all its components, as experienced by patients after different forms of open heart surgery. Earlier studies of open heart surgery patients have collected isolated medical information regarding late survival, symptoms, and physical capacity. Substantial but scattered data also exist on the mental abilities, emotional state, return to work, leisure-time activities, and personal, familial, and marital relationships before and after various operations, i.e., these represent only partial aspects of the term quality of life. Although almost all of these components, after the four types of open heart surgery, had been investigated to some extent by various experienced teams, this symposium (and book) brought the inter-relation of their work into focus.

As a result, some common strategies emerged which have been found to improve the quality of life of patients undergoing all kinds of open heart surgery. These include identification and earlier operation of premorbid personalities, psychological counselling before and after the operation, explanation of true risks and postoperative abilities, instruction to the family in change of roles, stressing the importance of returning to normal activities in education, employment, and society, financial support through health insurance to cover the high cost of open heart surgery, and formulating socioeconomic policies which encourage returning to work. Strategies specific to the different operations include: for heart valve replacement, patients must participate in deciding the kind of prosthesis according to their life-style and anticoagulation schedules must be improved and internationally standardised; coronary bypass patients benefit broadly through a dietary, exercise, and no-smoking rehabilitation. For congenital heart disease, emphasis was laid on the need to educate parents about the disease, the importance of open discussion between parents, the patient, and the pediatric cardiologist, and the function of parent self-help groups. For heart transplantation patients, the support of a cohesive family and of trained social workers before and after the operation can help the patient in adapting to the magnitude of the event.

The book will be of special interest to all those involved in comprehensive cardiac rehabilitation of patients undergoing open heart surgery, e.g., cardiologists, cardiac surgeons, psychologists, social workers, and general physicians. It is also intended to act as a reference guide to physicians, nurses, and para-medical staff involved in the care, general well-being, and occupational reintegration of these patients.

Heart patient groups, such as heart transplant patient groups and parent organisations of children with congenital heart disease, may find reassuring information and several useful suggestions, not only for the patients but also their spouses and their families, in the book. Health policy planners, like the WHO, and those responsible for allocating the budget to various forms of therapy, have also been interested in propagating the 'quality of life' aspect of medical treatment. Most importantly, the book intends to shift the attention to patient satisfaction, and to relieve the unseen mental anguish of patients in day-to-day clinical practice, which had hitherto been overlooked in counting the years of survival achieved by surgery.

I would like to thank Dr Nanette K. Wenger for accepting the task of being Honorary President of the symposium and for validating the value of the book through writing the Foreword. To all the authors who have contributed manuscripts and to those several sponsors whose names are not separately mentioned here, I express my deep gratitude, because without their help, the symposium or the book would not have been possible. Also, I thank Kluwer Academic Publishers for putting this book into print in such a thoughtful way.

PAUL J. WALTER

Foreword

Science has been described as the search for truth. Progress in this task is frequently accelerated when scientists from differing disciplines, in this instance a variety of specialists involved in the surgical care of patients with cardiovascular disease, meet to share newly acquired knowledge, to define areas of consensus and aspects with a clear need for additional information, and to display opportunities for cooperation in the acquisition of these data. The science of open heart surgery, in particular the exploration and assessment of its outcomes, has been propelled forward by Dr Paul J. Walter's organization of the spectacular 1991 international symposium, 'Quality of Life after Open Heart Surgery', in Antwerp, Belgium, and the subsequent publication of this volume.

The repeatedly emphasized recognition that virtually all open heart surgical procedures are palliative, mandates appreciation of the consequences of each procedure, its subsequent actual and feared complications, the requirements for care, and the overall impact on the subsequent quality of the postoperative patient's life. Equally exciting was the congruence expressed both by the cardiovascular surgical pioneers – and their medical counterparts – that serial and multifactorial outcome assessments were requisite, given the half-century of progress since the initial cardiac surgical corrections were undertaken for congenital heart disease. Surgery for congenital heart disease using extracorporeal circulation and surgery for heart valve replacement are now in the fourth decade; for coronary artery bypass surgery in the third decade of experience; and the newest of the undertakings – cardiac transplantation, has over two decades of experience.

Despite ample evidence of the high overall beneficial effects of most contemporary cardiovascular open heart surgical procedures, high priority was given to investigation of the impact of cardiopulmonary bypass – independent of the specific surgical procedure – on both short-term and late postoperative cognition and emotional function. Neuropsychologic deficits, presumably related to intraoperative microemboli to the brain, and more prominent at early age, mandate undertaking more precise mechanistic delin-

Paul J. Walter (ed.): Quality of Life after Open Heart Surgery, xv–xviii.
© 1992 Kluwer Academic Publishers.

eations needed for the development of preventive strategies and technology. Defined multifaced predictors of successful outcomes could form the basis for other recommendations for improved care; interventions could then be undertaken to favorably alter adverse predictors. The data bases underlying development of contemporary guidelines for cardiovascular open heart surgical interventions, derived from randomized clinical trials and from registry studies, related predominantly and appropriately to relevant mortal and morbid events. Guidelines for additional components of perioperative and late postoperative management in clinical practice will require comparable compilations of information, many related to life quality issues; however, these indices of quality of life are far more likely to vary among differing national social welfare and health care systems and in populations with heterogeneous cultural attributes. The patients' perceptions of health and disease, important contributors to outcome, are likely to have substantial sociocultural variations as well.

With expansion of the elderly population worldwide and their concomitant high prevalence of advanced and often highly symptomatic cardiovascular disease, those quality of life variables related to meaningful prolongation of life at advanced age must be systematically examined, given the limited potential to prolonged survival in elderly populations, coupled with their amply documented excess of morbidity. Focus on those aspects that give meaning to life at advanced age can contribute to resolving the complex ethical and socioeconomic decisions that confront all health care systems, faced with expanding expensive cardiovascular technology increasingly applied to a growing aged population. This increase in the numbers of elderly and otherwise high-risk patients who present for open heart surgical interventions will likely require expansion of the life quality attributes examined to address specific problems and needs of these newer cardiac surgical populations; these evaluations deserve particular emphasis, because of the consistently greater benefit derived from favorable interventions in populations at increased risk. Technologic advances in cardiovascular surgery and the increasing availability of less invasive therapeutic modalities will require that, given comparable resulting procedural morbidity and mortality, other outcome variables be compared with equal precision and rigor, with emphasis on those outcomes desired and valued by specific subgroups of high-risk patients and by individual high-risk patients.

Standardized performance assessments emanating from cohorts of children with surgically-corrected cardiac defects currently reaching adult life are only initially appearing; and data regarding their resultant life quality in mature years must be awaited (and corrected for extracardiac variables, particularly comorbid congenital defects). Survival, the need for reoperation, the occurrence of sudden death, and persisting symptoms provide only the gross brushstrokes to delineate the spectrum of outcome measures. Perceived self-image and health status; physical function; intellective and emotional function; education, occupation, and family life; and overall satisfaction with lifestyle constitute other outcome variables (that should be determined for families as well as for patients). These latter aspects may elucidate more subtle differences related to the timing of operations, operative techniques, issues of comorbidity and the like; and may help define more precise recommendations for surgery as well as guidelines for early and late postoperative care and counseling. For example, in the 1954–1960 University of Minnesota ventricular septal defect repair cohort, the above average educational achievements, the rewarding occupations that correlated with educational status, and the satisfactory reproductive histories provided an added positive dimension to previously available survival data, all of which have likely improved with the dramatic surgical and perioperative technologic advances. Comparable data collection is rapidly expanding for open heart surgical corrections of more complex cyanotic hypoxemic congenital cardiac defects, where associated intellectual impairment and other less well defined aspects of cerebral dysfunction must be systematically explored.

Along the over 16 000 heart transplantations performed worldwide for end stage cardiac disease, extensive multifaceted pretransplantation evaluation is undertaken of both patient and family owing to the anticipated lifelong burden of postoperative care; thus far more life quality data are currently available for this fledgling, yet most challenging procedure, in the spectrum of open heart surgery. Major attention has been accorded psychologic outcomes and social relationships, in addition to the usual occupational and independence assessments, because of concerns in these spheres related to the challenges of a transplanted heart and its care. Improvements in techniques and procedures for detecting and controlling transplant rejection, in mechanical circulatory support devices as bridges to initial and retransplantation procedures, and in long-term complications of immunosuppression, to name a few, have characterized the evolution of this procedure; but added problems have become evident as survival has lengthened, now a median of five years. The dramatic life quality improvement described postoperatively should not be surprising, given the terminally ill population at baseline, but maintenance of life satisfaction has appeared equally adequate to favorable. Nevertheless, identification of components that impose limitations, including insurance and other social welfare aspects, should lead to strategies to improve these outcomes. The excellence of education/employment/life status components likely reflects substantially the complexity and intensity of the preprocedural screening; however, is this screening adequate, excessive, or do additional aspects warrant examination to define the personal and family resources needed to cope with the demanding postoperative management, the psychologic burden, or to define additional rehabilitative needs? Heart transplantation in the pediatric age group requires a far more extensive and interdisciplinary range of assessments that should be planned prospectively; these relate to childhood development, to adolescence, to potential educational and occupational discriminations, to uncertainty about prognosis, to concerns about reproductive issues, and to specific later life transplantation-associated illnesses – coronary atherosclerosis, malignancies, etc.

The quality of life research agenda charted at this symposium, coupled with the currently available and newly compiled life quality data that can guide contemporary clinical cardiovascular decisions and care, should serve to enhance for patients the increasingly favorable mortality and morbidity outcomes characteristic of open heart surgery as we approach the twenty-first century.

NANETTE K. WENGER, MD

List of contributors

R. A. BORNSTEIN
Ass. Professor of Psychiatry, Neuropsychology Laboratory, The Ohio State University, 473 West 12th Avenue, COLUMBUS, OH 43210-1228, U.S.A.
Co-authors: R. C. Starling and P. D. Myerowitz

H. BOUDREZ
Cardiac Rehabilitation Centre, University Hospital, De Pintelaan 185, B-9000 GENT, Belgium.
Co-authors: J. Denellet, B. J. Amsel, G. de Backer, P. J. Walter, J. De Beule and R. Mohan

MONIKA BULLINGER
Institute of Medical Psychology, Ludwig-Maximilians University München, Goethestrasse 31, DW-8000 MÜNCHEN 2, Germany.
Co-author Chapter 8: D. Naber
Co-authors Chapter 4: Christiane E. Angerman and Bernard M. Kemkes

BRIGITTA BUNZEL
II University Clinic – Surgery, University Hospital Vienna, Spitalgasse 23, A-1090 VIENNA, Austria.
Co-authors: A. Gründbock and G. Wollenek

C. CABROL
Department of Cardiovascular Surgery, Hospital la Pitié-Salpétrière, 47–83, Boulevard de l'Hôspital, F-75651 PARIS Cedex 13, France.
Co-authors: I. Gandjbakhoh, A. Pavie, V. Bors, Ph. Leger, E. Vassier, J. P. Levaiseur, M. Desruennes and A. Cabrol

NOREEN CAINE
Transplant Unit, Papworth Hospital, Papworth Everard, CAMBRIDGE
CB3 8RE, U.K.
Co-authors: L. Sharples and J. Wallwork

ELIZABETH LORNA CAY
Rehabilitation Medicine Unit, Astley Ainslie Hospital, Grange Loan, EDIN-
BURGH EH9 2HL, U.K.
Co-author: Aine O'Rourke

MARLEEN DHONDT
Children's Clinic, University Hospital, De Pintelaan 185, B-9000 GENT,
Belgium.
Co-authors: E. De Wit, H. Verhaaren and D. Matthys

ROGER W. EVANS
Senior Research Scientist, Health and Population Research Center, Battelle-
Seattle Research Center, 4000 N.E. 41st Street, SEATTLE, WA 98105,
U.S.A.

O. H. FRAZIER
Texas Heart Institute, P.O. Box 20345, HOUSTON, TX 77225-0345, U.S.A.
Co-author: Nancy L. Abow-Awdi

UTA GERHARDT
Medical and Sociology Unit, Justus Liebig Medical School, Friedrichstrasse
24, DW-6300 GIESSEN, Germany.

BERNARD J. GERSH
Division of Cardiovascular Disease, Mayo Clinic, 200 First Street, SW1,
ROCHESTER, MN 55905, U.S.A.

ALICE GRUNDBÖCK
II University Clinic of Surgery, General Hospital Vienna, Spitalgasse 23,
A-1090 VIENNA, Austria.
Co-authors: B. Bunzel and M. T. Schubert

DIETER HORSTKOTTE
Division of Cardiology, Pneumology & Angiology, Heinrich-Heine-Univer-
sity of Dusseldorf, Moorenstrasse 5, DW-4000 DUSSELDORF, Germany.

C. DAVID JENKINS
Department of Preventive Medicine and Community Health, Department

of Psychiatry & Behavioral Sciences, University of Texas Medical Branch, GALVESTON, TX 77550, U.S.A.

BRETT M. JONES
National Cardiac Transplant Unit, St. Vincent's Hospital, Victoria Street, DARLINGHURST NSW 2010, Australia.
Co-authors: Frances Taylor, K. Downs and P. Spratt

J. KACHANER
Children's Hospital, 149, Rue des Sevres, F-75730 PARIS Cedex 15, France.
Co-authors: J. Le Bidois, D. Sidi, J. F. Pléchaud and P. Vouhé

H. KALLFELLZ
Department of Pedriatic Cardiology, Medical University, P.O. Box 610180, DW-3000 HANNOVER 61, Germany.
Co-author: H. Kaemmerer

R. P. KAMPHUIS
Department of Pediatric Cardiology, University Hospital Leiden, P.O. Box 9600, 2300 RC LEIDEN, The Netherlands.

TERENCE KAVANAGH
Medical Director, Toronto Rehabilitation Center, University of Toronto, 345 Rumsey Road, TORONTO, Ontario, Canada M4G 1R5.

JAN J. KELLERMANN
Sackler School of Medicine, Tel Aviv University, The Chain Sheba Medical Center, TEL HASHOMER 52621, Israel.

W. J. KEON
Director General, Heart Institute, Ottawa Civic Hospital, 1053 Carling Avenue, OTTAWA, Ontario, Canada K1Y 4E9.
Co-author: S. C. Menzies

W. LANGOSCH
Benedikt Cross, Rehabilitation Centre, Sudring 15, DW-7812 BAD KROZINGEN, Germany.
Co-author: H-P. Schmoll-Flockerzie

KATHY S. LAWRENCE
Division of Cardiology, Children's Hospital of Pittsburgh, One Children's Place, 3705 Fifth Avenue at DeSoto, PITTSBURGH, PA 15213, U.S.A.
Co-authors: F. Jay Fricker and Susan Cardillo

C. WALTON LILLEHEI
Professor of Surgery, 73, Otis Lane, ST. PAUL, MN 55104, U.S.A.
Co-authors: Ceeya Patton and James H. Moller

FRANK LOSKOT
Centre for Cardiology Rotenburg, Panoramastrasse, DW-6442 ROTEN-BURG/Fulda, Germany.
Co-authors: Bernd Hartmann, Petrus Novotny and Niklas Mouselimis

GUIDO MAGNI
European Clinical Research and Development, Wyeth Ayerst, 6, Rue Clisson, F-75013 PARIS, France.
Co-author: G. Borgherini

FRANCOIS M. MAI
Chief, Department of Psychiatry, Ottawa General Hospital, University of Ottawa, 501, Smyth, OTTAWA, Ontario, Canada K1H 8L6.
Co-author: F. Neil Mckenzie

RICHARD MAYOU
Clinical Reader in Psychiatry, Department of Psychiatry, Department of Psychiatry, Warneford University Hospital, OXFORD OX3 7JX, U.K.

F. J. MEIJBOOM
Department of Cardiology, Sophia Children's Hospital, Gordeweg 160, 3038 GE ROTTERDAM, The Netherlands.
Co-author: John Hess

CHARLES J. MULLANY
Division of Cardiothoracic Surgery, Mayo Clinic, 200 First Street SW, ROCHESTER, MN 55905, U.S.A.
Co-author: Bernard J. Gersh

CATHERINE A. NEILL
Professor of Pedriatics, Brady 516, Johns Hopkins Hospital, Helen B. Taussig Childrens Heart Center, 600, North Wolfe Street, BALTIMORE, MD 21205, U.S.A.
Co-author: Edward B. Clark

STANTON NEWMAN
Department of Psychiatry, UCMSM, Wolfson Building, Middlesex Hospital, Mortimer Street, LONDON W1A 8AA, U.K.

JOHN Y. M. RELLAND
Attending Surgeon, American Hospital of Paris, P.O. Box 109, Boulevard
Victor Hugo, F-92202 NEUILLY Cedex, France.

DONALD N. ROSS
Consultant Cardiac Surgeon, 25, Upper Wimpole Street, LONDON W1M
7TA, U.K.

MILAN SAMÁNEK
Director, Centre for Cardiology, University Hospital Motol, CSFR-150 18
PRAGUE 5, Czechoslovakia.
Co-authors: A. Zapletal, J. Šulc and B. Hučín

PETER A. SHAPIRO
Department of Psychiatry, Columbia University College, Presbyterian Hospital, 622, West 168th Street, Box 427, NEW YORK, NY 10032, U.S.A.

PAMELA J. SHAW
First Assistant in Clinical Neuroscience, University of Newcastle upon Tyne,
and Royal Victoria Infirmary, Queen Victoria Road, NEWCASTLE UPON
TYNE NE1 4LP, U.K.

KYÖSTI A. SOTANIEMI
Assistant Professor, Department of Neurology, University of Oulu, SF-90220
OULU, Finland.

FRANCO P. STOCKER
Division of Paediatric Cardiology, Children's Clinic and Polyclinic, Medical
University, Freiburgstrasse, CH-3010 BERN, Switzerland.

E. STUCKI
Division of Paediatric Cardiology, Children's Clinic and Policlinic, Medical
University, Freiburgstrasse, CH-3010 BERN, Switzerland.
Co-authors: F. P. Stocker, H. Hämmerli, V. Rütenacht, M. Stucki, J. W.
Weber and P. Schüpback

LARS I. THULIN
Department of Thoracic Surgery, University Hospital, S-221 85 LUND,
Sweden.

MARKO TURINA
Clinic for Cardiovascular Surgery, University Hospital Zürich, Rämisstrasse
100, CH-8091 ZURICH, Switzerland.
Co-authors: Miralem Pasic, Monika Fry and Ludwig von Segesser

ELISABETH M. W. J. UTENS
Department of Child Psychiatry, Sophia Children's Hospital, University of
Rotterdam, Gordelweg 160, Rotterdam, The Netherlands.

PAUL J. WALTER
Professor of Cardiac Surgery, University of Antwerp
Head, Department of Cardiovascular Surgery, University Hospital Antwerp,
Wilrijkstraat 10, B-2650 ANTWERP/Edegem, Belgium
Co-author: B. J. Amsel

NANETTE K. WENGER
Director, Cardiac Clinics, Emory University School of Medicine, Thomas
K. Glenn Memorial Building, 69 Butler Street, S.E., ATLANTA, GA 30303,
U.S.A.

ALLEN E. WILLNER
Department of Psychiatry, Hillside Hospital, Long Island Jewish Medical
Center, P.O. Box 38, GLEN OAKS, NY 11004, U.S.A.

VADIM P. ZAITSEV
Head, Department for Psychosocial Rehabilitation, The USSR Research
Centre for Medical Rehabilitation and Physical Therapy, Kalinina Prospekt,
50, 121099 MOSCOW, Russia.
Co-authors: Tatyana A. Aivazyan, Nataliya I. Gracheva and Dimitry S.
Dekin.

1. Quality of life: Why the burgeoning interest in the clinical and research cardiology communities?

NANETTE K. WENGER

This exciting and innovative volume, examining the quality of life outcomes following open heart surgery, opens yet another frontier in the dramatic saga of cardiovascular surgery. As an introduction to the topic, let me first address what is meant by quality of life in the medical care context and then explore some of the compelling reasons for the current prominence of this concept in the clinical, the research, and the health policy arenas.

Consideration of quality of life in the medical care context addresses the ways in which a patient's life is affected both by an illness and by its care. It includes the resultant comfort and sense of well-being; the maintenance of physical, emotional, and intellective function; and the ability to participate in valued activities in the family, in the workplace, and in the community [1,2]. Spitzer has characterized the quality of life concept well, terming it "clinically relevant human attributes" [3]. But it is important to appreciate, as will be discussed subsequently, that these clinically relevant human attributes are the factors that typically determine a patient's satisfaction with the outcomes of medical care. Therefore an evaluative component that addresses the way in which a patient's life is affected by the illness and its care, in addition to the traditional medical measures of morbidity and mortality, appears warranted and of value [4].

In contemporary cardiology, a major contributor to the emphasis on quality of life outcomes is the increased prevalence of chronic cardiovascular diseases. Quality of life is of particular importance in any chronic illness, in that the therapeutic goals, by definition, are not a cure but rather an alleviation of symptoms, an improvement of functional capabilities, limitation of the progression of the disease, and a lessening of the adverse psychologic consequences that may lead to unwarranted invalidism [5]. All of these, as can readily be seen, encompass quality of life attributes. Concern with these outcomes in chronic illness was described well by Mosteller and associates in stating that

Public impression to the contrary, the bulk of medical and surgical treatment is not life-saving,

Paul J. Walter (ed.): Quality of Life after Open Heart Surgery, 1–5.
© 1992 Kluwer Academic Publishers.

but aimed at improving the state or quality of life. Most diseases are not dramatically fatal, but chip away at comfort and happiness. At the same time, treatments for life-threatening diseases often have different impacts on patient comfort. To the extent that we are unable to measure and compare the effects of treatments on the quality of the patient's life, we are unable to document advantages of treatments as well as their defects [6].

But in a sense it is this documentation that raises concern, particularly in the research setting, in that quality of life attributes are intensely personal and subjective. They reflect an individual patient's personal value systems and judgements about his or her general health status, about well-being, and about life satisfaction. Nevertheless, this perceived health status is of importance in that in some studies it correlates well with the risk of mortality [7,9]. Perceived health status also often correlates better with actual work performance than does the objectively measured functional capacity. But perhaps of greater relevance is that perceived health status may be favorably altered by appropriate education and counselling. Let me return again to subjective versus objective features in quality of life outcomes; perhaps this is why return to work, which is readily quantifiable, has been used almost as a surrogate for quality of life in some research studies, despite the fact that it taps only one component of quality of life [10,11]. Even in the work sphere, return to work does not address job satisfaction, job performance, the opportunity for advancement, or the adequacy of income; and return to work is an inappropriate goal for many elderly or retired patients as well as for many medically-complex and severely impaired patients [12]. It is not my purpose here to discuss the techniques for measurement of quality of life. Rather I will assure you that there are well-validated global measures of life quality such as the Nottingham Health Profile [13], the Quality of Well-Being Scale [14], and the Sickness Impact Profile [15] among others; and that there are many established disease-specific measures, including the New York Heart Association Functional Classification [16], the Specific Activity Scale [17], the Rose Chest Pain Questionnaire [18], and the Canadian Cardiovascular Society Classification [19] for angina as examples of some measures used for cardiovascular diseases, as well as many others that will be discussed later in this book.

A second major driving force for the current prominence of quality of life outcomes is the contemporary increased emphasis on preventive cardiovascular care [5]. Two examples, familiar to all of us, are the detection and treatment of asymptomatic systemic arterial hypertension and of asymptomatic hypercholesterolemia, both of which, in recent years, have been targeted by nationwide public and professional educational programs in a number of countries. Let us review the characteristics of individuals to whom these preventive therapies might apply. They are ambulatory, and are typically well and asymptomatic. Their disorders are characterized by an excellent prognosis and a low incidence of complications, at least in the short-term; and often have a relatively low rate of individual complications even over months to years. Therefore morbidity and mortality data are typically not helpful in characterizing the outcomes of preventive treatments. However, since many therapies for these conditions may cause symptoms in an otherwise symptomless individual, it is important to consider those features that may adversely alter the subject's functional status and sense of well-being [20,21]. It has been said by Hoerr that it's hard to make an asymptomatic patient feel better. Stated another way, we must be concerned with a wide spectrum of benefit to harm ratios, and these include the outcomes as they are perceived by the patients or subjects. Remember that preventive therapies typically involve long-term recommendations for care [22]. We are thus involved in a vicious circle in that long-term adherence is likely to influence the outcome, but the patient's perceptions of the relative benefits and harms likely will influence his or her adherence. Many preventive therapies involve changes in lifestyle – in diet, in activity, in smoking, or in alcohol use. Because these are often nonpharmacologic interventions they cannot automatically be considered as without harm, because these nonpharmacologic measures may exert an adverse effect on the patient's desired lifestyle [22].

The third of the compelling reasons for interest in quality of life outcomes is the proliferation of comparably effective therapies, comparable in limiting morbidity and mortality, both for the management of chronic cardiovascular illnesses and for preventive efforts [5]. The efficacy of many of these therapies clearly depends on the patient's adherence to medication, to diet, and the like. Since compliance is likely to be influenced by a number of variables that affect the quality of the patient's daily existence, these aspects must be serially measured in both clinical and research encounters. The effect on life quality of medical versus surgical therapies, or among surgical therapies many vary substantially among different groups of patients.

In this regard, and closely related, is the contemporary emergence of what I have termed "enlightened consumerism" in health care [23]. Patients know that there are options for the treatment of many cardiovascular problems, and require information as to the outcomes of an intervention or of a plan of care so that they can participate with their physician in the selection of management strategies. Knowledge of the effects of treatments on quality of life attributes can improve the ability of both physicians and their patients to make meaningful choices among therapeutic options. Many aspects of outcome of therapy do not relate to morbidity and mortality, but can improve the outlook of patients in other meaningful respects, specifically improving their ability to live with the problems of a chronic illness. As physicians were charged to act in the best interests of our patients; but in order to do so, it is important that we become aware of a specific patient's individual judgements as to personal life plans, life satisfaction, sense of well-being, i.e., the values of importance to that particular patient. Does the patient want to survive or to completely recover? Does the patient want to feel better or to feel completely well? Does the patient want to resume an independent or possibly even an active lifestyle? Is return to work a desired option? Dr. Francis Peabody of Boston highlighted these differences in delineating that "the treatment of a disease may be entirely impersonal; the care of a patient must be completely personal".

This, in turn, leads to the last of the features fostering interest in quality of life, and that is the determinants of the cost-effectiveness of cardiovascular care. Just as quality of life attributes are appropriate considerations in assessing health care outcomes, they also appear appropriate in the determination of health-related public policy and the attendant costs. The Medical Outcomes Study (MOS) in the United States is currently using among its clinical endpoint outcomes: physical, social, and role functioning in everyday life; patients' perceptions of their general health and well-being; and satisfaction with treatment [24]. So much of the contemporary cardiovascular care is costly high technology care. Unquestionably morbidity and mortality data are important components of cost-effectiveness, but a number of quality of life attributes must also enter the equation: independence, productivity (including return to work); and life-satisfaction, to name a few. As noted earlier, unfortunately return to work has been inappropriately used as a surrogate for quality of life in many discussions of health-related policy, including how much expensive medical care any society can afford.

Let me summarize: many medical ethicists have applauded the consideration of quality of life outcomes as reflecting a substantial ethical progression in our methods of clinical evaluation. They cite life quality as a better correlate between the aims and goals of medical care and the ways in which we evaluate outcomes of medical care. Stated another way, the end result of medical interventions is considered to be a lessening of the morbidity and mortality of patients so treated, but it must also encompass efforts to help patients with chronic illness lead better and more meaningful lives. As I anticipate will be derived from this meeting, consideration of quality of life outcomes may help in the medical judgements of what is best for a specific patient in a specific situation, may help patients in their decisions for choice among therapeutic interventions, and may ultimately contribute to reasonable policy decisions in the allocation of health care resources.

References

1. Wenger NK, Mattson ME, Furberg CD, Elinson J (eds): Assessment of Quality of Life in Clinical Trials of Cardiovascular Therapies, LeJacq Publishing, New York, 1984.
2. Wenger NK: Quality of life: Can it and should it be assessed in patients with heart failure? Cardiology 1989;76:391–398.
3. Spitzer WO: Keynote Address: State of science 1986: Quality of life and functional status as target variables for research. J Chronic Dis 1987;40:465–471.
4. Patrick DL, Erickson P: What constitutes quality of life? Concepts and dimensions. Qual Life Cardiovasc Care 1988;4:103–127.

5. Wenger NK: Quality of life in chronic cardiovascular illness. [editorial] J Cardiopulmonary Rehabil 1990;10:88–91.

6. Mosteller F, Gilbert JP, McPeek B: Reporting standards and research strategies for controlled trials. Controlled Clin Trials 1980;1:37–58.

7. LaRue A, Bank L, Jarvik L, et al: Health in old age: How do physicians' rating and self-ratings compare? J Gerontol 1979;34:687–691.

8. Kaplan GA, Camacho TC: Perceived health and mortality: A nine year follow-up of the human population laboratory cohort. Am J Epidemiol 1983; 117:292–295.

9. Mossey JM, Shapiro E: Self-rated health: A predictor of mortality among the elderly. Am J Public Health 1982;72:800–808.

10. Russell RO Jr, Abi-Mansour P, Wenger NK: Return to work after coronary bypass surgery and percutaneous transluminal angioplasty: Issues and potential solutions. Cardiology 1986;73:306–322.

11. Walter PJ (ed): Return to Work after Coronary Artery Bypass Surgery. Psychosocial and Economic Aspects, Springer-Verlag, Berlin, 1985.

12. Wenger NK, Furberg CD: Cardiovascular disorders. In: Spilker B (ed.), Quality of Life Assessments in Clinical Trials, Raven Press, New York, 1990, pp. 335–345.

13. Hunt SM, McKenna SP, McEwen J: A quantitative approach to perceived health. J Epidemiol Community Health 1985;34:281–295.

14. Bush JW: General health policy model/quality of well-being (QWB) scale. In: Wenger NK, Mattson ME, Furberg CE, Elinson J, (eds.), Assessment of Quality of Life in Clinical Trials of Cardiovascular Therapies. LeJacq, New York, 1984, pp. 189–199.

15. Bergner M, Bobbitt RA, Carter WB, et al: The Sickness Impact Profile: Development and final revision of a health status measure. Med Care 1981;19:787–805.

16. Harvey RM, Doyle EF, Ellis K, et al: Major changes made by the Criteria Committee of the New York Heart Association. Circulation 1974;49:309.

17. Goldman L, Hashimoto B, Cook EF, et al: Comparative reproducibility and validity of systems for assessing cardiovascular functional class: Advantages of a new Specific Activity Scale. Circulation 1981;64:1227–1234.

18. Rose GA, Blackburn H. Cardiovascular Survey Methods. Geneva: World Health Organization 1986;56:1–188.

19. CASS Principal Investigators and their Associates: Coronary artery surgery study (CASS). A randomized trial of coronary artery bypass surgery. Quality of life in patients randomly assigned to treatment groups. Circulation 1983;68:951–960.

20. Jachuck SJ, Brierley H, Jachuck S, Wilcox PM: The effect of hypotensive drugs on the quality of life. J R Coll Gen Pract 1982;32:103–105.

21. Lefebvre RC, Hursey KG, Carleton RA: Labeling of participants in high blood pressure screening programs. Implications for blood cholesterol screenings. Arch Intern Med 1988;148:1993–1997.

22. Wenger NK: Quality of life issues in hypertension: Consequences of diagnosis and considerations in management. Am Heart J 1988;116(Pt 2):628–632.

23. Wenger NK: Keynote Address, NHLBI Workshop, 'Quality of Life and Cardiovascular Disease', Winston-Salem, North Carolina, June 7–9, 1988. In press.

24. Tarlov AR, Ware JE Jr, Greenfield S, et al: The Medical Outcomes Study. An application of methods for monitoring the results of medical care. JAMA 1989;262:925–930.

PART ONE

QUALITY OF LIFE AFTER HEART VALVE REPLACEMENT

A: Physiological State

2. Results after biological heart valve replacement

DONALD N. ROSS

An assessment of quality of life after open heart surgery presents a number of difficulties since we know that no one can precisely define quality of life. The problem is compounded by the fact that we have to rely more on the patients subjective symptoms than on medical and technological assessment.

My brief relates specifically to biological valve replacement and I should admit straight away that I have had a bias in favour of this type of valve since I inserted the first homograft valve in 1962 [1]. At that time we regarded it as a temporary expedient until we could import one of the newly developed mechanical valves from the United States. However, three months after insertion, our homograft patient was at home and living a normal life without medication or fear of embolism (which at that time was a major hazard). We forgot about importing the Starr Valve and this state of amnesia has persisted from that time. The story does, however influence my views on the quality of life after heart valve replacement and my belief that it is the patient's point of view, not the doctors', that should be paramount.

With this I would like to make the point that quality of life which is in many ways a psychological rather than a physiological concept is on the whole better when the valve is repaired and retained and the patient feels his heart is intact rather than when a new valve is in place. I readily acknowledge the many contributions made by my colleagues to valve preservation techniques but we are concerned here particularly with the patient after valve replacement. While recognising that as a form of treatment it is basically palliative rather than curative it is still fair to say that the quality of life for the patient is almost always improved and is often excellent.

It is only within recent years that valve replacement has become an acceptable form of treatment particularly because of the risk to life involved in the use of cardiopulmonary bypass 25 years ago. At that time cardiologists were also sceptical, and with justification, about the additional hazards and long-term prospects for the somewhat primitive valve replacements available and early experiences were certainly not encouraging.

Consequently the possibility of surgery and valve replacement was usually

Paul J. Walter (ed.): *Quality of Life after Open Heart Surgery*, 9–12.
© 1992 Kluwer Academic Publishers.

withheld till the last moment (or until the patient was 'sick' enough) which meant that by then the myocardial reserves were all but exhausted, digitalis and diuretics were no longer effective and the condition was largely irreversible. A lingering persistence of this attitude is probably the most important factor militating against an excellent functional result even today.

Once the myocardium has passed beyond the point of no return presenting as a dilated fibrous bag or as a muscle-bound mass with no cavity, there is usually additional multiple organ failure and electrolyte imbalance.

Having progressed beyond that desperate era, the onus now lies on the cardiologist, surgeon and referring doctors to be fully aware of the natural history of the disease untreated. Also they should be cognisant of the risks, advantages and disadvantages of the operation and the various valve options. In this way they will be in a position to choose a time when there is the best prospect of restoring a worthwhile functional status to the myocardium. Quality of life is largely predetermined by that feature for without an adequate cardiac output life is no longer tenable.

To be more specific my brief is to consider quality of life after biological valve replacement and here we need to define a biological valve. Unlike the mechanical valve the true biological valve has no supporting frame or stent but there is a compromise valve introduced by Carpentier which combines a biological valve with a frame. This is the bioprosthesis and incorporates most of the advantages of the true biological valve but with a few of the mechanical valve disadvantages. From our point of view we can consider biological and bioprosthetic valves together.

As has been mentioned when talking about quality of life the patient's point of view is paramount since he is the only one who can assess it accurately. My belief is that the mechanical valve is produced primarily with the surgeon and commercial valve manufacturer's interests in mind. While the surgeon glows with satisfaction at a job well done, the patients quality of life is profoundly and permanently altered from the moment the valve is in place.

Not only does he have a sword of Damocles hanging over him the threat of embolism, thrombosis and anticoagulant hemorrhages, there is also the need to attend regularly at haematology departments and readjust the daily medication. Additionally there are restrictions on sports, alcohol intake and the hazardous combination of peptic ulcer aspirin and anticoagulants. For women of course, pregnancy poses extra problems. Added to this is the knowledge that any failure of the mechanical device is likely to be catastrophic and sudden, none of which adds to mental or physical tranquility even though the mechanical efficiency of the heart may be greatly improved.

The biological valve, as typified by the aortic homograft, has presented a different picture over the years: Embolism and thrombosis have never occurred in our entire experience nor do the patients require anticoagulants with their attendant risks. In general they need neither medical supervision nor medication. The danger of sudden or catastrophic valve dysfunction is absent and the inevitable eventual failure of the valve is a slow process giving plenty of warning before an elective low risk reoperation is carried out and not as an emergency.

On the one hand you have a life confronted by a number of unknown eventualities and regular medical ministrations and on the other hand a 'normal' life but with the certain knowledge that the valve will have to be replaced usually between 10 and 15 years post-operatively.

Collateral evidence on the advantages to the biological valve patient comes from extensive comparative analysis on patients operated upon at the Cleveland Clinic over a 24 year period [2]. Comparing roughly equal numbers of mechanical and biological replacements, their conclusions were that patients with bioprosthesis had better event-free survival than those with mechanical valves and that applied particularly to patients over 40 years of age.

Given the facts objectively laid before them and knowing that either option will be haemodynamically satisfactory, patients will respond usually according to their personality and their current lifestyle. For example physically active people and frequent travellers find anticoagulants burdensome while older more sedentary patients readily accept medication and other limitations.

It is of some interest to me that only one of my homograft patients has asked for his second operation to be with a mechanical valve and he subsequently felt he had made the wrong decision.

If we keep the patient's point of view firmly in mind, we need to re-interpret the questions he puts to his doctor in the light of our usual clinical assessment. For example the patient will want to know: will I die; how long will I live and what sort of life will I lead? Translated into medical jargon this means: operative mortality, late deaths and complications.

The patients third question, what sort of life will I lead is the crucial one and although this becomes simplified as complications to us the patient is concerned with more subjective phenomena like general well being, vitality, zest for living and enthusiasm for his work none of which can be scientifically assessed. The nearest compromise offering a degree of objectivity and one which we can all understand is the N.Y.H.A. grading which again depends largely on subjective assessments.

We can of course do complex ventricular function and cardiac output studies and apply multivariate analysis to as many cardiac indices as we like but we come down to the fact that the ill-defined quality of life is not subject to actuarial analysis.

In summary on the simple basis of a return to normal or acceptable physical activity the valve replacement patient usually benefits very considerably. But if we have to define the improvement further to include abstractions like quality of life then I believe the biological valve patient has advantages over the mechanical heart valve patient plus a degree of mental tranquility which is of incalculable value and adds up to an improved quality of life.

Summary

Quality of life is difficult to define but relates more specifically to the patient's subjective symptoms rather than medical and technological assessment.

Quality of life after valve replacement is modified by the fact that virtually all of these procedures are palliative but in fact they nearly always result in an improved physical and psychological state.

An important factor in improving the patients prospects in this respect is for the patient's cardiologist and surgeon to be fully appraised of the risks involved and the potential advantages and disadvantages of the various valve substitutes.

Furthermore in order to achieve a maximum improvement in the patients condition the valve needs to be tackled surgically while there is still a reversible myocardial disability and we are not dealing with end-stage disease with incipient or overt secondary organ failure.

By offering a life virtually free from the threat of embolism, as far as the aortic valve is concerned, and with no regular medication and medical checks, the patient with a biological valve has virtually a normal lifestyle or quality of life.

References

1. Ross DN: Homograft Replacement of the aortic valve. Lancet 1962:2,487.
2. Lytle BW. Cosgrove DM et al: Primary isolated aortic valve replacement. Early and late results. J Thorac Cardiovasc Surg 1989:675–94.

3. Quality of life after mitral valve repair

JOHN Y. M. RELLAND

Quality of life after valve surgery should optimally approach if not equal quality of life in patients not needing cardiac surgery. As we all know, leading a normal life does not entail taking anticoagulants, does not mean living in constant fear of strokes and waking up hemiplegic and/or aphasic. It means not having to fear sudden death from catastrophic valve failure. It also means not having to put up with annoying clicking sounds which are upsetting to more than 50% of patients and frequently to their spouses and people in their immediate surroundings [1]. On a positive note, it also means being able to get pregnant and have children for women in the childbearing age range. And it allows the practice of sports or physically demanding and/or risky manual work both for men and women of all ages. In a word, quality of life following valve surgery should ideally lead to a normal life.

On the other hand, placing a prosthetic valve in the blood stream can be considered an iatrogenic disease. Although we are all familiar with the great advances brought about by the development of the first prosthetic valve introduced by Albert Starr in 1960 in treating mitral valve disease and the numerous other mechanical valves developed since then, we also know that in medicine, when multiple solutions are presented for a single problem, none of them is a panacea. It is with these complications in the use of prosthetic valves in mind that Alain Carpentier in 1968 pioneered the use of the first bioprosthesis fashioned from glutaraldehyde tanned porcine valves in order to render them non-antigenic as well long lasting. While this resolved some of the problems associated with artificial valves, it did not resolve all of them, notably it did not resolve the problem of longevity and the necessity of reoperation which can also adversely affect the quality of life of patients after valve surgery. That is the reason why, also in 1968, Alain Carpentier developed the semi-rigid annuloplasty rings designed to correct mitral and tricuspid insufficiency. By 1972, four additional techniques had been developed to correct mitral valve insufficiency: triangular resection of the anterior leaflet, shortening plasty of chordal structures, leaflet mobilization and quadrangular resection of the posterior leaflet. Since the introduction in 1982

Paul J. Walter (ed.): *Quality of Life after Open Heart Surgery*, 13–18.
© 1992 Kluwer Academic Publishers.

of transposition of chords, triangular resection of the anterior leaflet has virtually been abandoned. Whilst not wanting to burden the reader with these technical operative techniques, it is important to understand them since we are now in a position to evaluate the long term results using these various techniques which comprise the Carpentier valvuloplasty technique for correcting mitral valve insufficiency.

Concerning quality of life then, there exists an alternative to prosthetic valve replacement for the mitral valve: bioprosthesis or valve reconstruction. Harking back to our initial definition of the optimal quality of life, how do these three solutions compare? Several years ago, in an elegant study, one our clinical fellows, Patrick Perier compared the mid-term follow-up of patients having been subjected to one of four operations for mitral valve disease [2]. He analysed four groups of consecutive patients operated in the same time frame, in the same service and by the same surgeons and compared them using different parameters at the end of seven years. The four groups were comprised of 100 patients each having undergone mitral valve repair, mitral replacement by a bioprosthesis, mitral valve repair by mechanical prosthesis either a Starr–Edwards valve or a Bjork–Shiley valve. What this study showed when comparing various parameters at seven years was a statistically significant difference in the incidence of thromboembolic complications between the valve repair and bioprostheses groups on the one hand and the mechanical valves on the other and this in spite of a fifty percent atrial fibrillation rate in the first two groups. Also surprising was the fact that at seven years, there was no statistical difference between the reoperation rate in the four groups of patients.

While the previous study is interesting because it compares different procedures from a same center, it concerns only the midterm follow-up period. Quality of life also clearly must be evaluated in the long-term. For a patient undergoing open heart surgery today, the importance of being assured of a long term predictably stable result is of the utmost importance. Therefore, we investigated the long term results following mitral valve repair in a group of 195 consecutive surviving French patients operated in our center from 1972 through 1979 [3]. 1972 was chosen as the starting point of the study because by then all of the basic techniques utilized in the Carpentier valvuloplasty technique had been developed by that time and were in use. The study was limited to French patients exclusively because the follow-up period was long and it was necessary to contact either the patients themselves or their referring cardiologists. All patients underwent Echo–Doppler studies in order to evaluate valve function as well as myocardial function. Including foreign patients, many of whom come from North Africa of southern Italy, would have led to a statistically significant loss of follow-up. As it was, only three out of 197 French patients in our study were lost to follow-up.

The results of this study were deemed to be interesting not only because they were long-term results with an average follow-up period of 10 to 17

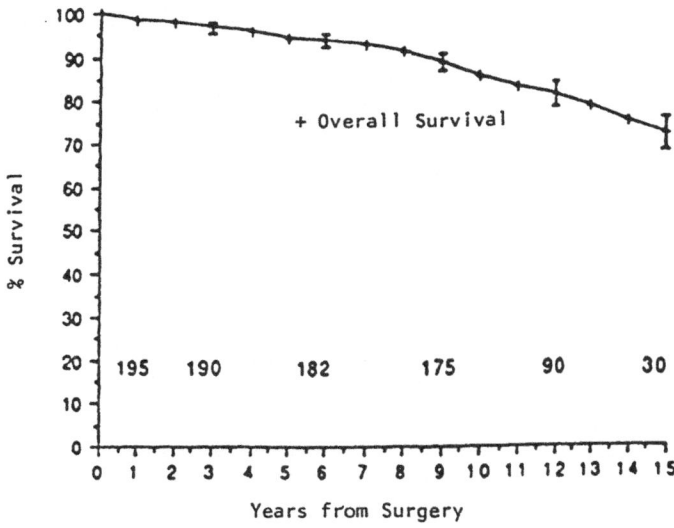

Figure 1. Overall mortality (hospital mortality excluded).

years (average 13.2 years) but because they could be analysed in the light of the quality of life of these patients. Without going into all of the results of the study, it is interesting to note that preoperatively, the majority of patients (97%) were in New York Heart Association Classification (NYHA) III & IV while post-operatively the great majority of patients were in NYHA class I & II. Freedom from death plays a role in the quality of life and the long term mortality rate showed that 81% of patients were alive at the end of the study period for an actuarial survival rate of 72.48% at 15 years (Figure 1). Thromboembolism is a constant specter for patients after valve surgery and the freedom from thromboembolism was 93.97% at 15 years in spite of the fact that atrial fibrillation was present in 48% of patients (Figure 2). Reoperation is also an important consideration and freedom from reoperation was 87.39% at 15 years. Interestingly enough, when this was broken down into two subsets, comparing the degenerative group with the rheumatic group, the degenerative group had a significantly lower reoperation rate: 92.73% free from reoperation versus 76.12% in rheumatic group (Figure 3). This is a reflection of the progressive nature of rheumatic valvular disease.

Combining all these factors, one can construct a long term symptom free survival curve which shows 65% of patients living and symptom-free at 15 years (Figure 4). Again, separating this group into two subsets one finds a significant difference between the rheumatic and the degenerative group, 54% versus 73%, free from valve related complications at 6 years (Figure 5); this because of the average age difference of patients in the degenerative group as opposed to the rheumatic group which tend to be operated at an earlier age.

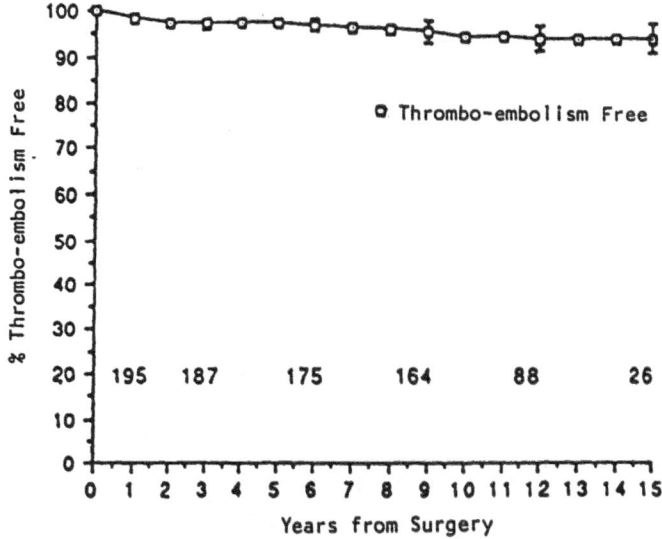

Figure 2. Survival free from thromboembolic events.

This long term study [3] then conclusively demonstrates that mitral valve reconstruction is both predictable because of the low rate of early reoperation and stable because of the low incidence of late reoperation. Moreover, the quality of life is further reflected in the low rate of thromboembolic complications and valve failure.

Our present therapeutic policy is to approach all aortic, mitral and tricuspid valves with an attempt at valve repair. Whenever valve replacement is

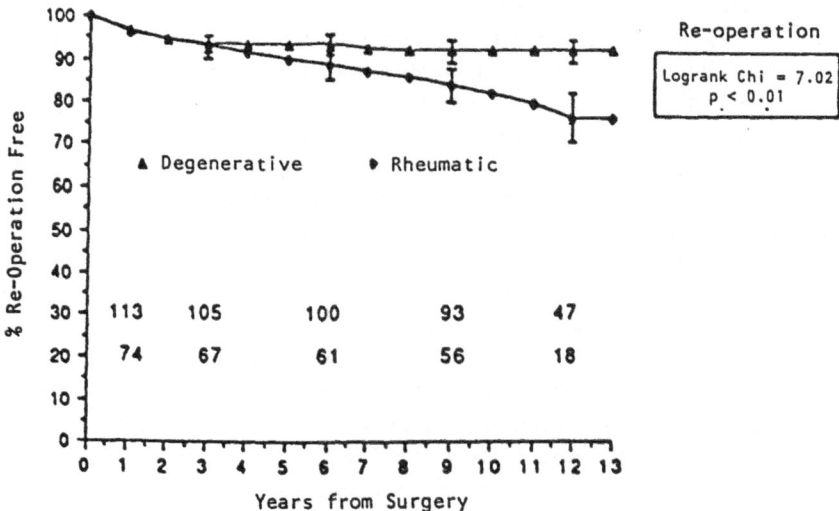

Figure 3. Comparison between rheumatic and degenerative diseases.

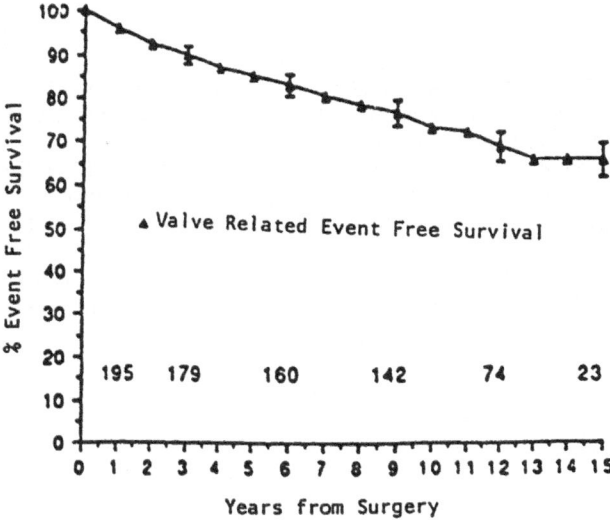

Figure 4. Survival free from valve-related mortality and other valve-related complication.

deemed necessary, either in valve surgery in the mitral position alone or in the aortic position in association with a mitral valve repair, we utilize a bioprosthesis whenever possible, naturally after having discussed the advantages and disadvantages with the patient, who should actively participate in the ultimate decision based on personality, life style, age and disease process. This therapeutic approach offers to each individual patient the best chance of achieving the highest level of quality of life following valve surgery.

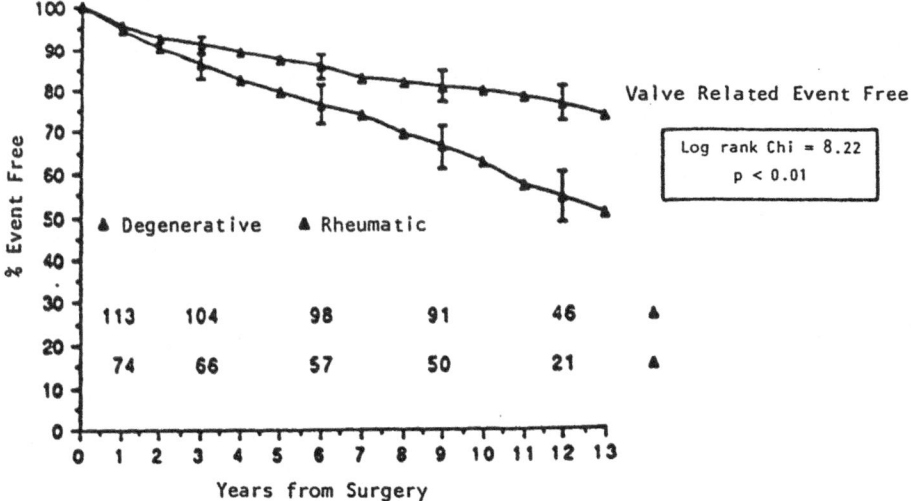

Figure 5. Comparison of rheumatic and degenerative diseases.

References

1. Limbs DL, Kay PH, Murday AJ: Problems associated with mechanical heart valve sounds. Presented at the XVIIth European Alpine Cardiology and Cardiac Surgery Meeting, March 18–20, 1991, Meribel-Mottaret, France.
2. Perier P, Deloche A, Chauvaud S, Fabiani JN, Rossant P, Bessou JP, Relland J, Bourezak H, Gomez F, Blondeau PC d'Allaines C, Carpentier A: Comparative evaluation of mitral valve repair and replacement with Starr, Björk, and porcine valve prostheses. Circulation 1984;70 (suppl I):1–187–191.
3. Deloche A, Jebara VA, Relland JYM, Chauvaud S, Fabiani J-N, Perier P, Dreyfus G, Milhaileanu S, Carpentier A: Valve repair with Carpentier techniques, the second decade. J Thorac Cardiovasc Surg 1990;99:6–990–1002.

4. Quality of life and prognosis following heart valve replacement

DIETER HORSTKOTTE, HAGEN D. SCHULTE, WOLFGANG
BIRCKS and BODO E. STRAUER

1. Introduction

Heart valve replacement, after more than three decades of continuous efforts
to improve the prostheses, has become a routine procedure. Apart from some
recent set-backs with a mono-tilting disc [1] and one bi-leaflet prosthesis [2],
the mechanical prostheses used today are reliable and durable for the period
for which they have been followed and likely for a much longer time. Thrombogenicity, the major disadvantage of all mechanical heart valve prostheses,
has also been reduced by designs allowing a more physiological transprosthetic flow profile and by use of the more biocompatible pyrolytic carbon
[3–5].

There is now sufficient evidence that with modern mechanical and biological heart valve prostheses, the optimum time for surgical intervention, as
well as the quality of the postoperative management, rather than the prosthetic device itself are the decisive factors to improve the overall prognosis
and the quality of life of patients with advanced valvular heart disease [6,7].

2. How can quality of life after heart valve replacement be determined?

From the beginning, the success of valve replacement surgery has been
measured mainly by event-free survival, while the improvement of the quality
of life has attracted little attention so far. One reason may be that, even
with insufficient follow-up techniques, it is not very difficult to count major
events of complications or deaths [8,9], while more sophisticated techniques
are necessary to make statements about a change in the quality of life by
valve replacement.

Quality of life after heart valve replacement is determined by the improvement of the prognosis when comparing it to the natural history of the lesion,
and the objective functional improvement after surgical intervention (10)

Paul J. Walter (ed.): Quality of Life after Open Heart Surgery, 19–35.
© 1992 Kluwer Academic Publishers.

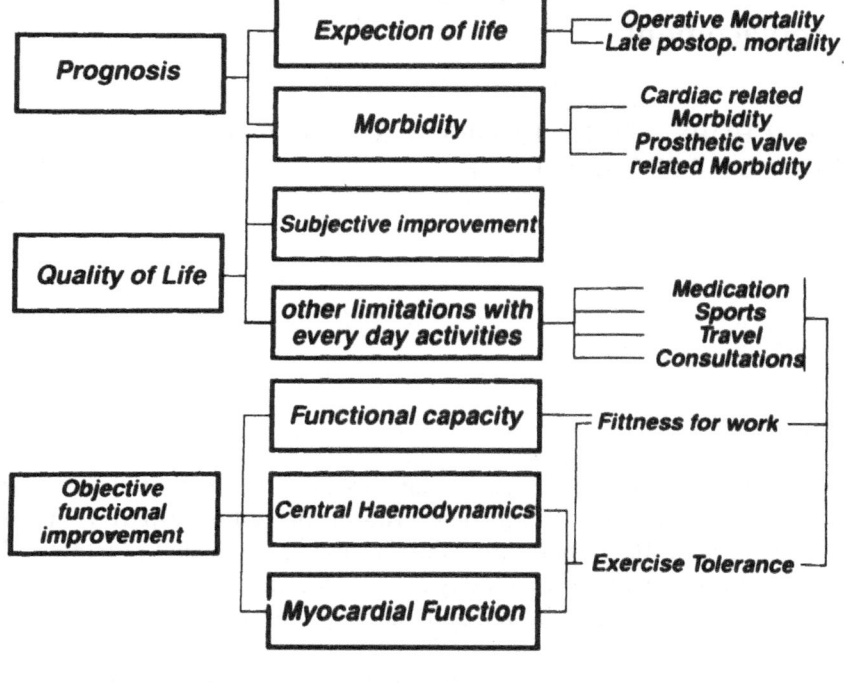

Figure 1. Factors influencing the various parameters that decide about quality of life and prognosis following heart valve replacement.

(Figure 1). Quality of life and objective function improvement are clearly related to each other. Late prognosis and functional improvement can be objectively measured by the residual life expectancy, morbidity and mortality following valve replacement, the functional capacity, the central hemodynamics and the improvement of a preoperatively impaired right or left ventricular function.

Despite some hundred publications every year, comparison between different types of heart valve prostheses are limited in view of the fact that most of these studies are retrospective or non-randomized, or both, and therefore biased and inappropriate to prove the influence of pre- and perioperative parameters on the late outcome [8]. Moreover, many complications occurring in the postoperative course and which are counted by definition as 'prosthetic-valve related', actually may not be related to the artificial device but to the underlying valve lesion with consequent atrial fibrillation, chamber dilation, impaired myocardial function, reduced cardiac output, increased pulmonary resistance, myocardial fibrosis or ventricular arrhythmias [11,12].

3. Prognosis following heart valve replacement

In the individual valve patient, besides patient-related factors, timing of surgery and the quality of the postoperative treatment may have a more significant influence on the long-term prognosis than the implanted device itself.

The cumulative survival as well as the event-free rates which are commonly used to assess long-term valve performances would have to be compared ideally to similar survival functions of an age- and sex-matched group of the general population and to the survival of those patients who received medical rather than surgical treatment. Unfortunately, the former is not always readily available and the latter could not be done in a randomized fashion for ethical reasons [10,13].

3.1. *Operative mortality*

As a result of the improved perioperative management, the operative mortality, which means death from any course within 30 days of operation or any in-hospital death, has significantly decreased in the last two decades. With the increasing numbers of older patients, who have been operated upon in the 1980s, the perioperative mortality for this group of patients also has fallen down and actually is only slightly higher for patients older than 70 years than for patients being 60 years or younger (Figure 2). Age is thus no longer a single decisive parameter to reject patients from valve surgery, especially from aortic valve replacement, or to use palliative non-surgical procedures (balloon valvuloplasty) in such patients.

3.2. *Late postoperative morbidity and mortality*

In contrast to the early years of valve replacement surgery, prosthetic valve-related causes for late death are now in the minority. Morbidity unrelated to the valve substitute is of growing importance, as there is a close correlation between this kind of morbidity and the optimal time for surgical intervention (Figure 3).

An analysis of the frequency and the incidence of different sources for postoperative mortality in large numbers of patients, demonstrates that myocardial failure is a major cause for late postoperative mortality. For aortic and mitral-aortic valve replacements, it is followed by unexpected sudden death or documented ventricular arrhythmias, while in the mitral valve re-

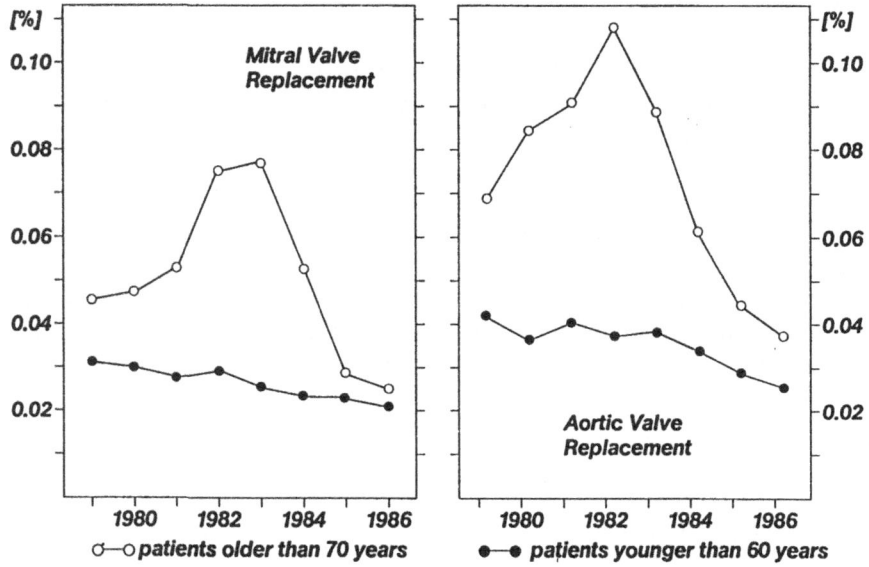

Figure 2. Perioperative mortality for all consecutive patients (all patients with additional procedures included) with isolated mitral (left) or aortic valve replacement surgery (right side). The mortality is given for patients older than 70 years in comparison to patients being younger than 60 years at operation. Unlike the early years when the indication for valve surgery had been widened to older age groups, along with the improvement of the perioperative management of older patients, perioperative mortality of patients being 70 years or older is now not significantly higher than for patients being 60 years or younger.

placement group, the second most frequent complication is thromboembolism and anticoagulant-related hemorrhage (Table 1).

Structural deterioration or non-structural dysfunction of the prosthetic device, the major source for morbidity in the early years of valve replacement surgery, is found today to be only of minor importance for the patient's overall prognosis. Within 10 to 20 years of follow-up these complications account for only 0.17 to 2.6% of morbidity per year.

3.2.1. *Prosthetic valve-related morbidity*
Prosthetic valve-related morbidity includes, by definition all structural and non-structural dysfunctions, prosthetic valve endocarditis and all thrombotic and thromboembolic complications, as well as bleedings related to an anticoagulant treatment.

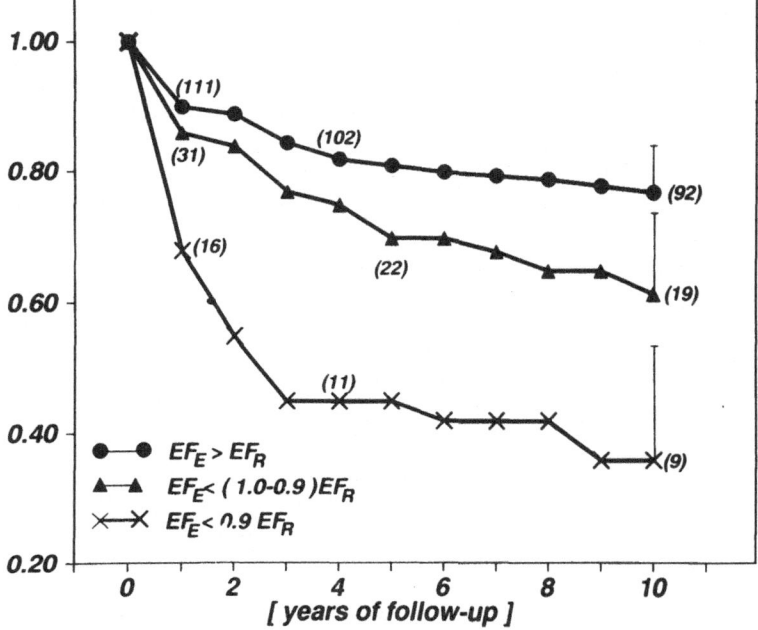

Figure 3. Influence of the left ventricular function on the actuarial survival of 178 consecutive patients operated upon for severe aortic stenosis (1978–1980). EF = left ventricular ejection fraction, E = Exercise, R = Rest. Patients with a physiological increase of their left ventricular ejection fraction during preoperative bicycle exercise had a much better long-term prognosis than patients in whom left ventricular ejection fraction dropped up to 10% with preoperative exercise. Patients in whom left ventricular ejection fraction dropped more than 10% by preoperative exercise had an even more unfavourable prognosis.

The linearized incidences for the most frequent prosthetic valve-related complications during two different time frames are given in Figure 4.

Improved designs and the use of new materials have reduced the incidence of thromboembolic events, but they are still significantly higher with mechanical prostheses than with tissue ones. Despite anticoagulant therapy and consequent high rates of bleeding complications, the long-term success after mechanical heart-valve replacement is thus influenced negatively by thromboembolic complications. The incidence of thromboembolic complications is obviously dependent on the intensity of the anticoagulation management. Consequently, it is necessary to give the cumulative linearized incidence for thromboembolic plus bleeding complications. Comparing the annual percentage of thromboembolic and bleeding complications in patients with mechanical heart valve prostheses using different intensities of oral anticoagulation, it can be clearly shown that a lower incidence for thromboembolic

Table 1. Long-term results after valve replacement for mitral stenosis[1]. Late postoperative mortality in 452 consecutive patients (Düsseldorf 1970–1975) compared to 386 consecutive patients with aortic prostheses[2,3]

Cause of death	MVR (n = 452)		AVR (n = 386)	
	n (%)	LI[4]	n (%)	LI[4]
Left heart failure	12 (8.5)	0.25	31 (25.0)	0.77
Right heart failure	16 (11.3)	0.34	3 (2.4)	0.07
Sudden death/arrhythm.	24 (16.9)	0.50	21 (16.9)	0.52
Acute MI	10 (7.0)	0.22	10 (8.0)	0.24
Thrombembolism	28 (19.7)	0.59	15 (12.0)	0.36
Bleeding	27 (19.0)	0.57	20 (16.0)	0.48
PV endocarditis	5 (3.5)	0.11	7 (5.6)	0.17
Non-cardiac	20 (14.1)	0.42	17 (13.7)	0.42
	142 (100.0)	2.99	124 (100.0)	3.09

[1]Pure or predominant; [2]prospective follow-up; [3]median follow-up 184.1 months, total follow-up 103.667 months.
[4]LI=linearized incidence; mortality per 100 follow-up years (%/y).

plus bleeding complications can be expected with an INR between 2.5 and 3.0 rather than with an INR of 3.5 to 4.5 routinely recommended for patients with mechanical protheses (Figure 5).

Such a very narrow target (INR 2.5 to 3.0) – for some very low thrombo-genetic devices like the St Jude Medical prosthesis, even INR 2.0 to 2.5 – would be ideal to achieve the lowest incidence of thromboembolic plus bleeding complications, can, however, be aimed for only highly compliant patients.

4. Subjective functional improvement

4.1. *Subjective and clinical improvement*

The subjective improvement after heart valve replacement depends on the postoperative status of the pulmonary circulation and the function of the left ventricle.

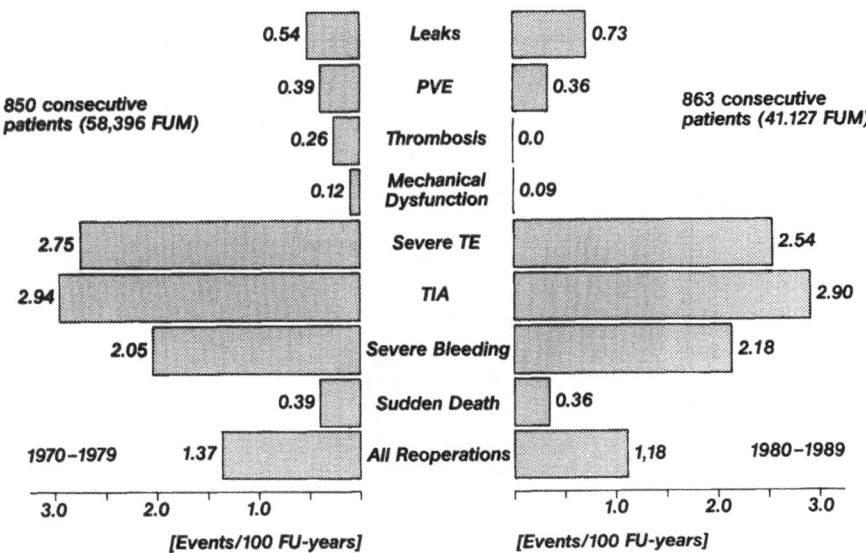

Figure 4. Late postoperative complications after valve replacement for mitral stenosis. This is a comparison of 850 consecutive patients (58,396 follow–up months) operated upon between 1970–1979 (left side) and 863 consecutive patients (total follow up months 41,127) who had been operated in the 1980s (1980–1989). PVE = Prosthetic valve endocarditis, TE = Thrombo-embolism, TIA = Transitory ischemic attacks.

If the preoperative diagnosis was mitral stenosis or mixed mitral valve disease, the pulmonary artery pressure will play a decisive role. In cases with pure mitral regurgitation or aortic valve disease indicating valve replacement, the postoperative left ventricular function will first of all determine the degree of subjective, as well as clinical, improvement. However, significant differences may exist between subjective and clinical improvement in individual cases, which may be due to nothing more than the patient's unrealistic expectations prior to surgery. An important factor in this respect is the preoperative functional status, which will serve as the point of reference for the patient.

Due to the residual transprosthetic gradients after mitral valve replacement, on average one can expect clinical improvement by one NYHA class (Figure 6). A more significant decrease in symptoms and increase in functional capacity can be expected in some patients with modern prostheses which create only a very low resistance to forward blood flow. Absence of symptoms after valve replacement for chronic mitral lesions that would allow

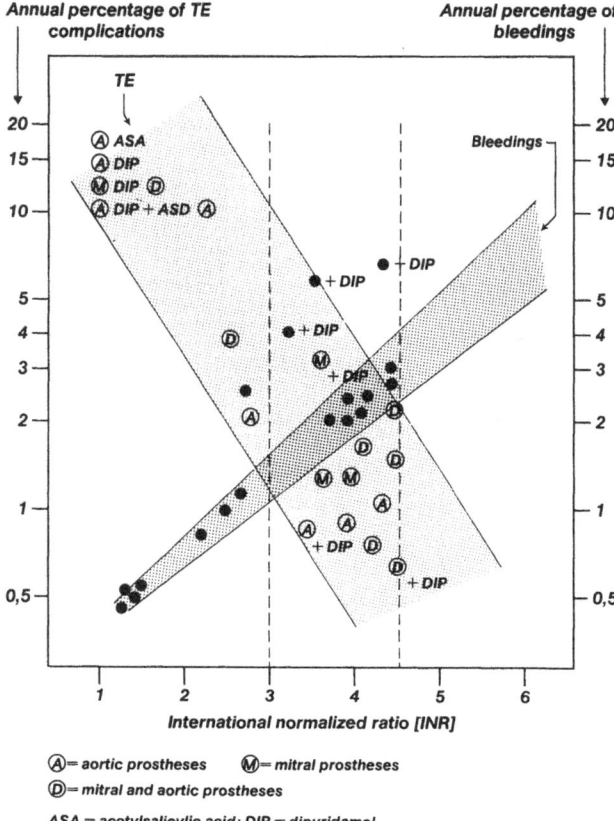

Figure 5. Optimum range for oral anticoagulation when comparing thromboembolic and bleeding complications. Data have been gathered from the literature. With more insensitive anticoagulation (increasing INR) the incidence of thromboembolic events (TE) is reduced, however the number of bleeding complications is increasing. According to these published results there is some evidence that the cumulative hazard for thromboembolic plus bleeding complications is lowest with an anticoagulation according to an INR of 3.0. A = Aortic prosthesis, M = Mitral prosthesis, D = Mitral and aortic prosthesis, ASA = Acetylsalicylic Acid, DIP = Dipyridamol.

patients to be placed in NYHA class I is rarely observed. In the majority of patients atrial fibrillation persists postoperatively. Moreover, many patients have symptoms during strain imposed by ordinary day-to-day activities, which are consistent with NYHA class II. Thus it is obvious that, in nearly all reports of subjective improvements of the majority of patients after mitral valve replacement up to NYHA class I, the criteria of the NYHA are poorly applied, which contributes to the confusion in comparing postoperative results in valve patients [14].

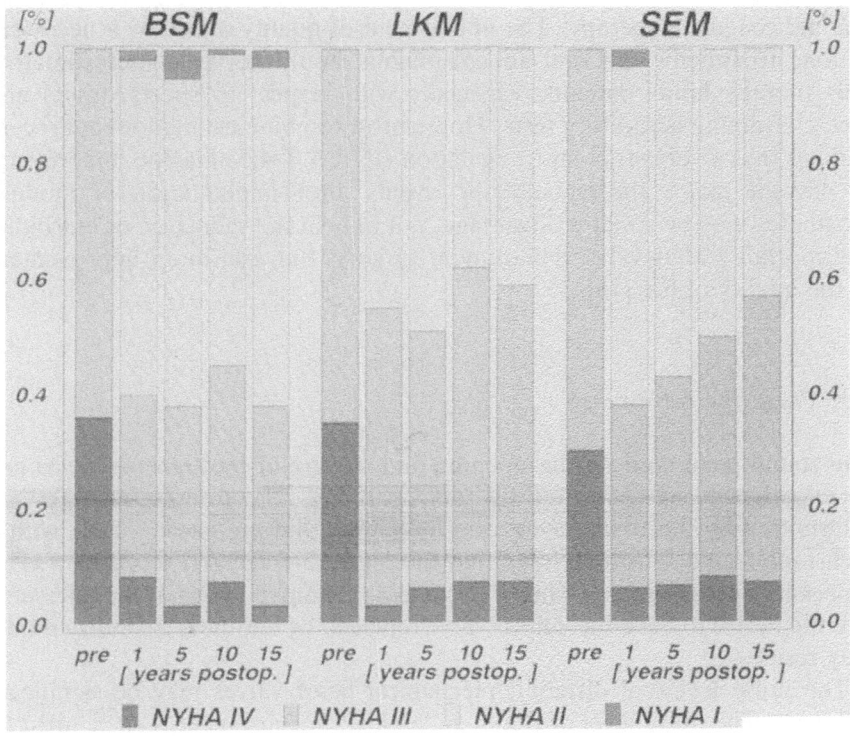

Figure 6. Functional results according to the classification of the NYHA following randomized mitral valve replacement with three different mechanical prostheses (BSM = Björk–Shiley mitral, LKM = Lillehei – Kaster mitral, SEM = Starr–Edwards mitral valves). Between the three valve types there are differences in the functional results, with a more significant decrease of NYHA functional classes in the Björk–Shiley group. NYHA functional class I is rarely observed in patients with mitral prostheses. Over the years, there is a slow but continuous increase in patients who had to be graded NYHA class III. This may be due to a compromised myocardial function following rheumatic fever.

4.2. *Limitations with day-to-day activities*

Functional improvement depends on the restoration of myocardial function, and the central hemodynamics. As the central hemodynamics, however, remain more or less disturbed in a substantial number of patients, subjective and functional improvement as well as work load may remain limited, especially after mitral valve replacement [15,16].

Besides the limited exercise tolerance, patients with heart valve prostheses are limited in their day-to-day activity by specific medications, primarily by oral anticoagulant therapy. The impairment of quality of life by a necessary lifelong treatment with oral anticoagulants should not be underestimated. This therapy limits patients, especially with respect to sports, travel and time-consuming laboratory tests. Home prothrombine estimation and recent findings that a very strict anticoagulation (INR 3.0–4.5) may be unnecessary to prevent major thromboembolic events after implantation of modern prostheses may be a major advantage, not only in the reduction of morbidity and mortality after valve replacement surgery, but also in an improvement of the quality of life [16].

4.3. *Prosthetic valve noise*

The sound generated by the opening and closing of mechanical valves can be experienced as disturbing by some patients. The prostheses clicks are transmitted by the tissue layers and airways within the chest. Those with a high tone sound sensitivity may find the high tone clicks (exceeding 8 kHz) especially unpleasant and cannot become accustomed to them. Sleeplessness and the desire to have the culprit valve replaced by another, less noisy model may result.

The noise levels of different mechanical heart valves may be significant different. The noise level of the St Jude valve, for instance, is $40 \pm 7dB$ (A) and that of the Edwards–Duromedics valve 47 ± 7 dB(A) at 10 cm distance from the chest, and it is 24 ± 4 dB(A) and 39 ± 6 dB(A), respectively ($p < 0.001$) at 1 meter distance. This 15 dB(A) difference between these two noise levels corresponds to a nine-fold increase in sound pressure on the logarithmic dB(A) scale [17]. This is an explanation as to why patients with the Edwards–Duromedics valve suffer sleeplessness three times as often as those with the St Jude Medical prosthesis, and 11% of them feel disturbed during daytime activities. Another major experience is the new Bicer mono-tilting disc prosthesis, in which the noise level at 10 cm distance from the chest is approximately as high as in the St Jude prosthesis; however, these clicks exeed 30 kHz and are thus inaudible to the patients.

5. Objective functional improvement

5.1. *Central hemodynamics*

In native mitral valves, clinical signs and symptoms of mitral stenosis are present if the mitral orifice area is reduced to less than 1.5 cm^2 in adults [18].

In most adult patients receiving mitral valve prostheses, a device with an outer diameter of 29 mm can be used. Depending on the type of the prosthesis, valve orifice areas measured in vivo for 29 mm prostheses vary between 1.7 and 3.2 cm^2 [15,16]. The design characteristics of the implanted device thus do have a decisive influence on whether a given prosthesis will produce signs and symptoms of mitral stenosis or not.

Unlike atrioventricular valve replacements, residual transaortic pressure gradients are of only minor importance if the usual valve sizes are used and normal prosthetic function is present.

Volume loss of prosthetic valves may vary significantly with heart rates, stroke volumes and valve design. There is, however, no evidence so far that volume loss (closing volume plus leakage flow) is of any clinical importance in modern prostheses.

Besides pressure and volume losses the hemodynamics of a prosthesis is described by its flow profile. More or less turbulent flows with consequent shear stresses to corpuscular blood elements and large recirculation areas behind the prosthesis are of major importance for late postoperative complications like prosthetic valve thrombosis, thromboembolism, tissue ingrowth and chronic intravascular haemolysis.

5.2. *Functional capacity and exercise tolerance*

After mitral valve replacement, an increase in the functional capacity as assessed by exercise tests has been reported to be 40 to 100% [15]. Differences in the increase may depend on hemodynamic properties of the implanted valve type and on increased pulmonary vascular resistances, which may persist postoperatively.

If one requests patients to climb stairs until dyspnea appears, one can measure differences in the functional capacities after implantation of various prostheses. In our patients the functional capacity one year after valve replacement was generally lower after implantation of a bioprosthesis (Ionescu–Shiley, Carpentier–Edwards) than after implantation of a bileaflet prosthesis. Postoperative increase was found to be only 74% in patients with Ionescu-Shiley, but 180% in patients with a St Jude Medical prosthesis. Although implantation of the different prosthetic types was performed only by clinical decision, there were no statistical differences in the preoperative hemodynamics, nor in the preoperative myocardial function. Nevertheless, conclusions drawn from these findings are restricted due to the fact that the comparison was not randomized. However, the more significant increase of

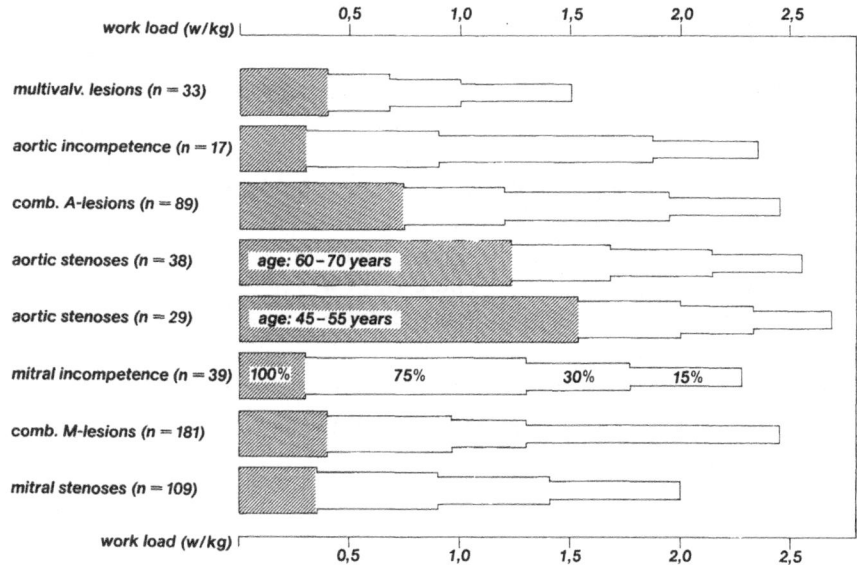

Figure 7. Functional capacity after heart valve replacement. The work load is given as W/kg body weight for the different preoperative lesions. For all these groups there is a wide scale of work loads (the figure gives the work load that 100%, 75%, 30% and 15% of the patients could experience).

functional capacity after implantation of modern mechanical prostheses rather than with pericardial tissue valves seem to be obvious [14,16].

5.3. *Functional improvement and timing of surgery*

There is no doubt that the predominant factor influencing functional capacity after heart valve replacement is the timing of surgery. The wide scale of work loads experienced by patients after mitral, aortic and double valve replacement reflects the fact that patients are operated upon under very different clinical conditions and at different time points during the natural history of their underlying lesions (Figure 7). In most of the patients with low postoperative exercise tolerance, operation was performed after irreversible damage of the myocardium had occurred. On the other hand, early operation, which means surgical intervention in a mitral (Figure 8) or aortic lesion (Figure 9) before myocardial function is compromised, usually results in work loads which are not significantly different from the general population in patients with isolate aortic valve replacement or with mitral valve replacement using a modern mechanical device.

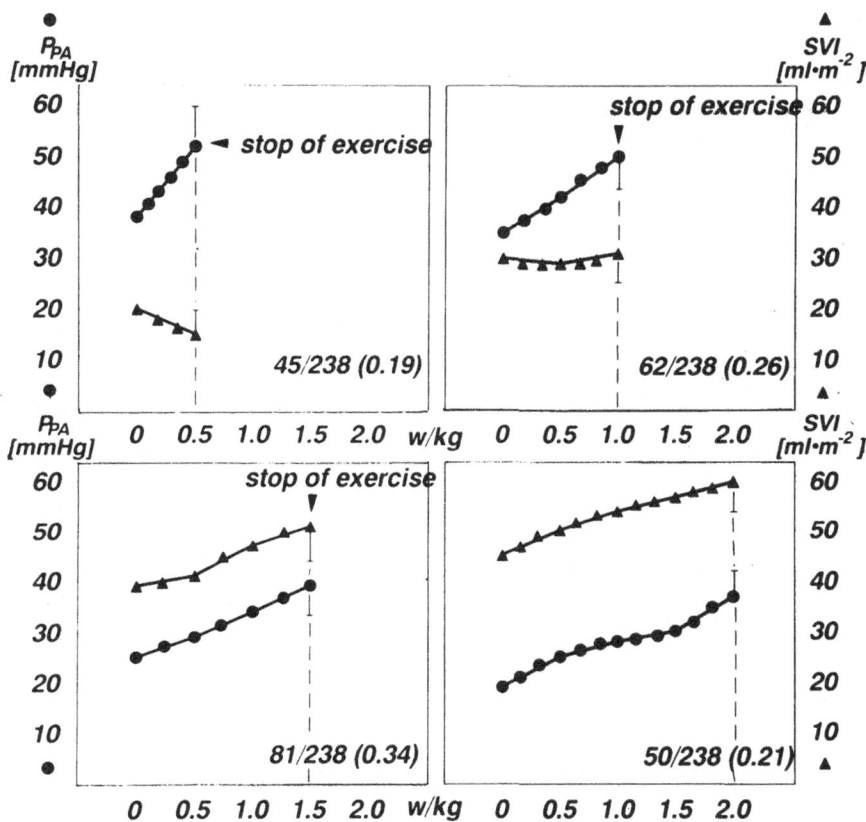

Figure 8. Exercise capacity (W/kg body weight) experienced by 238 consecutive patients one year after mitral valve replacement (with various prostheses) for mitral regurgitation between 1973–1990. Patients are subdivided into four groups: patients who stopped exercise at a level of 0.5 W/kg, at 1.0 W/kg, at 1.5 W/kg and who experienced 2.0 W/kg or more. It is obvious that patients with low postoperative exercise capacity had a significantly impaired left ventricular function with consequent unphysiological decrease of their stroke volume index (SVI) and consecutive increase of the pulmonary artery pressure (PPA). Patients with high exercise capacities, on the other hand, had significant increases of their stroke volume indexes and only relatively mild increases of their PPA.

6. Perspectives

6.1. *Optimal timing for surgical intervention*

To improve quality of life as well as prognosis of patients who have to undergo valve replacement surgery, it is of major importance to choose the

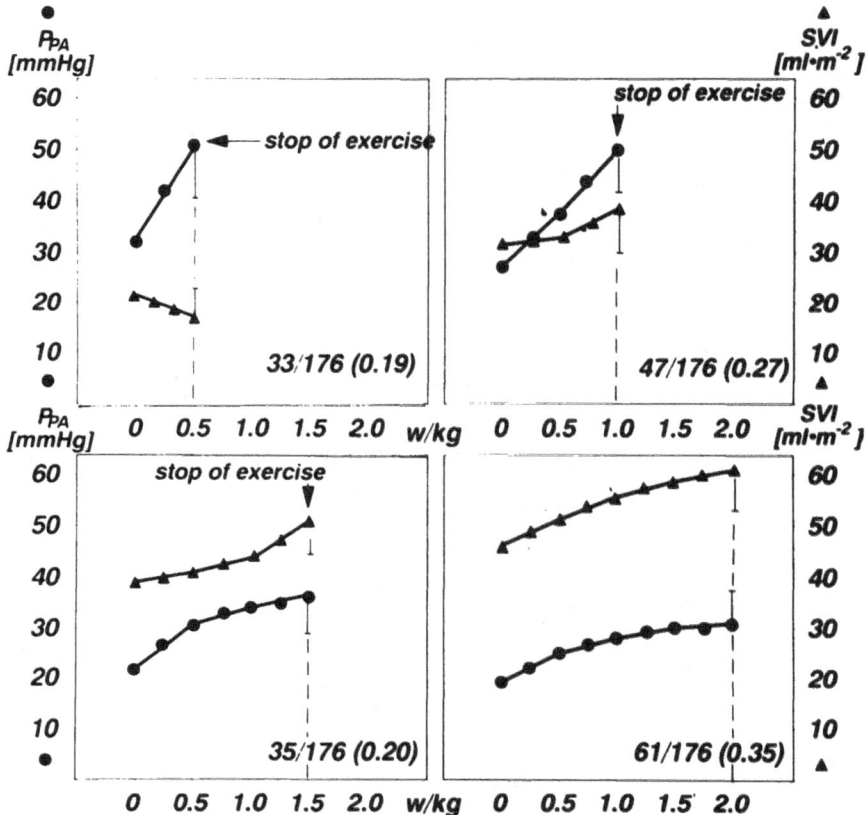

Figure 9. Exercise capacity following St Jude Medical aortic valve replacement (size 27 mm) in 176 consecutive one-year survivors who had been operated for aortic stenosis between 1978–1988. PPA = Mean pulmonary artery pressure, SVI = Stroke volume index. For more details see legend to Figure 8.

optimum time for surgical intervention. Determination of the optimum time for surgical intervention needs sophisticated diagnostic methods to detect early myocardial dysfunction. Usually, early myocardial compromisation can be detected only by invasive methods and exercise tests (Figure 10).

In mitral regurgitation early detection of myocardial dysfunction may be particularly difficult. Due to the given impedance, the left ventricle is able to eject a significant percentage of its end-diastolic volume into the left atrium. The low afterload in these patients is thus an important compensatory mechanism, serving to maintain a 'normal' ejection fraction. A normal left ventricular ejection fraction in these patients thus does not necessarily imply normal left ventricular function. This is the reason why imaging techniques

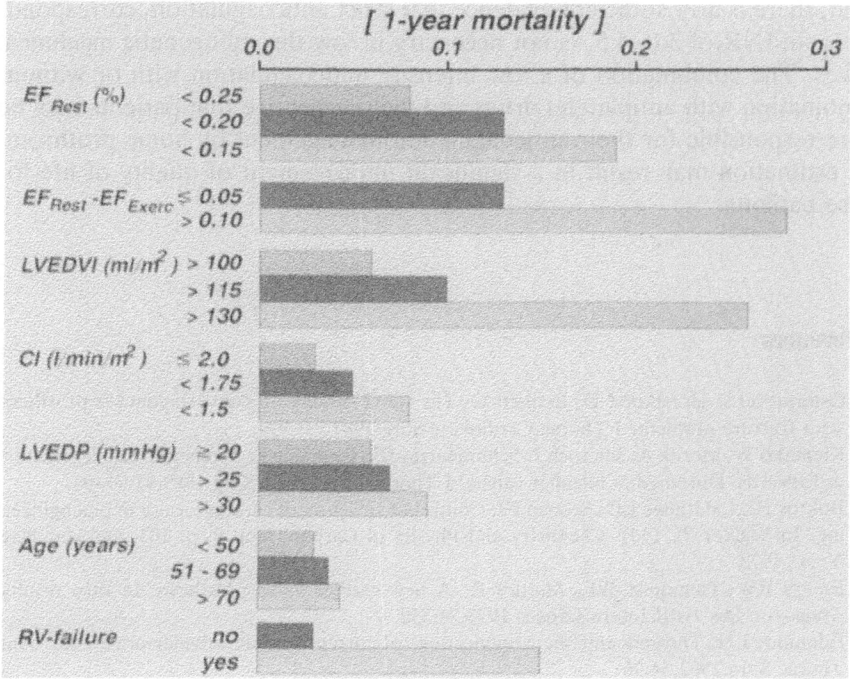

Figure 10. Central hemodynamics and other parameters influencing one year mortality after valve replacement for aortic stenosis (1975–1989). EF = Ejection fraction, LVEDVI = Left ventricular end-diastolic volume index (ml/m^2), CI = Cardiac index ($1/min/m^2$), LVEDP = Left ventricular end-diastolic pressure.

like angiography or echocardiography are unable to quantify the true hemo-dynamic severity of mitral regurgitation as far as the consequences for the left ventricular myocardium are concerned.

6.2. *Optimization of anticoagulation therapy*

Many postoperative complications after valve replacement surgery can be prevented, if anticoagulation therapy could be optimized. Efforts have been made to improve anticoagulation management in patients depending on a life-long anticoagulation therapy. One step is home prothrombin estimation for which apparatus and kits are now commercially available. On the other hand, there is now sufficient evidence that strict anticoagulation, corresponding to an INR of 3.0–4.5, is not necessary in low thrombogenetic mechnical valves. The combination of a low intensity anticoagulation with or without combination with antiplatelet drugs and the perspective that patients may be more responsible for their anticoagulation management by home prothrombin estimation may result in a significant improvement of quality of life for these patients.

References

1. Ostermeyer J, Horstkotte D, Bennett G: The Björk–Shiley 70° convexo-concave prosthesis strut fracture problem. J Thorac Cardiovasc Surg 1987;93: 999.
2. Klepetko W, Moritz A, Mlczoch J, Schurawitzki JH, Domanig E, Wolner E: Leaflet fracture in Edwards–Duromedics bileaflet valves. J Thorac Cardiovasc Surg 1989;97:90–94.
3. Bokros JC, LaGrange LD, Schoen FJ: Control of structure of carbon for use in bioengineering. In Walker PL (ed): Chemistry and Physics of Carbon, Vol. 9, p. 103. Dekker, New York, 1973.
4. Emery RW, Palmquist WE, Mettler E: A new cardiac valve prosthesis: in-vitro results. Trans Am Soc Artif Intern Organs 1978;24:550.
5. Edmunds LH: Thromboembolic complications of current cardiac valvular prostheses. Ann Thorac Surg 1982;34:96.
6. Butchert EG, Lewis PA, Combes J, Breckenridge IM: Moving towards prosthesis-specific anticoagulation. In Bodnar E (ed): Surgery for Heart Valve Disease, ICR Publishers, London 1990.
7. Horstkotte D, Loogen F: Operationsindikation bei erworbenen Herzklappenfehlern. In Horstkotte D, Loogen F: Erworbene Herzklappenfehler. Urban und Schwarzenberg, München, 1988, p. 170.
8. Horstkotte D, Trampisch HJ: Long-term follow-up after heart valve replacement. Z Kardiol 1986;75:641.
9. Edmunds LH, Clark RE, Cohn LH, Miller DC, Weisler RD: Guidelines for reporting morbidity and mortality after cardiac valvular operations. Ann Thorac Surg 1988;46:257.
10. Horstkotte D, Loogen F, Kleikamp G, et al: The influence of heart valve replacement on the natural history of isolated mitral, aortic and multivalvular disease. Z Kardiol 1983;72:494.
11. Lillehei CW: The St Jude medical prosthetic heart valve: results from a five-year multicentre experience. In Horstkotte D, Loogen F (eds): Update in Heart Valve Replacement, New York, Springer, 1986.
12. Horstkotte D: Thromboembolic hazard following heart valve replacement. Influence of patient-related and other non-therapy dependent factors. Austin, Silent Partners, 1992.
13. Blackstone EH: Methods and limitations of follow-up assessment of replacement heart valves. In Bodnar E, Frater RWM (eds): Replacement Cardiac Valves, Pergamon, New York, 1991.
14. Horstkotte D: Prosthetic valves or tissue valves – a vote for mechanical prostheses. Z Kardiol 1985;74 (suppl. 6):19.
15. Horstkotte D, Haerten K, Schulte HD, et al.: Hemodynamic findings at rest and during exercise after implantation of different mitral valve prostheses with equal tissue annulus diameter. Z. Kardiol 1983;72:385.
16. Horstkotte D, Friedrichs W, Schulte HD, Loogen F: Haemodynamik und Leistungsfähigkeit

von Patienten nach prothetischem Herzklappenersatz. In Loskot F (ed): Herzerkrankungen, Darmstadt, Steinkopff, 1986, pp. 387.

17. Moritz A, Kobinia G, Steinseifer U, et al: Subjective noise perception and sound pressure levels after valve replacement with St Jude medical and Duromedics–Edwards bileaflet heart valve prostheses. Z Kardiol 1989;78:784.

18. Horstkotte D, Loogen F: Histoire naturelle des cardiopathies valvulaires acquises: In Acar J (ed): Cardiopathies Valvulaires Acquises. Paris, Flammarion, 1985, pp. 225.

B: Intellectual Functioning

5. Cognitive function before and after cardiac surgery: a comparison of cardiac valvular replacement and coronary artery bypass surgery

ALLEN E. WILLNER

1. Summary

Cardiac valvular surgery patients have often been found to have poorer cognitive functioning than coronary artery bypass graft (CABG) surgery patients. Since studies of cardiac valvular surgery were usually reported in the 1970s and CABG studies in the 1980s, the finding, as Sotaniemi [1] suggested, could be attributed to:

(1) more severe pathology in the valvular surgery patients; or
(2) the studies having been done in two different decades. Surgical techniques had improved considerably by the 1980s and, with lower surgical stress, the CABG patients might appear to function better.

The results of 456 patients tested preoperatively at three time intervals (1972–73, 1980–85, 1985–88) were examined. Of these patients, 380 were also retested approximately a week postoperatively. Patients were examined pre- and post-operatively with the conceptual level analogy test (CLAT). No significant differences between CABG and Valve surgery patients were found overall or at any of the three intervals. The mean ages of the patients who had surgery did increase significantly over the three intervals (CABG 54, 58, 62; Valve 54, 56, 59). Some sex differences were found: women had significantly lower preoperative scores than men. Finally, patients who had a postoperative cognitive drop (of at least one standard deviation) were compared across the three time intervals. The percentages of valve patients with cognitive drop were: 18, 12, and 0%; the corresponding figures for the CABG group were: 7, 11, and 4%.

These data were derived from coronary bypass and cardiac valvular surgery patients selected from the same milieu at the same hospital, during three time intervals spanning seventeen years. They do not support the hypothesis of poorer cognitive functioning in valve than in CABG surgery patients.

Paul J. Walter (ed.): *Quality of Life after Open Heart Surgery*, 39–45.
© 1992 Kluwer Academic Publishers.

2. Introduction

Despite the general impression that cardiac valvular surgery has more severe consequences for cognitive functioning than coronary artery bypass graft (CABG) surgery, remarkably few studies have looked into the matter. Although several investigators have used sizable numbers of CABG and valve surgery patients [2–8], few if any have investigated any differences in cognitive functioning between them.

The general impression of greater severity of cognitive problems in valvular surgery may be related to the intrusiveness of this surgery in which the heart is opened with potential for release of surgical air, thrombi, calcium deposits and other debris into the circulation. It may also be related to the chronicity of the cardiac valvular disease. CABG surgery on the other hand, takes place on the surface of, rather than inside the heart, and therefore is less likely to provoke such problems. On the other hand, as Sotaniemi [1] has noted,

. . . it must be emphasized that most of the CABS studies have been published in the '80s and those dealing with valvular surgery during the '70s, which together with surgical and technical improvements may overestimate the hazards of modern valvular surgery.

There seem to be few if any studies conducted with samples of both CABG and valvular surgery patients carried out at the same time in the same setting. This issue was addressed here by examining several samples, each including both coronary bypass and cardiac valvular surgery patients. Each sample had its surgery in the same hospital during the same period of time. Thus, one would not expect differences to be a function of improvements in surgical technique over time. Three such samples, each consisting of CABG and cardiac valvular surgery patients studied in the same hospital over a period of 17 years, are reported here.

3. Methods

3.1. *Study sample*

Four hundred and fifty-six cardiac surgery patients were examined preoperatively during three intervals of time: 1972–73, 1980–85, 1985–88 (Table 1). Of these patients, 380 were also retested about a week postoperatively. The first sample (1972–73) consisted of 199 patients, 125 coronary artery bypass graft (CABG) patients (107 male and 118 female) and 74 cardiac valvular surgery (Valve) patients (42 male and 32 female). The second sample (1980–85)included 166 patients, 140 CABG (112 male and 28 female) and 26 Valve patients (11 male and 15 female). The most recent sample (1985–88)

Table 1. Demographic information for 456 coronary bypass and cardiac valvular surgery subjects operated on at three different periods of time.

N = 199(44%)	BYPASS		VALVE	
	MALE	FEMALE	MALE	FEMALE
N	107	18	42	32
X̄ AGE	54.1	57.6	52.9	56.5
X̄ CLAT	5.54	5.56	5.40	3.72

PERIOD 1
1972-1973

N = 166(36%)	BYPASS		VALVE	
	MALE	FEMALE	MALE	FEMALE
N	112	28	11	15
X̄ AGE	58.2	58.7	55.7	55.4
X̄ CLAT	6.73	4.39	7.55	4.80

PERIOD 2
1980-1985

N = 91(20%)	BYPASS		VALVE	
	MALE	FEMALE	MALE	FEMALE
N	50	23	5	13
X̄ AGE	63.4	64.4	62.0	57.5
X̄ CLAT	5.36	3.39	3.40	2.69

PERIOD 3
1985-1988

consisted of 91 patients, 73 CABG patients (50 male and 23 female) and 18 valve patients (5 male and 13 female).

The proportion of valvular surgery patients in the overall sample of 456 patients was 26% with the remaining 74% having CABG surgery. The proportion of valvular surgery patients in the three time periods sampled was: 37, 16, and 20%, with the remainder being CABGs. The overall sample was divided among the three time intervals as follows: 199 in period 1 (44%), 166 in period 2 (36%), and the remaining 91 (20%) in period 3.

3.2. *Neuropsychological tests*

An extensive battery of tests was administered at each time interval studied. Unfortunately, because of the length of the time interval (17 years) and the different aims of the investigations, only one test was used at all three periods of time, the conceptual level analogy test (CLAT). It was used so consistently because of the investigators' impression of its sensitivity to cognitive losses in cardiac surgery patients.

The CLAT is a 42-item, multiple-choice analogy test [6,9] constructed so as to be refractory to solution by word association, and in which the major variable is the difficulty of the analogical relationships, and not the vocabulary or information level of the items. The CLAT test has been used in several

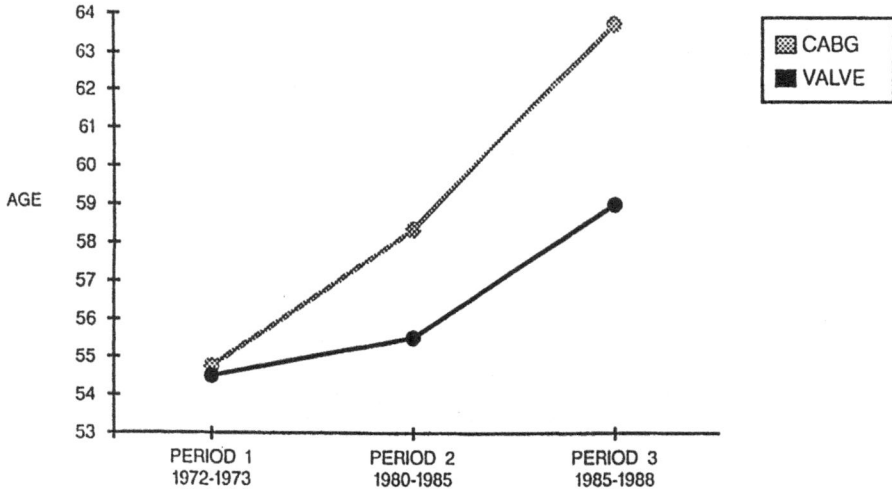

Figure 1. Mean age of CABG and valve surgery patients operated at 3 periods of time.

studies of cardiac surgery [6–7,9]. It was administered about a day or two preoperatively and about a week after the surgery.

4. Results

Figure 1 indicates the mean ages of CABG and Valve patients at each of the three periods of time. As one can see, the mean ages increase sharply with time ($p < 0.001$), especially in the case of the bypass patients. The mean age of the CABG patients was higher than that of the valve patients.

Figure 2 shows no significant change in preoperative CLAT scores over the time period studied. Preoperative CLAT scores rose from period 1 to 2, and declined from period 2 to 3. There was no significant difference between the preoperative CLAT scores of CABG and valve patients, either overall or at any one of the three time periods

Table 2 gives preoperative minus postoperative CLAT scores (difference CLAT scores) for 380 CABG and Valve patients. The remaining 76 patients were not retested for several reasons, because of: problems in scheduling, but also refusal to be retested, being too ill or expiring. In time period 1, 71% of the patients were retested, 78% of the CABGs and 59% of the Valves. This was the lowest proportion of patients retested in any time period. In time period 2, 99% of the patients were retested, and in period 3, 80% were retested.

An analysis of the data summarized in Table 2 shows no significant differences in mean CLAT scores between CABG and Valve patients either overall, or at any of the three time periods. Although there were no signifi-

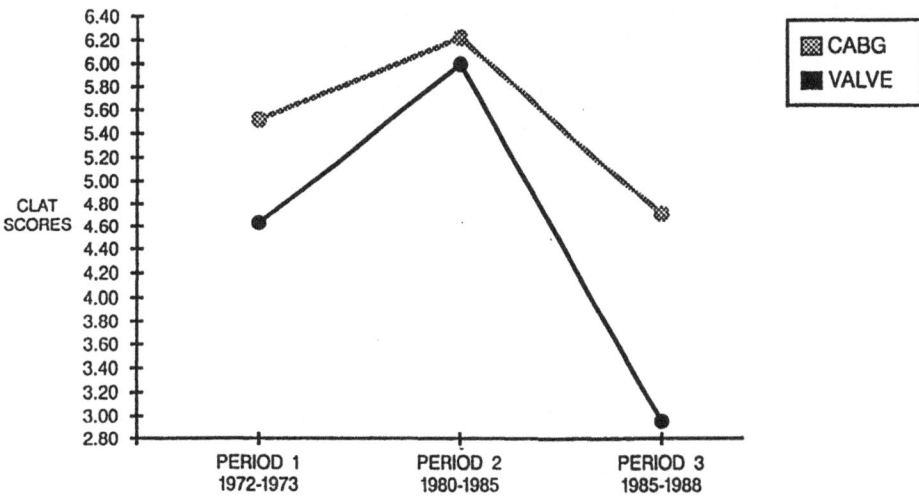

Figure 2. Comparison of pre-op CLAT mean scores in CABG and valve patients at 3 time periods.

cant changes in mean CLAT scores postoperatively it was possible that the cognitive losses of a minority of patients were overwhelmed by modest increases in a majority of patients. To evaluate this possibility, the number of cases with a postoperative 'cognitive drop' was calculated. Cognitive drop was defined as any instance in which the postoperative CLAT was one

Table 2. Preoperative minus postoperative CLAT scores for 380 coronary bypass and cardiac valvular surgery patients operated on at three periods of time.

	BYPASS		VALVE	
	MALE	FEMALE	MALE	FEMALE
N	84	14	27	17
X̄ AGE	53.8	57.4	51.6	57.1
X̄ DIFFCLAT	-0.46	0.36	0.22	0.47

PERIOD 1
1972-1973

	BYPASS		VALVE	
	MALE	FEMALE	MALE	FEMALE
N	111	28	11	15
X̄ AGE	58.1	58.7	55.7	55.4
X̄ DIFFCLAT	0.55	-0.43	1.36	-1.33

PERIOD 2
1980-1985

- CLAT = INCREASE POSTOP
+ CLAT = DECREASE POSTOP

	BYPASS		VALVE	
	MALE	FEMALE	MALE	FEMALE
N	39	17	5	12
X̄ AGE	61.7	61.4	62.0	57.0
X̄ DIFFCLAT	-0.21	0.12	0.20	-1.17

PERIOD 3
1985-1988

Table 3. Proportion of patients whose CLAT score drops postoperatively by at least 3 points arranged according to type of surgery and period of time in which the surgery was done.

	PERIOD 1	PERIOD 2	PERIOD 3
BYPASS	$\frac{7}{98}$ = 7%	$\frac{15}{139}$ = 11%	$\frac{2}{56}$ = 4%
VALVE	$\frac{8}{44}$ = 18%	$\frac{3}{26}$ = 12%	$\frac{0}{17}$ = 0%

CORRELATIONS (r) BETWEEN COGNITIVE DROP AND PERIOD OF TIME

FOR CABG PATIENTS r = −0.03, p = 0.64
FOR VALVE PATIENTS r = −0.20, p = 0.058

standard deviation or more below the preoperative CLAT. Table 3 shows that the incidence of cognitive drop across the three time periods was: for CABGs 7, 11, and 4%; and for Valves 18, 12, and 0%. The correlation between incidence of cognitive drop and time period was −0.03, for CABGs ($p = 0.64$), and −0.20 ($p = 0.058$) for Valves.

Figure 3 shows a strong trend for the incidence of cognitive drop in Valve patients to decline over the 17 year period, whereas there was no discernible relationship for CABG patients.

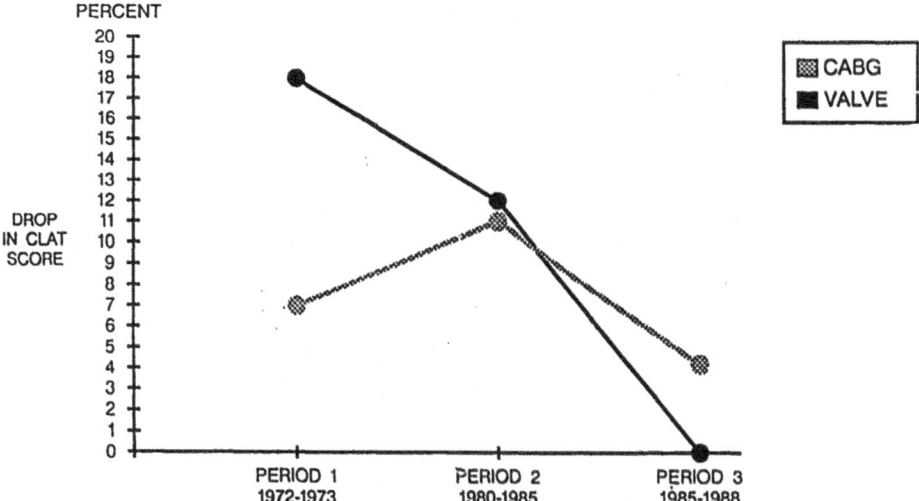

Figure 3. Proportion of patients whose CLAT score drops postoperatively by at least 3 points arranged according to type of surgery and period of time in which the surgery was done.

5. Discussion

The study investigated the general impression that cardiac valvular surgery patients were more cognitively impaired than CABG patients. The results in this study do not support that impression. No significant differences were found between CABG and Valve patients: preoperatively, postoperatively, across all time intervals, or at any of the three time intervals. These results call into question the general impression that valve surgery patients have more cognitive problems than CABG patients. That impression may be attributable to the fact that valve surgery was developed before CABG surgery. Surgical techniques had improved considerably by the 1980s and with reduced surgical stress the CABG patients might appear to do better than the valve patients of the previous decade. The second finding of the study – that there has been a significant increase in the mean age of both CABG and Valve surgery patients – corresponds with the general impression.

References

1. Sotaniemi KA: Prevalence and causes of cerebral complications in cardiac surgery. In: Willner, AE ed. Cerebral damage before and after cardiac surgery. Dordrecht: Kluwer Academic Publishers, in press.
2. Aberg T and Kihlgren J: Effect of open heart surgery on intellectual function. Scand J Thor Cardiovasc Surg (Suppl. 15), 1974.
3. Aberg T and Kihlgren M: Cerebral protection during heart surgery. Thorax 1977b;32:525.
4. Willner AE, Rabiner CJ, Wisoff BG, Fishman J, Rosen B, Hartstein M, Klein DF: Analogy tests and psychopathology at follow-up after open heart surgery. Biological Psychiatry 1976;11:687–696.
5. Garvey JW, Willner AE, Wolpowitz A, Caramante L, Rabiner CJ, Weiss D, Wisoff BJ: The effect of arterial filtration during open heart surgery on cerebral function. Circulation 1983(Suppl II);68:125–128.
6. Willner AE, Caramante L, Garvey JW, Wolpowitz A, Rabiner CJ, Weiss D, Wissoff BG: The relationship between arterial filtration during open heart surgery and impaired mental abstraction ability. Proceedings of the American Academy of Cardiovascular Perfusion, Volume 4 1983.
7. Willner AE, Rabiner CJ, Wissoff BG, Hartstein M, Struve FA, Klein DF: Analogical reasoning and postoperative outcome: predictions for patients scheduled for open heart surgery. Arch of Gen Psychiatry 1976;33:255–259.
8. Willner AE, Rabiner CJ: Psychopathology and cognitive dysfunction five years after open heart surgery, Comprehensive Psychiatry 1979;20:409–418.
9. Willner AE: Conceptual Level Analogy Test. Copyright, 1971.
10. Willner AE, Rodewald G eds: Impact of cardiac surgery on the quality of life. Neurological and Psychological aspects. New York: Plenum, 1990.

6. Neuropsychologic outcome after heart valve replacement

KYÖSTI A. SOTANIEMI

1. Introduction

The cardiac valve surgery patient faces the threat of a number of central nervous system (CNS) complications before, during and after operative procedures. The cardiac disorder itself often leads to various kinds of cerebral dysfunction; the necessary investigations preceding surgery carry their own risks, and the operation itself is a complex procedure with a vast variety of potentially hazardous factors; and finally, the postoperative phase brings the risk of further complications such as those associated with prosthetic infections and lifelong anticoagulant therapy. Although surgical skills, anaesthesiological equipment and standards of care and surveillance have improved enormously, the past three decades of reparative heart surgery have clearly shown that CNS dysfunction still remains a major challenge in all the mentioned phases of the treatment of cardiac valvular disease.

The occurrence of severe cerebral damage induced during operations has become rare which is, of course, of paramount importance, but at the same time improved cerebral investigatory methods have also clearly shown that what has previously been known of the postoperatively detected CNS disorders has been but a narrow view of the actual events. In addition to neurologic defects, intellectual and psychic complications have also been encountered and it is possible to find subclinical CNS damage much more often than has been supposed. This has been shown with the use of neuropsychologic, electroencephalographic (EEG), neuroradiologic and neurochemical investigations. Now, as the major operative technical and surgical problems seem to be in the process of being solved, increasing attention is paid to the impact of even the most subtle CNS complications in order to achieve further development in the operative safety thus improving the quality of life and long-term well being of the patient.

This chapter reviews the prevalence, causes, clinical features, prediction and prevention of neuropsychologic and organic mental disturbances related to cardiac valvular surgery.

Paul J. Walter (ed.): Quality of Life after Open Heart Surgery, 47–60.
© 1992 Kluwer Academic Publishers.

2. Prevalence of CNS complications in cardiac surgery

Because the neurologic and neuropsychologic disturbances are often, although not necessarily, interrelated, a review is given over both clinical neurologic and higher cerebral dysfunction associated with the cardiac investigations and treatments.

2.1. CNS complications related to investigatory procedures

The reported prevalence of cerebral complications associated with cardiac catheterization is low, from 0.03% to 0.23% [1–3]. In a large study on over 1000 catheterizations, 10 cases of cerebral dysfunction were described [2]. The mechanisms thought to be responsible for cerebral damage are: toxic reaction to contrast medium; thrombosis related to pre-existing disease; dehydration; hypotension; and embolization from the vessels, heart or catheters [1–4]. Stroke in catheterization is most probably caused by embolism [3,4]. The prevalence of brain stem stroke when compared with carotid territory stroke has been disproportionally high[2,3] which has led to suggestions that, as most emboli are known to be distributed in the carotid arteries, a large proportion of the carotid emboli must remain unrecognized in comparison with the emboli of the more symptomatic brain stem area [5].

2.2. Postoperative neurologic complications in valvular surgery

In cardiac valvular replacement surgery, overall neurologic complication prevalence values between 3% and 53% have been reported [6–10]. Considering the available studies with properly performed neurological assessment, 23% [8] seems to be the lowest value. The mentioned prevalences include all the clinically detectable abnormalities and therefore represent only the minimum percentage of actual cases with CNS involvement; the inclusion of subclinical disorders in the compilation of these prevalence values would naturally increase the percentage. The prevalence of fatal cerebral damage has decreased clearly since the early years of valvular replacement, being now of the order of 2% [10,11].

Motor deficits in the extremities or in the cranial nerve distribution, primitive reflexes, visual field defects, sensory disturbances and cognitive defects have been the most common CNS abnormalities [6–13]. The signs may be focal and single but may also form a complex variety of signs reflecting diffuse or multiple cerebral damage. Generally, the clinical signs have been found to show a good and rapid recovery, resulting in a favourable outcome; at the time of discharge from hospital 2% to 15% of survivors are reported to display residual signs of cerebral complications and the prevalence of persistent invalidizing abnormalities is well below 5% [10,12,14]. Most of the available studies have covered only the first postoperative weeks or months and information concerning any later outcome is scarce. In one five-year follow-up study [14] of 55 valvular replacement patient, two patients had persistent motor defects and two further patients who had initially fully recovered from their motor defects within the firt postoperative months were found to redevelop the same sign year after operation without any obvious neuroradiologic or other verification of cerebral infarction or any other specific cause. Thus, the influence of operation-related complications on the patient's well-being is not necessarily eliminated when the clinical signs have recovered.

Multiple valve replacements are known to be associated with cerebral complications more often than single valve replacements [8,10,15]. Moreover, mitral valve patients may run a higher risk of CNS damage than aortic patients [16]. These differences may be attributable to the more complex and more prolonged operative procedure needed for multiple valve reconstructions than that for single operations but they may also be attributable to the preoperative events and to the nature and duration of the cardiac disease itself [17,18]. Embolic complications are well known to be more frequent in mitral than in aortic procedures, and this factor may be reflected in the less favourable outcome of the former cases.

In addition to CNS complications, the valvular replacement procedures may entail various peripheral nervous disorders. Of these, brachial plexopathy which occurs in up to 5–12% [19,20] and peripheral neuropathies are the most common manifestations.

2.3. *Neuropsychologic dysfunction after valvular surgery*

2.3.1. *General considerations*
Assessment of the exact prevalence of cerebral dysfunction related to cardiac valvular replacement is difficult due to the heterogeneity of the patient materials and investigatory methods and timings. The reported prevalence values have varied throughout the range between 0% and 100% [7–9,16,21–23]. Some aspects require specific consideration. The detection of CNS dysfunction is essentially dependent on the investigatory methods used and on the timing of evaluations. Some authors have registered only obvious intellectual and cognitive defects while others consider any postoperatively detected decline in the psychometric scores to reflect CNS complications. Generally, the studies performed by non-neurologists and investigators without neuropsychological training have ended up with considerably lower prevalence values than those with appropriate training [17,24]. This difference is not limited just to the postoperative examination but obviously also

affects both the data available on the preoperative CNS events and the assessment of their role as the determinants of the outcome.

There is no reason to overlook even the most subtle disturbances detected postoperatively. Although some of the disorders found immediately or shortly after anaesthesia may be related to the used medications and be non-specific and rapidly resolve themselves, all kinds of disturbances should be considered as potential indices of brain damage regardless of the presence or absence of actual functional invalidity. There is indeed evidence that many varied subclinical events are associated with brain damage and that even the slightest postoperative signs of dysfunction, despite a usually rapid recovery, may predict later problems evident in the long-term outcome of the patient [18].

Further embarrassment in the evaluation of the reported complication frequencies is caused by the heterogeneous patient materials. In general, reparative heart surgery for congenital defects and for valvular disease seems to carry a higher risk of major cerebral complications than coronary artery bypass grafting (CABG). On the other hand, it must be emphasized that most of the CABG studies [25–31] have been published in the '80s and '90s and those dealing with valvular surgery [8–9,16,21–23] during the '70s and early '80s, which together with surgical and technical improvements may overestimate the hazards of modern valvular replacement surgery.

Another factor which has a great influence on the CNS complication values is the study methodology. Both in valvular and CABG surgery, studies with retrospective evaluations [15,31,32] have claimed that postoperative CNS disturbances are rare (from 1.3% to 5.6%) while prospective studies [8–10,16,25–31] report values of a quite different magnitude of up to 61–85%. Retrospective studies must be interpreted with caution, at least when any less severe complications than frank hemiplegia are considered.

2.3.2. *Nature of neuropsychologic complications in valvular replacement surgery*

The use of neuropsychologic tests a indicators of postoperative CNS dysfunction is based on their ability to distinguish emotional based task interference from interference due to structural or physiologic changes in the brain. Considering the post-operative effects, it is important to note that neuropsychologic disturbances are not unique to cardiac operations although they are far more common in open-heart surgery than in general thoracic and other major vascular surgery [23,26,27]. Extracorporeal circulation during the cardiopulmonary bypass is, however, the condition unique to open-heart surgery and, most commonly, the occasional postoperative CNS disturbances are clearly attributable to this particular procedure.

As mentioned earlier, neuropsychologic studies concerning the outcome of valvular surgery are not very recent, studies on CABG patients having been given the main attention presently. Most certainly, this must not be interpreted to indicate that the neuropsychologic problems related to valvular surgery have been solved but that the factors potentially harmful to the brain are far more numerous and complicated in valvular replacement than in CABG.

Gilberstadt and Sako (1967) [34] investigated 53 valvular replacement patients and reported a significant decline in speed of perceptual motor coordination, attention span and rote memory three weeks after surgery as compared with the preoperative performance. They stated that patients with least reserve due to old age, poor intellectual capacity, and presurgery neurological complaints had the highest surgical risks. Lee *et al.* (1969) [8] observed disturbances in higher cerebral functions to be still present three months after surgery. They emphasized the role of low cardiac output, diminished cerebral perfusion and cerebral hypoxia as the determinants of CNS dysfunction manifesting as postoperative decline in overall intellectual performance, object assembly, psychomotor speed and recent memory. The disturbances showed a beneficial outcome three months after the operation. The prevalence of postoperative disorders was 31% in their patient material of 71 patients with extracorporeal circulation, which contrasts to 0% in the control patients without such a procedure.

Frank *et al.* (1972) [35] evaluated 49 patients by psychometric tests immediately before and six months after valvular surgery and found an improvement in all measured areas of intellectual performance. They reported statistically significant improvements in the full scale of Wechsler Intelligence quotient as well as in the tests for visual and verbal functions. It was concluded that the observed improvement was only due to practice effects and that improved cerebral perfusion did not measurably enhance intellectual functions. In a further study with one year's follow-up, Heller *et al.* (1974) [36] stated that although over 90% of the patients showed improvement in their physical condition compared with preoperative evaluation, general psychologic adjustment declined.

In another study [23] 113 patients had a neuropsychological follow-up for two months and 45 patients up to one year after valve replacement. Patients without any obvious postoperative neurologic disorders showed a marked impairment in four of the used six psychometric tests about a week after surgery. Two months later this group still showed a pervasive difference when compared with the general thoracic surgery group which was used as a reference group. The tests howing the most marked changes were the ones measuring visual and spatial perception and perceptual speed whereas those measuring verbal comprehension, logical reasoning and short-term memory were more stable. Patients displaying obvious neurologic signs postoperatively showed an extreme fall in all six subtests one week after operation; the preoperative level of performance was regained within two months. The most important intraoperative parameters determining the neuropsychologic outcome were the length of the perfusion time and the presence of valvular calcification.

In contrast to a vast literature devoted to the short-term neuropsychologic outcome after valvular surgery, reports on the long-term postoperative outcome are scarce. Sotaniemi *et al.* (1981) [16] carried out a one-year follow-up in 49 valvular surgery patients and continued the follow-up to five years [18]. A battery of seven psychometric tests was used in the studies. Overall analysis of the postoperative results showed a statistically significant rise of the performance sum score of the tests. However, when the patients were divided according to the presence or absence of neurologic signs of operation-induced cerebral damage significant improvement was seen only in those without clinically detectable disorders, the others failing to reach in five years the level the uncomplicated patients had reached already in two months. In the long-term course, verbal and visual tests were the tests which differentiated the two patients groups from each other. Those patients whose first postoperative performance sum score was lower than the preoperative score never gained any improvement during the following five years. Of the intraoperative parameters, long perfusion time was found to be the most important one. The neuropsychologic outcome was significantly less beneficial after operations with perfusion times longer than two hours than after shorter perfusion times. Interestingly, the difference between the two perfusion time groups was most evident not early after operation but during the late phase of the follow-up. As in previous reports, the postoperatively seen improvement was interpreted to be due to the practice effect. However, some data were given to suggest that the possibility of even real enhancement of psychometric performance achieved by correcting the long-lasting circulatory disturbance should perhaps not be totally denied as has been done thus far. Any firm evidence of even more beneficial consequences of the treatment lacking, it was, however, clear-cut that the patients who had an uneventful operation could not only maintain their performance level but could also achieve benefit of the learning effect while those who developed CNS complications displayed the contrary. It is noteworthy that poor postoperative performance was not related to the presence or clinical complications only; also the patients with long perfusion times but without any clinically detectable disorders showed a poor neuropsychologic outcome.

2.3.3. *Relationship between neuropsychologic and other measures of postoperative outcome*

In contrast to some early papers on valve replacement [34,35], most of the available studies report a significant interrelationship between neuropsychologic and clinical outcomes [8,16,23,37]. In one study [16], impairment of the psychometric performance was seen in 8% of the patients without and in 85% of the patients with clinical signs of CNS damage. In particular, the visual tests and the tests for psychomotor speed, memory and attention correlated with the clinical measures both in the short-term and in the long-term follow-up as has been reported earlier [23,24]. This emphasizes that there is no reason to overlook even the slightest degree of clinical disturbance related to operation because it may indicate the presence of other disorders which may otherwise remain unrecognized but may even entail long-term consequences.

Relatively little attention has been paid to the investigation of the correlation between neuropsychologic measures and other subclinical indicators of postoperative outcome. Electroencephalographical (EEG) studies [16,18] have shown that neuropsychological dysfunction is more frequent in patients with EEG indicators reflecting diffuse rather than focal cerebral damage. Patients who had improvement in their psychometric scores after operation had a more beneficial EEG outcome than those whose scores declined. The prevalence values of abnormal EEG before and five years after operation were 47% and 19% in the former and 42% and 33% in the latter group [18]. Quantitative EEG analysis showed that the increase in slow wave activity and the decrease in alpha activity in the latter group between one year and five years after operation were both two times greater than in the former group. The value of EEG investigations performed simultaneously with clinical and psychometric testing is in providing objective evidence of cerebral involvement but a perfect parallelism cannot be expected because of the different levels of function that these methods measure.

3. Delirium after cardiac valve replacement

Delirium used to be a very common complication after valvular surgery in the '60s, the reported prevalence values ranging from 41–70% [38–40]. More recently, considerably smaller prevalence values have been reported, from 4% to 35% in prospective [7,9,19,34–36] and up to 13% in retrospective studies [12]. In CABG surgery, postoperative delirium has been reported to range from 1–31% in the available prospective studies [13,26,27] whereas the prevalence value in the retrospective evaluations has been claimed to be as low as from 0.3–2% [32,33]. One comparison between valvular replacement and CABG patients [41] revealed postoperative psyhiatric complications in 41% of patients with valvular surgery in contrast to 16% in CABG patients, the difference being statistically significant. In contrast to these relatively high prevalence values in adults, postoperative organic mental disorders are considered rare in children, the available reports claiming delirium to be virtually non-existent [42,43]. As regards to the detection of neuropsychologic dysfunction, also the detection of delirium is dependent on the methods used. Regular postoperative surveillance, despite all advances and all the available information concerning the cerebral complications of cardiac surgery, is still principally orientated to recognizing and registering the cardiac and respiratory measures of the patient. Thus, the severity of brain dysfunction still too often has to be disproportionally hight to be recognized when compared, for instance, to disorders of cardiac functions, the smallest details of which are monitored with devotion. An example of this methodological and surveillance problem is a report [40] which describes postoperative delirium as occurring in 27% of patients when judged from chart reviews, in contrast to 70% when judged after an adequate interview.

4. Causes of postoperative neurpsychologic dysfunction

CNS damage during and after valvular surgery is well recognized but poorly understood. Sometimes specific causes as clear-cut infarctions due to demonstrable emboli, cerebral hemorrhages, and border zone ischemia are identified. However, it is often the case that either the cause of CNS damage remains inexplicable or else, because of the variety of concomitant harmful factors, it is impossible to pinpoint the actual cause of CNS damage. Information concerning the determinants of intraoperative CNS damage is even more embarrassing than that concerning the occurrence of complications described previously in this chapter. This is obviously due not only to the differences in study designs, standards of care and surveillance and surgical and anaesthesiologic skills but also quite evidently to the individual patient's particular abilities to tolerate the conditions operant during cardiopulmonary bypass.

Embolism from the heart or the cardiopulmonary bypass apparatus is one of the most commonly suggested causes of cerebral injury and the most probable cause of severe stroke related to valvular surgery. Macroembolization may be caused by air or particulate matter (valve fragments, calcified debris, fat, mural thrombi) dislodged during manipulation of the heart or crossclamping of the great vessels and embolizing in the cerebral arteries [6–15]. Embolization of calcium particles from the excised valves used to be very common in closed-heart surgery but is rare in modern valvular replacements. Fat may be released during sternotomy or during excision of the mediastinal tissues. Fat emboli may also be formed when blood is exposed to a gas interface or when pooled blood contains free fat droplets. Macroembolization of air may occur when air trapped in the heart or in the proximal parts of the great vessels is pushed forwards when the ventricles begin to eject. Gaseous emboli may also be generated either from air suspended in stored cold blood or from foaming occurring in the cardiopulmonary bypass device, or by technical disturbances in the oxygenator.

Microemboli in the cerebral arteries may consist of aggregated blood elements, fibers from cotton gauzes or sponges, and small bubbles of air.

Microemboli of air are considered to be among the most common causes of cerebral complications resulting in cerebral microinfarction or hypoperfusion [12,44–47]. Oxygenation, particularly in bubble oxygenators, tends to produce bubbling and as the available debubbling methods are not perfect, large quantities of microbubbles can be detected in the carotid arteries [46,47]. Membrane oxygenators produce considerably smaller quantities of microbubbles than bubble oxygenators. Neuropsychologic deficits have been reported to be more common and more severe after bubble oxygenation than after membrane oxygenation [47].

Cerebral hypoperfusion resulting in disturbed neuronal metabolism may be associated with a number of causes of which embolization, low flow rate in cardiopulmonary bypass malposition or obstruction of cannulae, and pre-existing cerebrovascular disease are among the most common [1,6,8,10,12,25–28,47–49]. Most recently, emphasis has been put on the regulation of carbon dioxide tension during cardiopulmonary bypass and its importance in cerebral hypoperfusion and related postoperative consequences [50–54].

The type of blood flow during cardiopulmonary bypass may also be important at the cerebral capillary level; pulsatile flow has been considered to provide a more adequate capillary perfusion than can be achieved with nonpulsatile flow [23,55–57] but clinical and neuropsychological benefits possibly related to pulsatile flow remain to be verified [58].

The role of arterial blood pressure, perfusion pressure and hypotension during heart operations has remained controversial as regards neuropsychological outcome. Intraoperative hypotension has been considered one of the most important causes of CNS damage by some investigators [7,9,27] but less important by many others [6,7,10,12,16,45]. Although it is clear that severe hypotension is disastrous to the brain, moderate hypotension seems to be tolerated but no safe pressure limit can be stated [10,12].

The duration of cardiopulmonary bypass has been regarded as an overall index of all the cumulative risks operant during perfusion. Several studies have shown a positive correlation between the prevalence and severity of postoperative neuropsychologic, clinical and EEG deterioration [7,10,12,16,59] although this has not been the rule [25]. A critical time threshold of two hours has been stated in a number of reports. The influence of long perfusion times has already been referred to earlier in this chapter.

In addition to the cause of cerebral dysfunction described above, there always remains a variety of other factors potentially harmful to the brain in such a complex procedure as valvular surgery is. Anaesthetics may disturb neurotransmission, there is a continuous threat of unexpected occurrences, toxins may be liberated or generated during the procedure, haematological and immunological disturbances may develop, and even thus far unrecognized determinants of cerebral damage may be present. Furthermore, the patient's age, sex and cardiac measures may modify the influence of not only all the above mentioned potential single determinants of CNS damage but also their different combinations.

5. Prediction of CNS dysfunction in cardiac surgery

Realizing the frequent occurrence of CNS disorders and the marked role played by the intraoperative factors of damage, any preoperative predictive information would be of great interest The information would be of especial importance when alternative methods of treatment are weighed against each other. Prognostic correlates would also be useful in detecting cases with particularly high risks, indicating those patients needing special consider-ations for surveillance. However, predictive analyses have been given little attention in the otherwise extensive literature on cardiac surgery.

In the early years of open-heart surgery attempts were made to predict fatalities which were found to be associated with preoperative anxiety, psy-chasthenia and hypochondriasis [60–62] but these analyses have a limited practical value in modern heart surgery which has a very much lower case fatality rate than that seen in the early '60s.

In another study, 50 valvular replacement patients were investigated using a multidimensional approach with simultaneous clinical, neuropsychologic, conventional EEG and computerized quantitative EEG (QEEG) evaluation to assess the preoperative prediction of the postoperative outcome [63]. The presence of one or more of the following indices was prognostically unfavourable: a history of cerebrovascular accidents; delta or sharp wave EEG abnormalities; low mean frequency in QEEG analysis; a poor perfor-mance score in one of the used psychometric tests (Stroop color test). Using these measures, 28 cases with presumably high risks were indicated, and 24 (86%) sustained cerebral complications attributable to the operation. The findings suggest that pre-existing, even slight, cerebral dysfunction may indi-cate not only the consequences of earlier events but also vulnerability and susceptibility to dysfunction in exceptional conditions such as, for example, the cardiopulmonary bypass is.

Unfortunately, the present knowledge of the predictive measures is inade-quate and more research is needed if we are ever to learn whether a practi-cally significant level of prediction for at least the more severe cases can be achieved.

6. Summary

Cardiac valvular disease patients are in danger of neuropsychologic dysfunc-tion related both to the disease itself and, particularly, to the intra- and postoperative conditions. Neuropsychologic complications are not unique to but continuously frequent in open-heart surgery despite all advances in surgical and anaesthesiological skills and techniques. It seems evident that cardiopulmonary bypass which includes a variety of more or less known, or perhaps still unknown, factors harmful to the brain is the main cause of postoperative intellectual disorders. The present cardiopulmonary bypass methods are still too imperfect to replace the physiological cardiorespiratory functions which challenges development, e.g. in microfiltration and in the control of cerebral acid–base balance. Progress in multidimensional investigatory procedures comprising psychometric, neurologic, psychiatric, EEG, microcirculatory and neurochemical measures has shown that the extracorporeal circulation almost invariably results in a certain amount of cerebral dysfunction of which the neuropsychologic disorders are among the most sensitive indicators. Whether or not the harmful consequences are detected, detectable or recognized, depends on the investigatory methods and timings and, of course, on the individual patient's compensatory mechanisms. The ability to tolerate the intraoperative conditions has been shown to be affected by preoperative cerebral events which, in turn, are often related to the cardiac disease itself. Therefore, further research is also needed to understand better the preoperative indices warning of operative risks and, particularly, from the cerebral point of view and not considering the cardiac well-being and outcome only. As higher cerebral functions, after all, determine the quality of life of the years achieved with successful surgery, very high priority should be given to the investigation, surveillance and care of cerebral well-being in cardiac disease and in all the phases of its operative treatment.

References

1. Adams DF, Fraser DB, Abrams HL: The complications of coronary arteriography. Circulation 1973;18:609–617.
2. Dawson DM, Fischer EG: Neurologic complications of cardiac catheterization. Neurology 1977;27:496–497.
3. Lockwood KI, Capraro J, Hanson M: Neurologic complications of cardiac catherization. Neurology 1983;suppl.2:143.
4. Dimmick JE, Bove RE, McAdams AJ: Fiber embolization: A hazard of cardiac surgery and catheterization. N Engl J Med 1975;292:685–689.
5. Hart RG, Sherman DG, Miller VT, Easton JD: Diagnosis and management of ischemic stroke. In: Harvey WP (ed.) Current problems in cardiology. Vol 7, No 7, New York: Year Book Medical Publishers, 1983.
6. Gilman S: Cerebral disorders after open-heart operations. N Engl J Med 1965;272:489–498.
7. Javid H, Tufo HM, Najafi H, Dye WS, Hunter JA, Julian OC: Neurological abnormalities following open-heart surgery. J Thorac Cardiovasc Surg 1969;58:502–509.
8. Lee WH, Brady MP, Rowe JM, Miller WC: Effects of extracorporeal circulation upon behaviour, personality and brain function. Ann Surg 1971;173:1013–1023.
9. Tufo HM, Ostfeld AM, Shekelle R: Central nervous system dysfunction following open-heart surgery. J Am Med Ass 1970;212:1333–1340.

10. Sotaniemi KA: Brain damage and neurological outcome after open-heart surgery. J Neurol Neurosurg Psychiatry 1980;43:127–135.
11. Larmi TRI, Kärkölä P, Kairaluoma MI, Sutinen S, Partanen-Talsta AL: Calcium microemboli and microfilters in valve operations. Ann Thorac Surg 1977;24:34–37.
12. Branthwaite MA: Neurological damage related to open-heart surgery. Thorax 1972;27:748–753.
13. Kolkka R, Hilberman M: Neurologic dysfunction following cardiac operation with low-flow, low-pressure cardiopulmonary bypass. J Thorac Cardiovasc Surg 1980;79:432–437.
14. Sotaniemi KA: Five-year neurological and EEG outcome after open-heart surgery. J Neurol Neurosurg Psychiatry 1985;48:569–575.
15. Branthwaite MA: Prevention of neurological damage during open-heart surgery. Thorax 1975;30:258–261.
16. Sotaniemi KA, Juolasmaa A, Hokkanen TE: Neuropsychologic outcome after open-heart surgery. Arch Neurol 1981;32:2–8.
17. Sotaniemi KA: Neurological complications of open-heart surgery. In: Silverstein A (ed.) Neurological complications of therapy. Selected topics. New York Futura Press, 1982:293–315.
18. Sotaniemi KA, Mononen H, Hokkanen TE: Long-term cerebral outcome after open-heart surgery. A five-year neuropsychological follow-up study. Stroke 1986;17:410–416.
19. Wander Salm TJ, Cereda JM, Cutler BS: Brachial plexus injury following median sternotomy. J Thorac Cardiovasc Surg 1982;89:447–452.
20. Sotaniemi KA: Brachial plexus lesion complicating sternotomy. J Neurol Neurosurg Psychiatry 1982;45:568.
21. Patrick RT, Kirklin JW, Theye RA: The effects of extracorporeal circulation on the brain. In: Allen JG (ed.) Extracorporeal circulation. Springfield: Charles C. Thomas, Ill, 1958:272.
22. Sachdev NS, Carter CC, Swank RL, Blachly PH: Relationship between post-cardiotomy delirium, clinical neurological changes and EEG abnormalities. J Thorac Cardiovasc Surg 1967;54:557–563.
23. Åberg T, Kihlgren M: Effect of open-heart surgery on intellectual function. Scand J Thorac Cardiovasc Surg 1974, supp. 15.
24. Silverstein A, Krieger HP: Neurologic complications of cardiac surgery. Arch Neurol 1960;3:601–605.
25. Breuer AC, Furlan MJ, Hanson MR et al: Central nervous system complications of coronary artery bypass graft surgery: prospective analysis of 421 patients. Stroke 1983;14:682–687.
26. Shaw PJ, Bates D, Cartlidge NEF et al: Early neurological complications of coronary artery bypass surgery, Br Med J 1985;291:1384–1387.
27. Smith PL, Treasure T, Newman SP: Cerebral consequences of cardiopulmonary bypass. Lancet 1986;i:823–825.
28. Shaw PJ, Bates D, Niall EF et al: Neurologic and neuropsychological morbidity following major surgery: comparison of coronary artery bypass and peripheral vascular surgery. Stroke 1987;18:700–707.
29. Harrison W, Schneidau A, Ho R et al: Cerebrovascular disease and functional outcome after coronary artery bypass surgery. Stroke 1989;20:235–237.
30. Carella F, Travaini G, Guzzetti S, Botta S, Pieri E, Mangoni A: Cerebral complications of coronary artery bypass surgery. A prospective study. Acta Neurol Scand 1988;77:159–163.
31. Ferry PC: Neurologic sequelae of open-heart surgery in children. Am J Dis Child 1990;144:369–373.
32. Gonzáles-Scarano F, Hurtig HI: Neurologic complications of coronary artery bypass grafting: case-control study. Neurology 1981;31:1032–1035.
33. Coffey CE, Massey EW, Roberts KB, Curtis S, Jones RH, Pryor DB: Natural history of cerebral complications of coronary artery bypass graft surgery. Neurology 1983;33:1416–1421.

34. Gilberstadt H, Sako Y: Intellectual and personality changes following open-heart surgery. Arch Gen Psychiatry 1967;16:210–214.
35. Frank KA, Heller SS, Kornfeld DS, Malm JR: Long-term effects of open-heart surgery on intellectual functioning. J Thorac Cardiovasc Surg 1972;64:811–815.
36. Heller SS, Frank KA, Kornfeld DS *et al*: Psychological outcome following open-heart surgery. Arch Intern Med 1974;134:908–914.
37. Willner AE, Rabiner CJ, Wisloff BG *et al*: Analogy tests and psychopathology at follow-up after open-heart surgery. Biol Psychiatry 1976;11:678–696.
38. Blachly PH, Starr A: Post-cardiotomy delirium. Am J Psychiatry 1964;121:371–375.
39. Egerton N, Kay JH: Psychological disturbances associated with open-heart surgery. Br J Psychiatry 1964;110:443–439.
40. Kornfeld DS, Zimberg S, Malm JR: Psychiatric complications of open-heart surgery. N Engl J Med 1965;273:287–292.
41. Rabiner CJ, Willner AE, Fishman J: Psychiatric complications following coronary artery bypass surgery. J Nerv Ment Dis 1975;160:342–348.
42. Stevenson JG, Stone EF, Dillard DH, Morgan BC: Intellectual development of children subjected to prolonged circulatory arrest during hypothermic open-heart surgery in infancy. Circulation 1974;49:suppl 2:459.
43. Messmer BJ, Schallberger U, Gattiker R, Senning A: Psychomotor and intellectual development after deep hypothermia and circulatory arrest in early infancy. J Thorac Cardiovasc Surg 1976;79:495–502.
44. Brierley JB: Neuropathological findings in patients dying after open-heart surgery. Thorax 1963;18:291–304.
45. Åberg T, Kihlgren M: Cerebral protection during open-heart surgery. Thorax 1977;32:525–533.
46. Deverall PB, Padayachee TS, Parsons S, Theobold R, Battistessa SA: Ultrasound detection of micro-emboli in the middle cerebral artery during cardiopulmonary bypass surgery. Eur J Cardiothorac Surg 1988;2:256–260.
47. Blauth C, Smith P, Newman SW *et al*: Retinal microembolism and neuropsychological deficit following clinical cardiopulmonary bypass: comparison of a membrane and a bubble oxygenator. A preliminary communication. Eur J Cardiothorac Surg 1989;3:131–138.
48. Branthwaite MA: Detection of neurological damage during open-heart surgery. Thorax 1973;28:464–472.
49. Reed GL, Singer DE, Picard EH, DeSanctis RW: Stroke following coronary-artery bypass surgery. A case-control estimate of the risk from carotid bruits. N Engl J Med 1988;319:1246–1250.
50. Henriksen L: Brain luxury perfusion during cardiopulmonary bypass in humans. A study of the cerebral blood flow response to changes in CO_2, O_2 and blood pressure. J Cereb Blood Flow Metab 1986;6:366–378.
51. Murkin JM: Cerebral hyperfusion during cardiopulmonary bypass: the influence of PaO_2. In: Hiderman J (ed.) Brain injury and protection during heart surgery. Boston: Martinus Nijhof, 1988:47–66.
52. Nevin M, Adams S, Colchester ACF, Pepper JR: Evidence for involvement of hypocapnia and hypotension in aetiology of neurological deficit after cardiopulmonary bypass. Lancet 1988;ii:1943–1945.
53. Prough DS, Rogers AT, Stump DA, Mills SA, Gravlee GP, Taylor C: Hypercarbia depresses cerebral oxygen consumption during cardiopulmonary bypass. Stroke 1990;21:1162–1166.
54. Gravlee GP, Roy RC, Stump DA, Hudspeth AS, Rogers AT, Prough DS: Regional cerebrovascular reactivity to carbon dioxide during cardiopulmonary bypass in patients with cerebrovascular disease. J Thorac Cardiovasc Surg 1990;99:1022–1029.
55. Wright G, Sanderson JM: Brain damage and mortality in dogs following pulsatile and non-pulsatile flows in extracorporeal circulation. Thorax 1972;27:738–749.

56. Kritikou PE, Branthwaite MA: Significance of changes in cerebral electrical activity at onset of cardiopulmonary bypass. Thorax 1977;32:534–538.
57. Andersen R, Waaben J, Husum B *et al*: Nonpulsatile cardiopulmonary bypass disrupts the flow-metabolism couple in the brain. J Thorac Cardiovasc Surg 1985;90:570–579.
58. Henze T, Stephan H, Sonntag H: Cerebral dysfunction following extracorporeal circulation for aortocoronary bypass surgery: no differences in neuropsychological outcome after pulsatile versus nonpulsatile flow. Thorac Cardiovasc Surg 1990;38:65–68.
59. Sotaniemi KA, Sulg IA, Hokkanen TE: Quantitative EEG as a measure of cerebral dysfunction before and after open-heart surgery. Electroenceph Clin Neurophysiol 1989;50:81–95.
60. Henrichs TF, MacKenzie JW, Almond CH: Psychological adjustment and acute response to open-heart surgery. J Nerv Ment Dis 1969;148:158–164.
61. Kimball CP: A predictive study of adjustment to cardiac surgery. J Thorac Cardiovasc Surg 1969;58:891–896.
62. Kilpatrick DG, Miller WC, Allain AN, Huggins MB, Lee WH: The use of psychological test data to predict open-heart surgery outcome: A prospective study. Psychosom Med 1975;37:62–73.
63. Sotaniemi KA: Prediction of cerebral outcome after extracorporeal circulation. Acta Neurol Scand 1982;66:697–704.

C: Emotional State

7. Psychosocial state of patients after heart valve surgery

C. DAVID JENKINS

Cardiac valve surgery began over 30 years ago. The earliest procedures involved merely surgical opening of valves that had been damaged by infectious processes and their sequelae. Subsequently, artificial valves and porcine valves were developed and this ushered in the era of cardiac valve replacement. During the 1970s and 1980s approximately 30 000 to 40 000 cardiac valve operations were performed each year in the United States. Taken together with the many thousands of these procedures performed in Europe, one can estimate that over a million such open-heart procedures have been performed thus far.

In contrast with the intense debate for nearly a decade about whether medical management or surgical management of obstructed coronary arteries was the better course of procedure, there has not been a similar debate over the value of cardiac valve surgery. These procedures have a dramatic effect in removing the symptoms of shortness of breath and physical disability as well as extending life expectancy. The major issue currently under discussion is the extent of additional benefits to other aspects of the quality of life. This report will concentrate on both psychological health and social role function.

Before entering into specific results, I would like to emphasize that cardiac valve patients should not be considered as just a single clinical group. This category involves many kinds of surgical interventions and combinations of interventions. For example, in the Recovery Study, a prospective consecutive series of both CABG and cardiac valve patients, the latter category included patients having surgery on the mitral valve only, aortic valve only, more than one valve (including tricuspid valve) [1]. In addition, over 35% had valve

This research was supported by a grant HL20637: "Recovery after Heart Surgery: Bio-Behavioural Factors" from the U.S. National Heart, Lung, and Blood Institute.

Table 1. Procedures provided to 104 patients receiving cardiac valve surgery.

Cardiac Valve		Valve plus CABG	
Follow-up		*Follow-up*	
Aortic Valve	21	Aortic & CABG	5
Mitral Valve	39	Mitral & CABG	16
Aortic & Mitral	4	Aorta, Mitral, CABG	2
		Other & CABG	2
Sub-total	64		25
Lost to Follow-up		*Lost to Follow-up*	
Died	6	Died	2
Lost to follow-up	1	Lost to follow-up	2
Missed, Seen later	3	Missed, Seen later	1
Total	74	Total	30

surgery in various combinations plus one or more coronary artery bypass grafts done at the same time (Table 1).

Another interesting feature of valve surgery patients is the association with gender. In a systematic random sampling of the members of a patients self-help group in North America, called the Mended Hearts, we found that about twice as many males as females had aortic valve surgery whereas about twice as many females as males has mitral valve surgery [2]. The sex ratio of coronary bypass surgery was 6 to 1 favoring males.

In this same survey, we studied quality of the recovery process over a period of time ranging from 1–15 years across the sample. We found that among valve patients women tended to have better emotional recovery pattern than men whereas among coronary bypass patients women did significantly worse in the recovery process than men. With regard to rehospitalization in the average $3\frac{1}{2}$ years since surgery, women having 2 + 3 vessel bypass and aortic valve surgery had an average of 16% more frequent rehospitalization than men whereas for mitral valve and 1 vessel bypass women had a lower percent of rehospitalization than men. The survey data, of course, maybe be biased by selective entry and drop out from the membership of the organization as well as selective survival of the original cohort.

Our prospective research, The Recovery Study, did not risk these sources of bias. Table 1 shows the distribution of our original entry cohort of 104 valve surgery patients and the reasons for drop out in the first six-months post-operatively, which yielded our final sample of 89 patients whose recovery will be reported in detail.

We were helped in our study design and decisions regarding measures of quality of life by the pioneering work of J.K. Ross and colleagues in Wessex, England who published the first really broad ranging quality of life reports on valve surgery patients in 1976 and 1978 [3].

The Recovery Study placed heavy emphasis on such measures as emotional status, psychoneurological function, social satisfaction, physical activity and

Table 2. Scores on psychological scales before and six months after cardiac valve and combination surgery in 89 patient.

Scale	Pre-op Mean	Post-op Mean	Change	p
Depression	8.68	5.88	−2.80	0.01
Hostility	5.89	6.06	0.17	−
Vigor	10.09	14.51	4.42	0.0001
Fatigue	7.14	5.81	−1.33	−
State-Anxiety	44.53	35.50	−9.03	0.0001
Positive well-being	4.41	5.00	0.59	−
Trouble sleeping	4.27	2.85	−1.42	0.01

social role function. We emphasized quantitation of results and data collection using rigidly structured interviews and patient-completed questionnaires.

We administered the same interviews and questionnaires 1 to 3 days before surgery and again six-months later. We inferred change by comparing scale scores on these two occasions. We believe that is an approach which is more valid than asking patients postoperatively whether or not they are feeling better or in what way their emotions or daily activities have changed. The latter approach is too vulnerable to the patient's desire to please the surgeon or rationalize that given the drastic nature of the intervention, something good must have come from it. It was this same desire to avoid bias that lead us to hire interviewers who were not a part of the clinical care team so that patients would not feel a need to please the interviewer with their responses.

One of our sets of emotional measures came from the Profile of Mood states [4]. This is basically an adjective check list on which respondents indicate the degree to which they felt each of the moods and feelings listed in the last week. Table 2 shows that only 2 of the 4 scales, depression and vigor, showed significant improvements. Fatigue also improved, but much less than expected. Hostility was not expected to change and it did not.

Table 2 also shows the changes occurring in scales for anxiety, well-being, and trouble sleeping. State anxiety, measured by the Spielberger Scale [5], showed a dramatic improvement. This may have been in part because patients were unusually anxious in the few days before they experienced valve surgery. An important addition to this finding is that this lower level of anxiety was also present at 12 months postoperatively. So the gains shown were not transient. Well-being did not improve from pre to post surgery, but there was considerable reduction in trouble sleeping.

We have found that our four-item scale for sleep problems is a strong predictor of physical recovery in the first six-months after surgery. Patients who are free of sleep problems before surgery are much more likely to have complete remission at six-months of dyspnea, angina, and other physical symptoms of cardiac disease. (Manuscript submitted for publication.)

Table 3. Frequency of psychosocial problems reported to have occurred in the first six months after heart surgery.

	Valve & combo	Coronary bypass
Fatigue or weakness	44%	48%
Sadness, depression or crying	39%	40%
Feeling anxious, worried or afraid	39%	38%
Feeling angry or resentful	26%	35%
Difficulty accepting reduced activity	36%	36%
Sample Size	89	318

We also administered scales before and after surgery to measure hopefulness, helplessness, independence and self-esteem. We anticipated that these will improve in persons recovering well from their operation. At six months, we found that none of these scales showed significant improvement. Upon thinking further about these results, we are pleased with the findings. There is really no reason to expect cardiac valve surgery to change feelings of independence, self-esteem and well-being. The fact that our respondents showed no change in averages on these scales over time, confirms that they were not just trying to make us happy by saying everything had improved. Thus, our findings seem not to be distorted by an overall response bias. This gives us greater assurance that our respondents were answering with caution and discrimination and that we can take the positive findings at face value.

From pilot studies we identified a number of psychological complaints that our advisory panel of heart surgery patients had told us were very common in the first six-months after surgery. Table 3 shows the percentage of valve patients who identified each of the five problems as being difficult for them postoperatively. Fatigue or weakness was the most commonly identified difficulty, but the general area of depression, anxiety and worry were also endorsed by 39% of patients. Difficulty accepting reduced activity was also common. The frequency of these complaints among 318 bypass surgery patients is shown in the same table. The two groups have very similar complaint rates despite the different natures of the underlying cardiac diseases and different gender composition.

These data are different than what is implied by the earlier scale scores. It must be remembered, however, that the earlier scales each referred only to the week preceding the examination. What these data say is that 35 to 40% of these patients had episodes of anxiety, depression, fatigue and difficult adjustment to the limitations on their activity, but that most of these were episodic and had cleared up before the one week period covered by the scales at six-month follow-up.

The Recovery Study also included measures of psychoneurological functioning, but these were kept to a minimum due to the large number of variables we felt it important to measure both before and after surgery [6].

We administered the Trailmaking Test and two sub-tests from the Wechsler Memory Scale, logical memory, and visual reproduction – these are the two subscales from this longer test which have the best track record of validity for detecting minor levels of neurological dysfunction. Not all psychoneurological studies of cardiac patients have measured patients both before and 2 times after surgery. We therefore defined normal function for each patient based on what he or she had scored preoperatively. This is a much safer procedure than using published norms because these norms often do not take into consideration the effects of the older age and prior medical history of cardiac valve patients. We arbitrarily selected one standard deviation of the distribution of scores of this patient group as a 'normal range of variability'.

At our reexamination 9 days after surgery, we found that about 1/4 of our patients had shown a decline in scores greater than one standard deviation from their preoperative level. However, by the time of our six-months follow-up examination, all but a very few patients had returned their scores to within one standard deviation of their preoperative level [7]. In fact, the group as a whole did better at six-months on the times for the Trailmaking B Test. This is probably due to a practice effect, but it also underlines the finding that with modern surgical and life support techniques cardiac valve surgery patients generally do not have psychoneurologic deficits which last for six-months.

Return to gainful employment is another commonly used indicator of psychosocial recovery after cardiac valve surgery. The best predictor of whether a patient will go to work after surgery is whether he or she was employed preoperatively and whether they are substantially below the usual retirement age. Of our 89 patients 65% were employed preoperatively. Of these about 2/3 returned to work within the first six-months. Most people resumed work either in the third or the fourth postoperative month. It was interesting to note that of those persons returning to employment, about 1/3 worked part-time, about 1/3 worked full-time, and the final third reported working overtime – more than 40 hours per week.

Interesting differences occurred with changes in disability levels and changes in physical activity levels in the six-months following surgery. There was a substantial reduction in days of disability as part of the recovery process and this occurred both for patients who had simple valve surgery and those who had a combination of valve and bypass grafting in the same operation. Preoperatively, 35% of the patients reported an inability to pursue their usual activities on 5 or more days in the preoperative month, whereas only 8% had this amount of disability six-months postoperatively. A short scale for the amount of daily activity showed no significant change before and after surgery. Both those patients having valve surgery only and those having combination surgery were similar in their daily physical activity levels both before and after their valve operation.

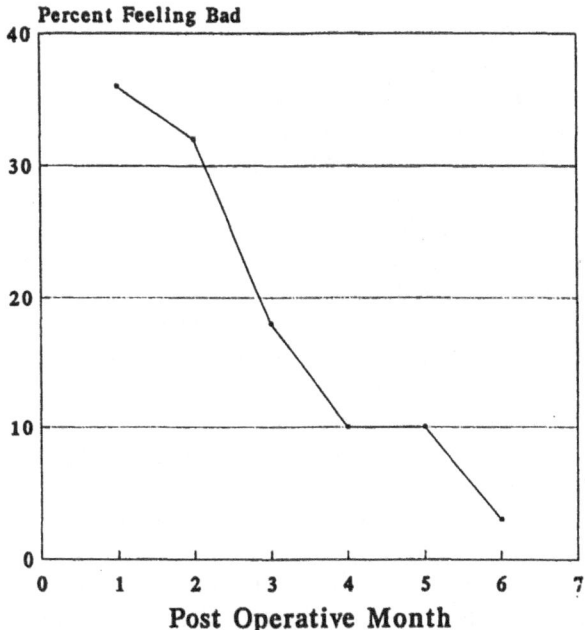

Figure 1. Frequency of 62 cardiac valve surgery patients reporting that they 'Felt particularly bad, physically or other otherwise' by specific post-operative months.

We were interested in the speed at which the recovery process took place after surgery. Was there an immediate improvement? Was it slow and gradual over the full six-months of follow-up? We asked each patient, "Were there any months when you felt particularly bad, physically or otherwise, since your surgery? Let's see now, in what month did you have your surgery?" The interviewer then took the name of the month of surgery and followed by asking specifically about each of the six succeeding months individually and by name. "Was this a month when you felt particularly bad physically or otherwise?" From this style of questioning we could plot a curve showing the speed of recovery. The rapid and regular decline of symptomatic impairment is shown in Figure 1. More importantly, we see that more than 60% of the patients reported no single month particularly troublesome, physically or otherwise, after surgery.

Table 4 shows the severity of dyspnea both before and after surgery. We used the London School of Hygiene Dyspnea Scale to estimate the level of this condition. The table shows substantial improvement in breathing, which is one of the main purposes of cardiac valve surgery. Of the patients having dyspnea preoperatively, 69% were completely relieved at the postoperative interview.

Some colleagues involved in the planning of this study said that dyspnea was the key problem for cardiac valve patients and that angina was not a

Table 4. Changes in level of dyspnea in 89 patients undergoing cardiac valve surgery.

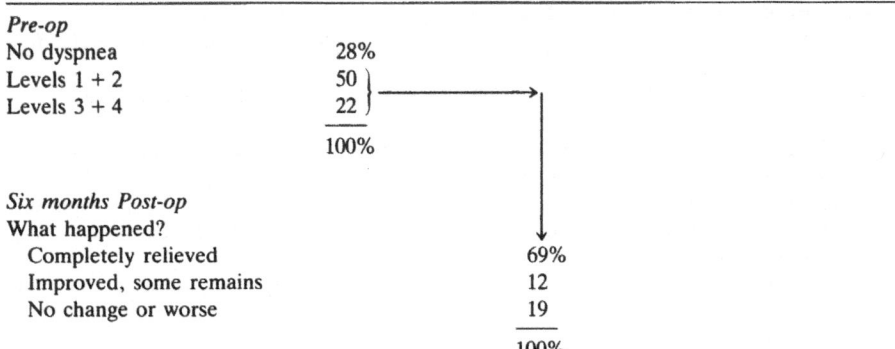

Pre-op	
No dyspnea	28%
Levels 1 + 2	50
Levels 3 + 4	22
	100%

Six months Post-op	
What happened?	
Completely relieved	69%
Improved, some remains	12
No change or worse	19
	100%

frequent symptom. We administered The London School of Hygiene Angina Scale also to valve patients and were quite surprised with the frequency of angina. Of the patients having valve surgery only, 39% reported exertional angina in the month before their operation. This could have been at levels 1, 2, 3 or 4 of the London Angina Scale. Of patients having both valve and bypass surgery, 54% reported exertional angina. This would be expected inasmuch as these patients also receive CABG surgery.

Valve and combination surgery were extremely effective in reducing angina postoperatively. Sixty-five percent of patients having only valve surgery reported complete relief of angina postoperatively, whereas 77% (i.e., 10 of 13 patients having preoperative angina within the smaller group of 25 combination surgery patients) reported complete relief from angina.

Considering the remarkable relief, both of angina and dyspnea symptoms, we conclude that there is ample reason for the total improvement in quality of life physical, emotional and social as a function of cardiac valve surgery.

One final question best summarized the patients overall evaluation of their surgery experience. We asked them, "In the light of what you know now, would you undergo surgery again if it were recommended?" The response was strongly positive with 70% giving an unqualified yes, 22% saying that it depended on the circumstances and only 8% giving a fully negative answer. In summary, we can conclude that cardiac valve surgery as it is now practiced has a tremendously high success rate and that the various dimensions of success include the psychological, psychoneurological, social, physical, and biomedical aspects of the patient's lives.

References

1. Jenkins CD, Stanton BA, Savageau JA, Ockene IS, Denlinger P, Klein MD: Physical, psychological, social and economic outcomes six months after cardiac valve surgery. Arch Int Med 1983;143:2107–2113.

2. Zyzanski SJ, Stanton BA, Jenkins CD, Klein MD: Medical and psychosocial outcomes in survivors of major heart surgery. J Psychosom Res 1981;25:213–221.
3. Ross JK, Diwell AE, Marx J et al: Wessex cardic surgery follow-up: the quality of life after operation. Thorax 1978;33:3–9.
4. McNair DM, Lorr M, Droppleman LF: Profile of Mood States: Manual. San Diego: Educational and Industrial Testing Service. 1971.
5. Spielberger CD, Gorsuch RL, Lushene RE: Manual for the state-trait anxiety inventory (self-evaluation questionnaire) Palo Alto, Calif.: Consulting Psychologists Press 1970.
6. Savageau JA, Stanton BA, Jenkins CD, Frater RWM: Neuropsychological dysfunction following elective cardiac operation. 1. Early assessment. J Thorac Cardiovasc Surg 1982;84:585–594.
7. Savageau JA, Stanton BA, Jenkins CD, Frater RWM: Neuropsychological dysfunction following elective cardiac operation. II. A Six-month reassessment. J Thorac Cardiovasc Surg 1982;84: 595–600.

8. Emotional state of patients one year after heart valve replacement: clinical, functional and psychosocial correlates

M. BULLINGER and D. NABER

1. Introduction

The emergence of the quality of life discussion in cardiology has prompted the inclusion of psychosocial endpoints also into cardiovascular surgery [1]. While outcomes such as return to work [2], mental function [3], psychopathology [4] and psychological adjustment [5], had already been considered in previous research, the explicit focus on the patients quality of life in terms of well-being and function is a more recent development.

Existing studies can be distinguished with regard to the type of quality of life assessment used, the research design chosen and the heart-surgical population considered. Especially in the larger outcome studies such as CASS [6], quality of life information is expert-based, i.e. gathered from physician ratings or inferred from medical ratings. However, patient self-ratings of quality of life are also increasingly included in cardiovascular research. In assessing quality of life from the patient's perspective, the use of standardized instruments increasingly replaces the use of methodologically less satisfying ad hoc measures [7]. In terms of design the original prevalence of cross-sectional studies is now supplemented by longitudinal studies with sufficient sample sizes for statistical analyses [8]. As regards the patient population, bypass surgery has been the predominant focus of quality of life research [9–11] while data on patient well-being and function after valve replacement are rare [12,13].

In general studies either do not differentiate between bypass and valve patients or they do not focus on the latter group. Existing research suggests, that patient well-being improves from pre-to-postoperative measure points in valve patients, while cognitive function might be negatively affected, and return to work is problematic in the majority of patients [14]. Referring to the notion of a better outcome in bypass patients, comparisons between both patient groups would be of interest. However, empirical support to assume differences between groups is virtually nonexistent since valve and bypass

Paul J. Walter (ed.): Quality of Life after Open Heart Surgery, 71–87.

patients have rarely been directly compared with regard to their quality of life.

Furthermore, it is unknown to what extent operative techniques such as aortic versus mitral valve replacement or the use of biological versus artificial material affects the outcome for the patient. Thus, research assessing the psychosocial effects of valve operations seems necessary. Such research profits from the inclusion of patient-based, standardized instruments for quality of life assessment which might be supplemented by external ratings through the patients' family. It also profits from the use of a longitudinal design in order to take into account the time perspective of potential psychosocial differences within and between patient groups.

Taking this perspective, the following paper presents results from a prospective study on the quality of life of valve and bypass patients from two weeks before until one year after the operation [15].

Research questions with regard to the patients emotional state related to:

(a) short-term psychiatric symptomatology during the inpatient phase;
(b) the course of emotional state from before to one year after surgery
    – as rated by patients
    – as rated by their family;
(c) differences in emotional state between patient groups one year after surgery
    – as regards types of valve operations
    – as regards bypass patients;
(d) correlates of overall postoperative well-being
    – as concerns indicators of emotional state
    – as concerns patient's psychosocial, clinical and functional state.

2. Methods

A prospective study on the quality of life of patients scheduled for valve replacement or bypass graft surgery was performed in cooperation with the German Heart Centre in Munich. Inclusion criteria were indication for either operation, surgery being scheduled during the 6-month recruitment period, patient age from 18 to 65 years, and informed consent. Exclusion criteria pertained to emergency operations, private health insurance and lack of fluency in German.

Within a multifactorial approach to quality of life the patient's self-rated emotional, physical, functional and social state was assessed. In addition external ratings of patient's quality of life by his or her family were obtained. Psychosocial background measures on coping, social support, health locus of control and personality were available as were psychiatric ratings of the

Table 1. Overview assessments.

Time			Pat Qol	Fam Qol	Psycho-soc	Psychiatr. rating	Neuro psych	Clin. data
Pre 1	−14	days home	X	X	X			X
Pre 2	− 1	day clinic				X	X	
Post 1	+ 4	days clinic				X		X
Post 2	+ 7	days clinic				X		X
Post 3	+10	days clinic				X	X	X
Post 4	3	months home	X	X				
Post 4	6	months home	X	X				
Post 6	12	months home	X	X				

inpatient psychopathology, assessments of neuropsychological functions and clinical data (see Table 1).

Since an extensive description of the assessment methodology can be found in published papers [15,16], the following information focuses on the description of the variables relevant for the analyses presented.

Patients rated their emotional state with a 35-Item German short form of the Profile of Mood States (POMS [17,18]), a translated and tested 22–item version of the Psychological Well-being Index (PGWB [18,19]), as well as a newly developed and tested Every-Day-Life Questionnaire (EDLQ [20]) and a five-point global rating of quality of life from 1 = excellent to 5 = miserable. These measures were obtained at home two weeks prior to the operation, as well as 3, 6 and 12 months after surgery. At the identical points in time, the families assessed the patient well-being using the POMS.

Patients' psychopathological symptoms during the inpatient phase were rated by trained doctoral students using the AMDP system [21]. This standard German rating scale yields six syndrome scores for apathy, depression, hostility, mania, paranoid-hallucinatory and psycho-organic states, as well as a total score. It was administered in the hospital one day prior to the operation as well as 4, 7 and 10 days thereafter. On the basis of seven neuropsychological tests performed, an index was formed representing the overall degree of cognitive impairment one day before and 10 days after the operation.

Two weeks before surgery, patients completed mailed questionnaires on coping styles (FEKB [22]), health locus of control (SKF [23]), social support (SSF [24]) and personality (FPI [25]).

Sociodemographic information, including vocational status, was available, as were clinical data during the preoperative (e.g. diagnosis, waiting time), perioperative (e.g. type of operation, extracorporal circulation), and postoperative phase (e.g. medication, complications).

For the present paper, the patients' emotional state as assessed via the AMDP system as well as with POMS, PGWB, EDLQ and global rating was analysed for change over time and differences between groups using *t*-tests or corresponding nonparametric tools. Relationships between variables were analysed using correlation techniques. Specifically, Spearman correlation coefficients were used to determine associations within variables assessing emotional state, as well as between emotional state and clinical, functional and psychosocial baseline data. All statistical analyses were performed using the SPSS-PC program.

3. Results

3.1. *Patient sample*

During recruitment, 172 patients fulfilled the inclusion criteria. Of these, 20 did not enter the study for reasons of exclusion, voluntary retreat or hospital-related organizational problems, and six patients rejected participation. In-patient clinical and psychopathological data were available on the 146 study patients. Since 34 patients did not respond to the home-mailed questionnaire preoperatively, the sample size of the present analysis had to be reduced to 112 patients. Of these, 48 received a valve operation and 59 a bypass procedure, the remaining 5 patients had mixed procedures that did not allow an inclusion in the present analysis. Regarding the majority of sociodemographic and clinical data, valve and bypass patients were comparable (see Table 2).

A higher percentage of female patients was found in the valve group, and a tendency toward younger age and correspondingly more health- as compared to age-related retirement was present. With regard to clinical data, the groups did not differ in NYHA status, but valve patients appeared to have had a slightly longer waiting time, shorter operation time, longer stay in intensive care and a higher percentage of postoperative complications, but comparable AMDP-pathology. However, only differences with regard to female sex, operation time and postoperative complications had any statistical significance.

3.2. *Short term Psychiatric symptomatology*

During the inpatient phase, the patients' emotional state was expert-rated using the AMDP total score and subscores for apathy, depression, hostility,

Table 2. Patient characteristics.

	Valve $n = 48$	Bypass $n = 59$
Age	56.6 + 11.5	60.0 + 8.9
% Female	56.3	13.6
% Married	70.8	78.0
% Employment		
full time	19.1	15.4
sick-leave	10.5	30.5
retired health	29.8	22.0
retired age	17.0	25.4
% NYHA II	29.2	27.1
III	60.4	66.1
Waiting time (weeks)	15.1 ± 3.5	13.9 ± 3.2
Operation Aorta	77.8	Grafts: 2.6 ± 0.8
Mitral	22.2	% >2: 63.4%
Operation time (min)	181.6 ± 54.7	232.3 ± 52.5
Intensive care (days)	3.2 ± 3.4	2.9 ± 1.4
% Post-op Complications	91.7	79.7
% Pre-op Psychopathology	25.5	27.7

mania, paranoid-hallucinatory and psycho-organic syndromes. A comparison of the postoperative syndrome scores at days 4, 7 and 10 to the preoperative level one day before the operation yielded significant increases only for the hostility subscale at day 10 ($t = -2.55$, $Df = 44$, $p = 0.02$). Furthermore, a tendency toward deterioration was apparent at day 4 as compared to day -1 in the paranoid-hallucinatory and psycho-organic syndromes, as well as in the total score, which failed to reach significance.

In comparison to the valve patients, the bypass patients showed an increase from the preoperative level to 10 days postoperatively in the total score ($t = 3.56$, $Df = 52$, $p = 0.001$) as well as in apathy ($t = -2.45$, $Df = 52$, $p = 0.018$) and depression ($t = 2.20$, $Df = 52$, $p = 0.032$). Increases in the scores of hostility, paranoid-hallucinatory and psycho-organic syndromes failed to reach significance. Regarding the clinical significance of these changes, it should be noted that apathy and depression were more prominent, both in the valve and bypass groups before the operation as well as thereafter, as were paranoid hallucinatory and organic syndromes (see Table 3).

As regards the patient psychopathology as examined by the AMDP-system, no significant differences between valve and bypass patients were found for the total score or either syndrome score before, as well as 4, 7 or 10 days after the operation. Thus, in terms of psychopathology both patient groups appeared comparable.

Table 3. Psychopathology.

AMDP	Psychopathology*			
	Pre-op −1 day		Post-op +10 days	
	Valve	Bypass	Valve	Bypass
Total score	25.5	23.7	31.9	33.9
Apathy	29.8	23.7	27.7	40.7
Depression	27.7	27.0	23.4	30.5
Hostility	6.4	3.4	23.4	13.6
Mania	8.5	5.1	6.4	6.8
Paranoid-hallucinatory	0	0	2.1	0
Psycho-organic	0	0	3.4	3.4

* Percentage of high score for valve (bypass) patients.

3.2. *Emotional state over time and differences between groups*

3.2.1. *Profile of Mood States (POMS)*
Within the valve patient group, improvements from the preoperative (−14 days) to the postoperative outpatient phase at month 3, 6 and 12 were identified with the POMS which measures four mood states during the preceding week (see Table 4).

Here depression scores dropped significantly from the preoperative to each postoperative time point, as did the fatigue and irritability scores, while vigor scores remained essentially unchanged. With regard to the family ratings a similar time course was found with regard to the significant drops in depression, fatigue and irritability, however, predominantly three months after surgery. From the family perspective, vigor levels increased especially at 6 and 12 months after the operation.

However, as Table 4 shows, slight but nonsignificant discrepancies in patient and family ratings were seen in the assessment of preoperative fatigue and vigor levels as well as postoperative in irritability ratings, with a tendency to a less positive outlook on patient's well-being by the family.

In general, the comparison between the patients' and the families' scores shows a high correspondence in ratings. This correspondence is stressed by high intercorrelations between patient and family ratings of 12-month postoperative mood. High correlations were found for valve (in brackets: bypass) patients and their respective relatives in depression: $r = 0.87***$ $(0.77***)$, fatigue: $r = 0.63**$ $(0.49**)$ and vigor: $r = 047*$ $(0.64*)$. These correlations, however, were lower and nonsignificant for irritability ratings in valve $(r = 0.10)$ and bypass patients $(r = 0.38)$.

As concerns group differences (see Table 4), a comparison of the 12-month postoperative POMS-scores of valve and bypass patients did not yield significant differences between groups. Neither was a comparison of scores

Table 4. Profile of mood states.

		Valve								Bypass	
		−14 days pre-op		3 months post-op		6 months post-op		12 months post-op		12 months post-op	
	Healthy persons	PAT	FAM	PAT	FAM	PAT	FAM	PAT	FAM	PAT	FAM
	n = 52	n = 36	n = 23	n = 36	n = 23	n = 28	n = 22	n = 32	n = 20	n = 45	n = 35
Depression 0–56 x	6.4	24.4	23.7	20.5*	19.0*	19.1*	22.3	20.2*	220.3*	20.3	21.1
sem	1.2	0.9	2.2	1.0	1.8	0.9	1.5	1.2	1.4	1.3	1.3
Vigor 0–28+ x	16.4	17.5	16.0	17.9	17.7	17.9	18.3*	18.2	18.7*	16.6	15.5*
sem	0.8	1.1	1.1	0.8	1.3	1.0	1.2	1.0	1.1	0.7	0.8
Fatigue 0–28 x	8.6	14.8	16.4	11.7***	13.1 ***	10.2***	12.6**	11.2***	11.3***	11.8	13.8*
sem	0.8	0.7	1.0	0.5	1.8	0.5	0.7	0.6	0.8	0.5	0.9
Irritability x	6.1	10.0	11.1	8.7**	8.6	8.0	10.6	8.8	9.6	9.4	11.3
sem	0.8	0.5	0.8	0.3	0.8	1.6	0.7	0.4	0.6	0.4	0.9

+ High score indicates positive well-being.
* $p < 0.05$, **$p < 0.01$, ***$p < 0.001$.

Comparisons were made within the valve patient group from each postoperative measure point to the preoperative level. The same was performed within the valve family group. Bypass patients were compared at 12 months to the valve patients. The same was done for bypass and valve patients families.

Table 5. Psychological general well-being index (PGWB).

			VALVE			Bypass
PGWB		Healthy controls n = 52	−14 days pre-op n = 36	3 months post-op n = 36	6 months post-op n = 28	12 months post-op n = 32	12 months post-op n = 45
Anxiety	x	16.1	15.5	16.6**	15.6	16.3	16.1
0–25[+]	sem	0.7	0.5	0.5	0.6	0.6	0.4
Depression	x	12.0	11.0	12.0*	11.5	11.7	11.8
0–15[+]	sem	0.6	0.4	0.4	0.5	0.5	0.4
Well-being	x	12.1	10.1	10.8	11.3*	11.3*	11.0
0–20[+]	sem	0.9	0.4	0.4	0.5	0.4	0.3
Self-control	x	11.3	8.1	7.8	7.1 ***	7.4**	7.9
0–15[+]	sem	0.4	0.2	0.2	1.6	0.3	0.2
Health	x	11.5	7.6	7.8	8.0*	8.5*	8.1
0–15[+]	sem	0.5	0.2	0.3	0.3	0.2	0.2
Vitality	x	12.8	10.5	9.5*	9.3*	9.4*	9.7
0–20[+]	sem	0.6	0.3	0.3	0.5	0.4	0.3

[+] Range of scores, high scores indicate positive well-being (i.e. lack of anxiety and depression).
* $p < 0.05$ as compared to valve pre-op scores, no significant differences were detected between valve and bypass patients 12 months post-op.

in subgroups of valve patients having received mitral vs. aortic valve replacement or biological vs. artificial valves significant. Bypass families, however, rated their relatives' well-being less favorably than valve families, with differences in fatigue and vigor reaching significance.

In summary the Profile of Mood states suggested an improvement in emotional state in valve patients which was reflected in the family ratings. Bypass and valve patients did not differ in their 12-month postoperative scores. However, only postoperative vigor scores were comparable to a healthy control group. Fatigue, irritability and depression scores tended to be substantially higher in patients as compared to healthy persons.

3.3.2. *Psychological general well-being Index (PGWB)*

More long-term changes during the four weeks preceding each measurepoint were picked up with the Psychological General Well-Being Index (PGWB) (see Table 5).

Here, anxiety scores decreased significantly three months after the operation, as compared to before, as did depression scores. Increases in well-being and in health were apparent 6 and 12 months after the operation, while self-control decreased at these measure points in comparison to the preoperative level. A slight but significant decrease in vitality was noted 3, 6 and 12 months after the operation, as compared to before.

Bypass patients did not differ from valve patients in their 12-month postoperative PGWB scores (see Table 5); they also did not differ at any other time

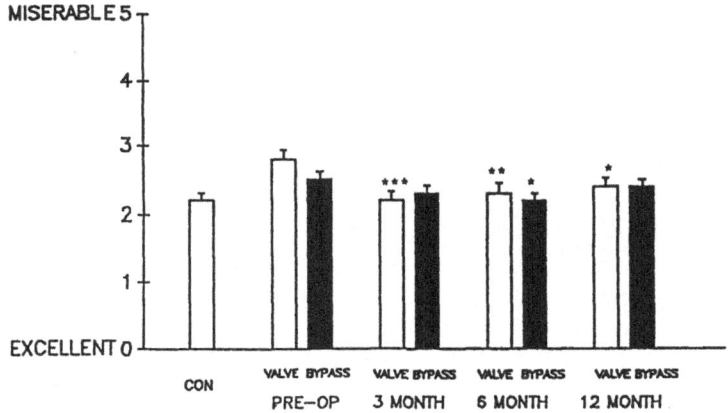

* p < 0.05, ** p < 0.01, *** p < 0.001

Figure 1. Global quality of life rating. Comparisons were made within the valve patient group from each postoperative measure point to the preoperative level. The same was performed with the bypass patients. No differences were found between valve and bypass patients at either measure point.

point. Furthermore, no significant differences in pre- and either postoperative PGWB score were detected between patients having received aortic versus mitral replacement or between patients with biological versus artificial valves.

Within the EDLQ the two subscales measuring psychological function are 'personal assertion' and 'joy of living'. In both subscales significant improvements over the preoperative level were apparent for 3, 6 and as shown 12 months after the operation (personal assertion: $t = 3.43$, $Df = 34$, $p = 0.002$; joy of living: $t = 3.16$, $Qf = 31$, $p = 0.003$). No significant differences in EDLQ were found for valve subgroups or for valve as compared to bypass patients. The general pattern of improvement in emotional state was also reflected in the global quality of life ratings.

3.3.3. *Global quality of life rating*
In the global quality of life rating (see Figure 1), valve patients showed a significant decrease from the pre-operative level as compared to 3, 6 and 12 months post-operatively, indicating a better quality of life. A similar decrease was found in bypass patients for whom – starting from a slightly better preoperative level – a significant improvement was only found three months after the operation. No difference between valve and bypass patients was noted at either measure point. With regard to healthy subjects, both patient groups rated their quality of life at comparative levels.

Table 6. Emotional correlates of one-year postoperative global quality of life ratings.[1]

	Valve n = 32	Bypass n = 45
POMS		
Depression	0.55**	0.70**
Vigor	-0.50**	-0.51 **
Fatigue	0.66***	0.37**
Irritability	0.20	0.32*
PGWB		
Anxiety	0.12	0.51 **
Depression	0.48**	0.68***
Well-being	-0.61***	-0.59***
Self control	0.05	0.31
Health	-0.01	0.03
Vitality	-0.33*	-0.56**
EDLQ		
Assertion	-0.57**	-0.55**
Joy of life	-0.45**	-0.74***

[1] High scores reflect low quality of life.
* $p < 0.05$, **$p < 0.01$, ***$p < 0.001$.

3.4. Correlates of postoperative quality of life

3.4.1. Indicators of emotional state
Relationships of the global rating of quality of life to indicators of emotional state 12 months after the operation were examined via Spearman correlation coefficients (see Table 6). High correlations were found to POMS depression, vigor and fatigue subscales for valve and for bypass patients. For the PGWB, correlations to well-being, depression and vitality were apparent in valve patients, with bypass patients additionally showing correlations to anxiety and to self-control. In the EDLQ, both subscales reflecting emotional state correlated significantly with global quality of life in valve and bypass patients.

Using the global quality of life rating as an overall indicator of patient's emotional state, psychosocial as well as clinical and functional correlates were examined.

3.4.2. Psychosocial correlates
Within the psychosocial data (see Table 7) three of the twelve personality traits, as measured by the FPI, showed significant correlations to the one-year postoperative quality of life rating in valve patients indicating that a high achievement orientation, low inhibition and high extraversion, as well

Table 7. Psychosocial correlates of one-year postoperative global quality of life.[1]

	Valve n = 32	Bypass n = 45		Valve n = 32	Bypass n = 45
Personality (FPI)			*Coping (FEKB)*		
Life satisfaction	−0.26	1.23	Denial and wishful thinking	−0.10	0.05
Social orientation	0.07	0.01	Depress.processing	−0.04	0.14
Achievement orientation	−0.38***	0.13	Rational problem solving	−0.12	0.02
Inhibition	0.28*	0.01	Religiosity	−0.68***	0.16
Irritability	−0.07	0.04	Joy of living	−0.22	0.07
Aggressiveness	−0.01	0.11	Social withdrawal	0.36**	0.01
Stress	−0.09	0.01	Self assertion	−0.23	0.07
Physical complaints	0.12	0.14	Social support seeking	−0.37**	0.01
Health worries	−0.03	0.04			
Openness	−0.09	0.10	Self reinforcement	−0.19	0..05
Extraversion	−0.31*	0.15	Relative comparison	−0.15	0.05
Emotionality	−0.04	0.24	Acceptance	−0.33*	0.28
Health Locus of Control (SKF)			*Social Support (SSF)*		
Internal	−0.03	0.07	Sumscore	−0.33**	−0.14
External others	−0.26	0.08			
External chance	0.14	0.13			

[1] High scores reflect low quality of life.

* $p < 0.05$, $p < 0.01$, $p < 0.001$.

as potentially high life satisfaction, are associated with a good quality of life outcome of valve operations. In bypass patients associations with life satisfaction and emotionality failed to reach significance. As regards the health locus of control questionnaires an external control orientation – i.e. health being mainly influenced by powerful others, such as medical experts – was associated with a high quality of life rating in valve patients. No such association was identified in bypass patients. Coping styles, as assessed by the FEKB, show the beneficial effect of religiosity, social support seeking and acceptance, while social withdrawal is negatively associated with the quality of life rating.

A further reinforcement of the social support concept comes from the respective questionnaire, which yielded a significant correlation between the sum score and the global rating. In bypass patients correlations of the global rating with coping and social support only yielded insignificant relationships.

3.4.3. *Functional and clinical correlates*

While psychosocial variables were related to global quality of life in valve patients, functional impairments in terms of to psychopathology (AMDP - rating) and neuropsychological performance (index of seven tests) were not

Table 8. Functional and clinical correlates of one-year postoperative global quality of life.[1]

	Valve n = 32	Bypass n = 45		Valve n = 32	Bypass n = 45
Psychiatric Ratings			*Clinical*		
Total score	0.17	0.22	Age	0.20	0.10
Apathy	0.07	0.13	NYHA	0.16	0.13
Depression	0.07	0.03	Waiting time	0.02	0.01
Hostility	0.15	0.16	Operation time	0.08	0.03
Mania	0.09	0.19	Days intensive care	0.07	0.32**
Paranoid-					
hallucinatory	0.09	0.19			
Psycho-organic	0.10	0.23			
Neuropsychology					
Index pre-op.	0.08	0.42			
Index post-op.	0.10	0.22			

[1] High scores reflect low quality of life.
* $p < 0-05$, **$p < 0.01$.

(see Table 8). Similarly, clinical data with regard to 4 pre-, peri- and postoperative data were not significantly correlated with the one-year post-operative quality of life score.

In contrast, for bypass patients the number of days in intensive care, as well as the degree of functional neuropsychological impairment, were related to a low postoperative quality of life. Psychopathological symptomatology as reflected by the AMDP-total score and the six subscores however, did not bear a significant relationship to the long-term quality of life outcome of surgery in bypass patients, as was the case in valve patients.

4. Discussion

The data presented suggest that in the hospital, patients confront emotional problems both after surgery as well as before it. The incidence of inpatient's postoperative total psychopathology and, especially, the depressive syndrome in valve and bypass patients', is comparable to previous findings, ranging around 30% [26–28]. In addition to changes in total psychopathology, depression and apathy in the bypass group, increases in hostility were noted in both groups. Syndromes reflecting exogenous psychoses did occur in both groups, but involved few patients. The psychopathology identified in the present study will be included in the following discussion with regard to its impact on long-term emotional outcome.

With regard to the emotional outcome, the results indicate a general improvement in mood (POMS) as well as in indices of overall well-being (PGWB, EDLQ) and global quality of life from before to one year after valvular surgery. However, a comparison of the psychological state of valve patients with a healthy reference group shows that one year after surgery the patients still suffer from substantial emotional impairment mainly in terms of depressive mood but also irritability and fatigue (POMS). Such differences are less pronounced in the PGWB indices, in which the depression, levels of healthy and valve surgical groups are comparable. Nevertheless, patients tend to have lower levels of health, vitality and self control than the reference group. In addition, in the latter two subscores a decrease from pre- to postoperative levels was noted in patients, indicating less self-control and vitality after the operation.

Thus, a complex picture of changes emerges which, on the one hand, suggests that in spite of short-term depressive mood fluctuations, patients emotional state (e.g. anxiety, well-being) after surgery is comparable to that of a healthy group. On the other hand, more physically related well-being measures either do not change over time (POMS-vigor), are above the healthy average (POMS-fatigue), improve only slowly (PGWB health), or might even slightly deteriorate over time (PGWB-vitality). Furthermore, indicators of emotional regulation suggest postoperative problems with regard to irritability (POMS) and self-control (PGWB). Taken together these findings only partly support the published results, in which the postoperative emotional improvement of valve patients [12–14] as well as bypass patients are stressed [9,11,29]. The lack of studies with standardized assessments of emotional state, however, makes comparative discussions difficult. This also applies to the findings with regard to family ratings of mood and to the group-differences in postoperative quality of life.

As concerns the family ratings, a high correspondence to patients self ratings was found in terms of the actual score values, the pattern of changes over time and the high correlations between patients' and family ratings.

This finding suggests the potential use of family assessments as additional or even substitute information on patients' well-being. It also suggests that debates on who should rate the quality of life [7,30] might profit from the inclusion of the family, not only as a reflection of patient evaluations, but also with regard to its own stress and strain. Such spouse emotions might underly the slightly more conservative ratings of patients' function that were found in the present study.

A last remark regarding patients' emotional state over time pertains to differences in postoperative scores with regard to subgroups of valve patients and in comparison to bypass patients. One year after surgery, no significant differences between valve and bypass patients were found in all indicators of emotional state (see Tables 5 and 6). Since this comparability of groups in emotional state also was found three and six months after the operation, the results suggest that the emotional effects of heart surgery do not vary with the type of surgery.

Hypotheses on how types of valvular surgery might affect the patients' well-being, or which differences could be expected between valve and bypass patients, seem to be based on medical knowledge with regard to clinical outcome. Either such psychosocial differences might in the long run be less dramatic than the clinical data would suggest [31], or survivors are similar in their psychosocial response to treatment [32], or the progress in surgical techniques, as well as the process of patient selection, is such that differences are not to be expected [33]. However, this issue cannot be resolved without the conduct of clinical trials with quality of life assessment, in which different types of surgery are systematically examined. As regards differences in quality of life between valve and bypass patients, further research is mandatory. In contrast to available quality of life assessments in prospective studies, as well as clinical trials, with regard to bypass surgery, longitudinal comparisons of both groups within one study are needed.

Correlational analysis with regard to patients' global quality of life one year after surgery showed strong associations with indicators of emotional state with the exception of self control and health (PGWB). Thus, in both patients' groups, the positive emotional well-being component of quality of life is reflected by the global rating. Factorial studies also isolated a strong emotional factor associated with general well-being [34]. Using the global rating as an overall indicator of quality of life, correlations with psychosocial data were examined. Here associations were most prominent in the valve group. Specifically, personality traits such as extraversion, a low inhibition and a high life satisfaction were associated with a high quality of life, as were coping styles such as religiosity, social support seeking, acceptance and low social withdrawal. Several studies have addressed the issue of personality [35] and coping strategies [36,37] as predictors of psychosocial outcome, as yet with inconclusive results. The role played by social support as well as a low external control orientation in achieving a good quality of life is a relatively novel finding in evaluative studies on cardiovascular surgery [38].

In contrast to the findings for the valve patients, associations between global quality of life and psychosocial variables did not reach statistical significance in the bypass group. This finding does not support of the numerous studies on the role of coping styles such as denial [39] for postoperative adjustment in bypass patients.

Negative results were also found with regard to functional correlates of quality of life. In neither the valve nor the bypass groups was a significant association with AMDP-psychopathology apparent. This suggests that inpatient psychopathology is unrelated to the long-term psychosocial outcome. This was also the case for postoperative neuropsychological function, while high preoperative scores were predictive of a lower quality of life in bypass patients. Finally, clinical variables were not significantly related to psychosocial outcome with exception of a negative effect of a long inpatient stay in bypass patients. Thus, the potential negative effect of inpatient psychopathology and mental dysfunction does not seem to be related to the psychosocial long-term outcome of valve or bypass surgery. While detrimental effects of clinical and functional status have been reported for the shorter postoperative phases (e.g. Ref. [40]), massive longer-term effects seem to occur less frequently.

In summary, the results presented stress the usefulness of the quality of life concept in evaluating the quality of life of treated patients. Although advocated [41], but most recently also debated, as an outcome criterion, especially in clinical trials [42], the increase of quality of life information in long-term clinical trials [10,31], as well as in prospective cohort studies, will provide a rich data pool from which to arrive at conclusive information on patients' emotional state. As does present the study, the results so far available indicate that, despite the favourable outcome of cardio-vascular surgery, improvement in patient information, psychotherapeutic support for patients and family, as well as rehabilitative efforts in terms of return to work are needed [43–45]. A consensus on indication, methodology and application of quality of life measures in cardiovascular surgery would greatly enhance the empirical basis on which recommendations for improved care can be made.

Acknowledgement

This study was conducted with the support of U. Preuss, R. Holzbach, G. Oliveri, T. Schmitt, E. Simon, B. Söllner and P. Schmid-Habelmann.

References

1. Wenger NK, Mattson ME, Furberg CD, Ellinson J: Assessment of quality of life in clinical trials of cardiovascular therapies. Am J Cardiol 1984;54:908–913.
2. Walter PJ: Return to work after coronary artery bypass surgery. Berlin: Springer, 1984.
3. Hammeke TA, Hastings JE: Neuropsychological alterations after cardiac operation. J Thorac Cardiovasc Surg 1988;96:326–331.
4. Heller SS, Kornfeld D: Psychiatric aspects of cardiac surgery. Adv Psychosom Med 1986;15:124–139.
5. Bass C: Psychosocial outcome after coronary artery bypass surgery. Brit J Psychiatry 1984;145:526–532.
6. CASS Principal Investigators: Coronary Artery Surgery Study (CASS) – A randomized trial of coronary artery bypass surgery. Quality of life of patients randomly assigned to treatment groups. Circulation 1987;68:951–960.
7. Patrick DL, Erickson P: Assessing health-related quality of life for clinical decision making. In: Walter SR, Rosser RM (eds.) Quality of life: assessment and application. Lancaster: MTP Press, 1988;44–94.
8. Eriksson J: Psychosomatic aspects of coronary artery bypass graft surgery. Acta Psychiatr Scand 1988;77:99–106.
9. Bunzel B, Eckersberger F: Veränderung der Lebensqualität nach aortakoronarem Bypass und Klappenersatz: Ein Gradmesser des subjektiven Operationserfolges. J Thorac Cardiovasc Surg 1987;35:242–247.

10. Folks DG, Blake DJ, Fleece L, Sokol RS, Freeman AM: Quality of life six months after coronary artery bypass surgery: A preliminary report. South Med J 1986;79:397–399.
11. Mayou R, Bryant B: Quality of life after coronary artery surgery. Quart J Med, New Series 1987;62:239–248.
12. Jenkins CD, Stanton D, Savageau JA, Ockene IS, Denlinger P, Klein MD: Physical, psychologic, social and economic outcomes after cardiac valve surgery. Arch Intern Med 1983;143:2167–2113.
13. Gregori AN, Hetzer R, Schwarz B, Mayer B, Buser K, Lichtlen PR, Borst HG: Veränderung der Lebensqualität nach Koronarrevaskularisation. Z Kardiol 1983;72:12–17.
14. Schönberg B, Zürcher M, Baur HR: Lebensqualität nach Herzklappenersatz. Schweiz Med Wschr 1985;115:239–241.
15. Bullinger M, Naber D: Quality of life after bypass and valvular surgery: results of a prospective study. In: Rychlik P (ed.) Heart failure: quality of life (Vol 1), Berlin: Springer 1991: 92–104.
16. Bullinger M, Holzbach R, Oliveri G, Schmitt T, Klein E, Preuß M, Schmidt-Habelmann P: Psychopathological symptoms in open heart surgery effects of a major stressor. In: Puglisi-Allegra S, Oliverio A (eds.) Psychobiology of stress, Dordrecht: Kluwer Academic Publishers 1989;241–250.
17. McNair D, Lorr M, Droppelman LF: EITS manual for the Profile of Mood States. San Diego: Educational and Industrial Testing Service, 1971.
18. Bullinger M, Heinisch M, Ludwig M, Geier S: Studien zur Erfassung des Wohlbefindens – psychometrische Analysen zum Profile of Mood States (POMS) und zum Psychological General Well-Being Index (PGWB). Z Diff Diagn Psychol 1990;11:53–61.
19. Du Puy HJ: The Psychological General Well-being (PGWB) Index. In: Wenger NK, Mattson ME, Furberg CD, Ellinson J: Assessment of quality of life in clinical trials of cardiovascular therapies. New York: LeJacq Publishers 1984;170–183.
20. Bullinger M, Gross M, Kirchberger I: The Every-day-life Questionnaire – Psychometric analyses. (In preparation.)
21. Arbeitsgemeinschaft für Methodik und Dokumentation in der Psychiatrie: Das AMDP-System. Manual zur Dokumentation psychiatrischer Befunde. Berlin: Springer, 1971.
22. Muthny FA: Krankheitsverarbeitung bei chronisch körperlich Kranken. Prax Psychother Psychosom 1989;34:64–72.
23. Klauer T: Gesundheitsbezogene Kontrollüberzeugungen: Skala für Patienten. Arbeiten aus dem Forschungsprojekt 'Psychologie der Krankheitsbewaltigung'. Unveröffentlichtes Manuskript, Universität Trier.
24. Donald CA, Ware JE: The quantification of social contacts and social resources. Santa Monika: Rand Corporation, 1982 (Report No. R-2937-H HS).
25. Fahrenberg H, Hampel R, Selg H: Die revidierte Form des Freiburger Personlichkeitsinventars FPI-R. Diagnostica 1985;31:1
26. Meyendorf R: Psychische und neurologische Storungen bei Herzoperationen. Fortschr Med 1976;94:315–320.
27. Rabinger C, Willmer AE, Fishman J: Psychiatric complications following coronary bypass surgery. J Nerv Ment Dis 1975;200:334–341.
28. Naber D, Bullinger M: Neuroendocrine and psychological variables relating to postoperative psychosis after open-heart surgery. Psychoneuroendocrinology 1985;10:315–324.
29. Caine N, Harrison, SCW, Sharples LD, Wall-Work J: Prospective study of quality of life before and after coronary artery bypass grafting. BMJ 1991;302:511–516.
30. Bullinger M, Hasford J: Testing and evaluating quality of life measures for German clinical trials. Cont Clin Trials 1991;12:195–1055.
31. CASS Principal Investigators: Ten year follow-up of quality of life in patients randomized to receive medical therapy or coronary artery bypass graft surgery. Circulation 1990:82:1647–1658.
32. Zyzanski SI, Stanton BA, Jenkins CD, Klein MD: Medical and psychosocial outcomes in survivors of major heart surgery. Psychosom Res 1981;23:213–221.

33. Montalescot G, Thomas D, Drobinski G, Evans JI, Vicant E, Chatellier G, et al.: Clinical and ultrasound results after aortic valve replacement: Intermediate term follow up with the St Jude medical prosthesis. Am Heart J 1989;118:104–113.

34. Jenkins CD, Stanton BA, Savageau JA, Denlinger P, Klein MD: Coronary artery bypass surgery – Physical, psychological, social and economic outcomes six months later. JAMA 1983;250:782–788.

35. Kilpatrick DG, Miller WC, Allain AN, Huggins MB, Lee WH: The use of psychological test data to predict open-heart surgery outcome: A prospective study. Psychosom Med 1975;37:62–73.

36. Bruce EH, Bruce RA, Hossak KF, Kusumi F: Psychological coping strategies and cardiac capacity before and after coronary artery bypass surgery. Int J Psychiatry Med 1983;13:69–84.

37. Meffert HJ, Dahme B, Flemming B, Goetze P, Huse-Kleinstoll G, Rodewald.G, Speidel H: Open-heart surgery from the psychological point of view and resulting therapeutic considerations. Psychother Psychosom 1979;23:148–156.

38. Flynn MK, Frantz R: Coronary artery bypass surgery quality of life during early convalescence. Heart and Lung 1987;16:159–167.

39. Folks DG, Freeman AM, Sokol RS, Thurstin AG: Denial: Predictor of outcome following coronary bypass surgery. Int J Psychiatry Med 1 988;18:57–66.

40. Gundlee HJ, Reeves BR, Tate S, Raft D, McLauren LP: Psychosocial outcome after coronary artery surgery. Am J Psychiatry 1980;137:1591–1594.

41. Fletcher AE, Hunt BM, Bulpitt CJ: Evaluation of quality of life in clinical trials of cardiovascular disease. J Chron Dis 1987;40:557–566.

42. Offerhaus L: Measurement of the quality of life in clinical trials: in pursuit of the unapproachable? Eur J Clin Pharmacol 1991;40:205–208.

43. Anderson EA: Preoperative preparation for cardiac surgery facilitates recovery, reduces psychological distress and reduces the incidence of acute postoperative hypertension. J Consult Clin Psychol 1987;55:513–520.

44. Kendall PC: Stressful medical procedures: cognitive behavioural strategies for stress management and prevention. In: Meichenbaum D, Jahremko ME (eds.) Stress Reduction and Prevention. New York: Plenum Press, 1982;159–191.

45. Walter PJ: Return to work after coronary artery bypass surgery. Eur Heart J 1988;9:58–66 (suppl.).

D: General Satisfaction

9. Aspects of quality of life in patients with mechanical heart valves

LARS I. THULIN

Heart valve surgery is in no way unique in the respect that treatment aimed to improve patient status may also lead to consequences which can result in the opposite. This is true in spite of the fact that the design and materials of artificial heart valves have been considerably improved since 1952 when the first mechanical valve was implanted in man. The 'ideal' substitute for native heart valves has not yet been taken into clinical use. Therefore whenever possible, valve repair should be considered the method of choice for heart valve reconstruction. Whatever the method used, all surgical interventions in heart valve disease will affect the natural course and thus it will influence the patient's quality of life.

The patients' satisfaction with the outcome of surgery is crucial and cannot be evaluated only in terms of survival and valve-related complications. All three dimensions of quality of life have to be assessed; subjective perception, objective function and treatment-related symptoms, and the influence of all these on daily life. Quality of life in patients with mechanical heart valves should be evaluated both in relation to what life would be like without heart disease and to what life would be like, were some other medical or surgical procedures to have been used. Some of the things that are of importance to these patients are (Figure 1): (1) freedom from early and late postoperative complications leading to prolonged hospital stay/or transient or permanent disability/discomfort; (2) medication, medical care or laboratory controls; (3) postoperative improvement of general health and physical activity; (4) limitations in eating and drinking habits; (5) not having to undergo, or worry about, a late reoperation due to valve failure; (6) the possibility to undergo desired or necessary medical investigations or operations; (7) freedom to travel; and (8) valve sound disturbances.

In this chapter I shall address some of these aspects, reflecting my view on the quality of life after implantation of mechanical prostheses.

Chronic anticoagulation seems to be mandatory in patients with mechanical heart valves, regardless of the valves' design and the materials used [1–3]. Attempts to manage these patients without anticoagulants have resulted in

Paul J. Walter (ed.): Quality of Life after Open Heart Surgery, 91–97.
© 1992 Kluwer Academic Publishers.

1. Freedom from early and late postoperative complications leading to prolonged hospital stay/or transient or permanent disability or discomfort for the patient.
2. The need for medication, medical care or laboratory controls.
3. Postoperative improvement of general health and physical activity.
4. Limitations in eating and drinking habits.
5. Not to have to undergo, or worry about, a late reoperation due to valve failure.
6. The possibility to undergo desired or necessary medical investigations or operations.
7. Freedom to travel.
8. Valve sound disturbances.

Figure 1. Quality of life

unacceptable rates of valve thrombosis and embolic complications [4–6]. Adequate treatment seems to be of great importance. It is a lifelong therapy that might be the one most important factor influencing the individual patient's long-term morbidity. The therapeutic range is very narrow and regular check-ups are necessary to monitor the treatment (Figure 2). Thus we have introduced a new iatrogenic disease in patients who have received a mechanical prosthesis. Comparatively little has been done over the years to improve

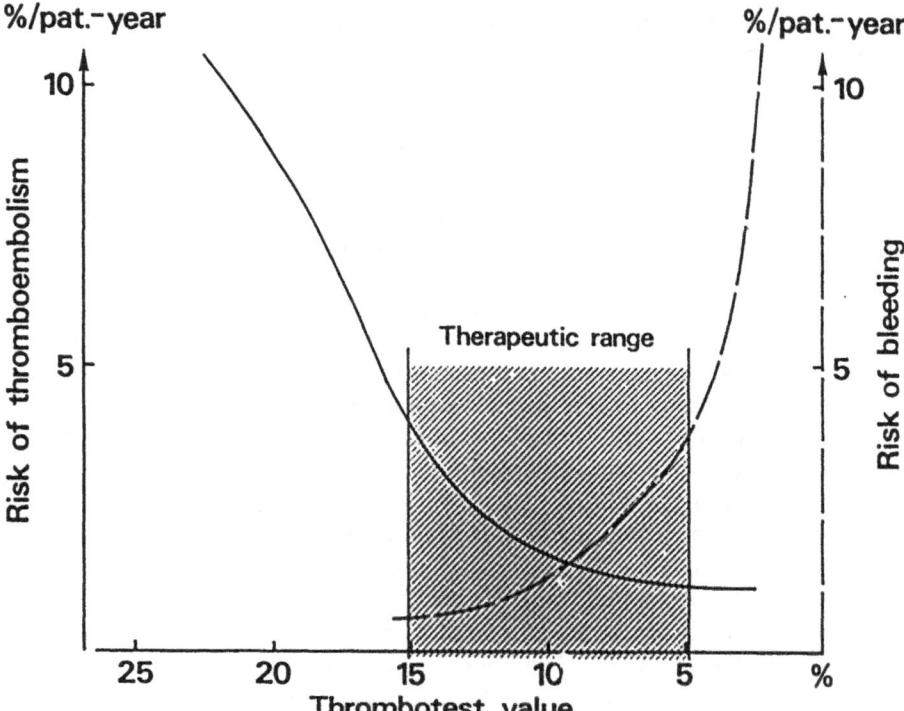

Figure 2. Schematic concept of the close therapeutic interval of oral anticoagulants (Warfarin sodium and Dicumarol) measured by the Thrombotest method.

patient education in this field, and to facilitate treatment control. Many patients suffer from complications and restrictions in their daily life: matters that could have been avoided with proper education. The patient must be allowed to take an active part in the treatment and the only way to ensure this is through education. Educational programs have been available for patients with diabetes, chronic renal disease and many other lifelong diseases. The time must now come for patients on chronic anticoagulant treatment to get the same chance to take full or partial responsibility for their therapy. Devices for self-control of the prothrombin value, or corresponding parameters, must be further developed, making it possible to perform these tests at home [7]. Adjustments of the treatment can then easily be done by the educated patient himself. This will also allow for more freedom in both eating and drinking habits.

Patients on chronic anticoagulation are sometimes advised not to travel abroad since different food, changes in alcohol intake and alterations in the degree of physical activity may well influence the anticoagulation therapy. One major obstacle to overcome, enabling patients to travel more freely, is the fact that different medical systems exist all over the world. Steps must be taken to seek international agreements and laboratory standards making it possible for patients to receive medical care on the same conditions when visiting a foreign country as when in their home country. Standardization of methods to determine the prothrombin time in oral anticoagulant control is desired to achieve a common language [8]. Adoption of the International Normalized Ratio (INR) will provide a universal scale for prothrombin times, easy for all to understand [9]. The INR will make it feasible to compare the therapeutic ranges recommended, and further improve the continuity of anticoagulant treatment of travelling patients. The INR standard is now gradually being adopted in many countries, often parallel to the old control index. This must be further encouraged.

Ischemic stroke in patients with mechanical heart valves is often considered to result in a high rate of mortality and morbidity. Thus many surgeons hesitate to implant mechanical prostheses, especially in elderly patients, since this group of patients is known to experience more difficulties with anticoagulation therapy. This may be due to poor patient compliance, drug interactions and differences in drug metabolism in elderly patients. In a consecutive series of patients with mechanical heart valves operated at our institution between 1974 and 1988 we studied stroke events during a six-year period (1983–1988). In all, 182 patients were followed and 16 patients (8.8%) experienced an ischemic stroke. Mean age at the time of operation was 63 years. During the same observation period only one patient (0.55%) experienced a cerebral hemorrhage. The outcome of this event was fatal. All patients with ischemic strokes were adequatly anticoagulated at the time of the event (INR 2.1–4.8). The diagnosis of stroke was verified with CT scan on either the first or the second day. Eight patients were considered to have very mild symptoms, seven had mild, and one patient had moderate symptoms. Thus there were no fatal strokes in this material. This is in sharp contrast to the grave short- and long-term prognosis in patients with cardiac embolism in non-anticoagulated patients [10]. The suggested conclusion of this study is that, in contrast to hemorrhagic infarctions, ischemic stroke in patients on anticoagulants are often mild,and a fatal outcome is rare. Furthermore, adequate anticoagulation does not prevent these episodes in patients with mechanical prostheses.

Mechanical failure is a well-known complication of both mechanical and biological artificial heart valves [11,12]. Whether it is a change in ball characteristics leading to ball escape in ball valves, leaflet escape in bileaflet valves or strut fractures in tilting disk valves, especially focused on the Björk–Shiley 60 and 70° CC valve, this complication may well result in a major event leading to death or disability. Considerable attention has been directed to the problem by news media and juridicial authorities. Both concern and confusion have been evoked among both patients and physicians. In particular, the strut fracture problem among patients with the Björk–Shiley 60 and 70° valves have resulted in concern, not only for patients who have received these valves, but for all patients with mechanical heart valves. The strut fracture problem has to be dealt with on the basis of individual risk evaluation. Patients must receive appropriate information from their physician and, in case of significant risks of mechanical failure, steps must be taken to avoid such an event.

In order to place the problem with strut fractures in Björk–Shiley 70° CC valves into its proper perspective I would like to present our experience in this matter. Between 1982 and 1983 we implanted 107 Björk–Shiley 70° CC valves in 90 patients. Follow up was performed in February 1990 and the total follow-up time was then 550 patient-years. There were four mechanical strut fractures (two in the aortic position and two in the mitral position). All events were fatal. Total mortality was 25%. The autopsy rate in the total material was 74%. There were no valve thromboses, endocarditis or paravalvular leaks. Four patients were re-operated with explantation of their 70° CC valve. All were elective cases. Re-operation was based on individual risk evaluation.

At the time of follow up, in February 1990, 65 patients were still in the study group. A questionnaire was sent to these patients asking about their actual status. In spite of a relatively high age, 77% were satisfied with their general state of health. Seventy percent were satisfied with their physical activity and 84 percent were in NYHA groups I or II. Improvement of cardiac symptoms were experienced in 81%. Major bleedings had been experienced by 17% (2.0 events/100 pt.-years). Cerebral emboli had been experienced by 14% (1.6 events/100 pt.-years) Sixty-six percent had been able to travel abroad for longer or shorter periods. Thirteen percent had undergone major surgery without complications and 61 percent were satisfied with their sex life. Of those hearing the valve clicking, 55% claimed that they were never disturbed by the closing sound. Eighty-three percent of the patients were satisfied with the information they had got concerning the strut fracture problem. Some patients, especially younger ones, wanted to get better updated information on actual risks.

We conclude that eight years after having had an implantation of the Björk–Shiley 70° CC valve, most surviving patients live a rich and active life. Mechanical failures have been experienced, but other cardiac causes of death were four times higher.

Most mechanical heart valve prostheses produce a distinct sound when closing [13,14]. This is in sharp contrast to the native heart valve. The closing sound may be perceived by the patient and thus it may affect the quality of life. Many factors, both patient-related and valve-related, may affect the sound generated by the closing valve and its perception. When discussing the effects of the closing valve sound on the individual patient, we have to be aware of the fact that actually hearing the valve sound, does not imply that the patient is being disturbed. In this respect, important roles are played by the patient's personality, emotional stability, heart rhythm and probably many other factors. It is also important to remember that loudness is not necessarily directly related to the intensity of a sound. We have performed a comparative study of closing valve sounds during standardized conditions in patients. Four different valve types were studied; Duromedics (Baxter–Edwards), St Jude Medical, Björk–Shiley Monostrut and the Carbomedics heart valves. All patients were males with single aortic valve replacement. Valve size was 25 mm and body index was equal. All patients were in sinus rhythm. There were seven patients in each group. Recordings were made in a 'silent room' at the department of audiology used normally for acoustic laboratory work. Recordings were made with patients sitting down and lying down with a microphone 5 cm from the chest wall. From the recordings we computerized 10–15 valve closures and established a mean valve sound loudness in each patient. The illustrations show the four valve groups with the seven different patients plotted against the dB(A) value. Both sitting down and lying down there are some significant differences (Figures 3 and 4). There are no significant differences between the Carbomedics and the St Jude Medical heart valves. The Duromedics heart valve is significantly louder than the Carbomedics and the St Jude Medical heart valve, but significantly less loud than the Björk–Shiley Monostrut heart valve ($p < 0.05$).

The conclusions I would like to make are the following.

Patients with mechanical heart valves seem to have a relatively high quality of life without restrictions and valve- and anticoagulation-related complications.

Implantation of mechanical heart valves puts special emphasis on management of the anticoagulant therapy. Standardization of anticoagulation is of outmost importance.

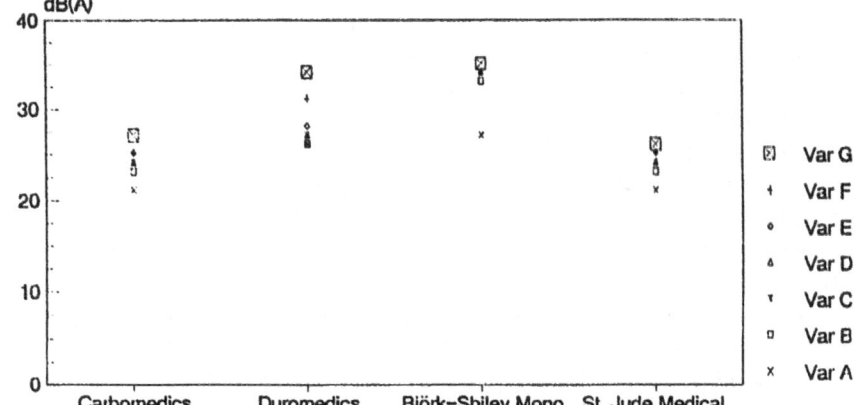

Figure 3. Heart valve sound. A comparative study. Lying down. Each variable represents one patient.

Patient education and responsibility for the anticoagulant treatment must be emphasized.

The choice of artificial heart valve to be implanted must be based on individual, patient-related factors.

The surgeon must be aware of the fact that the type of valve implanted or the type of surgery performed may well affect the patient's quality of life both early and late postoperatively.

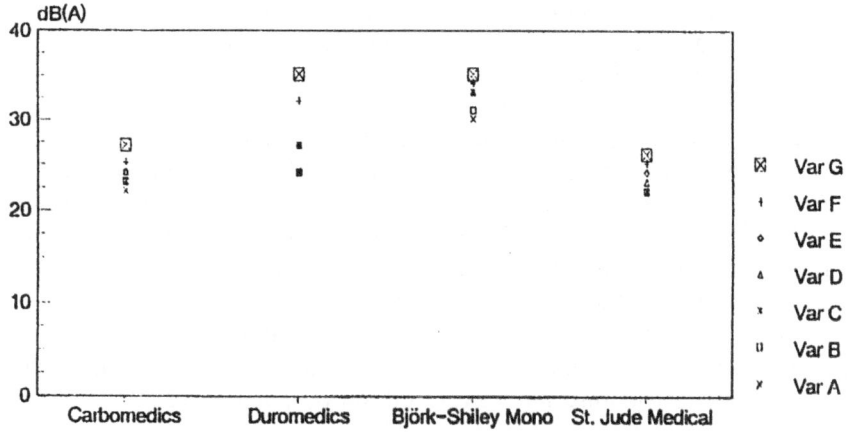

Figure 4. Heart valve sound. A comparative study. Sitting down. Each variable represents one patient.

References

1. Edmunds LH: Thromboembolic complications of current cardiac valvular prostheses. Ann Thorac Surg 1982;34:96–106.
2. Gössinger H, Niessner H, Grubeck B, et al: Thromboembolism in patients with prosthetic heart valves. An adequately controlled intense anticoagulant therapy and its influence on the occurrence of thromboembolism in relation to valve type. Thorac Cardiovasc Surg 1986;34:283–286.
3. Mok CK, Boey J, Wang R, et al: Warfarin versus dipyridamole-asprin and pentoxifylline-asprin for prevention of prosthetic heart valve thromboembolism: a prospective randomized clinical trial. Circulation 1972;5:1059–1063.
4. Boncheck L, Starr A: Ball valve prosthesis: Current appraisal of late results. Am J Cardiol 1976;35:843–854.
5. Limet R, Lepage G, Grondin CM: Thromboembolic complications with the cloth covered Star–Edwards aortic prosthesis in patients nor receiving anticoagulants. Ann Thorac Surg 1977;23:529–539.
6. Björk VO, Henze A: Management of thromboembolism after aortic valve replacement with Björk–Shiley tilting disc valve. Scand J Thor Cardiovasc Surg 1975;9:183–191.
7. White RH, McCurdy SA, von Marensdorf H, et al: Home prothrombin time monotoring after the initiation of warfarin therapy. A randomized, prospective study. Ann Intern Med 1989;111:730–737.
8. Butchart EG, Lewis PA, Kulatilake ENP, Breckenridge IM: Anticoagulation variability between centers: implications for comparative prosthetic valve assessment. Eur J Cardio-thorac Surg 1988;2:72–91.
9. van den Besselar AMHP: Standardization of the prothrombin time in oral anticoagulant control. Haemostasis 1985;15:271–277.
10. Snyder M, Renaudin J: Intracranial hemorrhage associated with anticoagulation therapy. Surg Neurol 1977;7:31–34.
11. Lindblom D, Björk VO, Semb BKH: Mechanical failure of the Björk–Shiley valve. J Thorac Cardiovasc Surg 1986;92:894–907.
12. Horstkotte D, Korfer R, Siepel L, Bircks W, Loogen F: Late complications in patients with Björk-Shiley and St Jude Medical heart valve replacement. Circulation 1983;68:175–84.
13. Thulin LI, Reul H, Giersiepen M, Olin CL: An in vitro study of prosthetic heart valve sound. Scand J Thor Cardiovasc Surg 1989;23:33–37.
14. Kupari M, Harjola A, Mattila S: Auscultatory characteristics of normally functioning Lillehei–Kaster, Björk–Shiley and St Jude heart valve prostheses. Br Heart J 1986;55:364–370.

E: Concluding Remarks

Quality of life after heart valve replacement

D. HORSTKOTTE

Most questions of the early days of valve replacement surgery have sufficiently been answered by now. Following the first successful replacement of
the aortic valve by Dwight E. Harken [1] and of the mitral valve by Albert
Starr [2] it soon became apparent that the overall prognosis of patients with
advanced valvular lesions could significantly be improved by the implantation
of an artificial device, despite the high rate of prosthetic valve related complications at that time [3,4]. During the 1960s emphasis was placed on valve
durability by testing new designs and a variety of materials. The following
decade focused on reducing specific complications associated so far with
prosthetic heart valves [5]. Although the two main types of prostheses –
mechanical and tissue valves – each brought about continues improvement
in design, so far no replacement valve meets all requirements of the ideal
heart valve substitute. Nevertheless, the overall beneficial effect of replacing
diseased human heart valves is now well documented (Figure 1) [6,7].

The major task for the future will be to further improve the prognosis and
the quality of life of patients who are candidates of valve replacement or
have undergone valvular surgery.

This concerns three periods in the clinical course of valvular patients:

1. Preoperative treatment and timing of the surgical intervention

It is uncertain how many patients are operated during the relatively short
period that is optimum to achieve the best postoperative prognosis and the
best quality of life by a maximum improvement in their condition. It is
assumed that, due to ignorance or a lack of operative capacity, this percentage is relativly small.

Obviously, a postponement of valve replacement that is indicated, may
have significant, sometimes even disasterous consequences regarding myocardial function and complications like arrhythmia or the potential for
cardioembolism. The findings that the best predictor for postoperative return

Paul J. Walter (ed.): Quality of Life after Open Heart Surgery, 101–104.

Mitral Valve Lesions   Aortic Valve Lesions

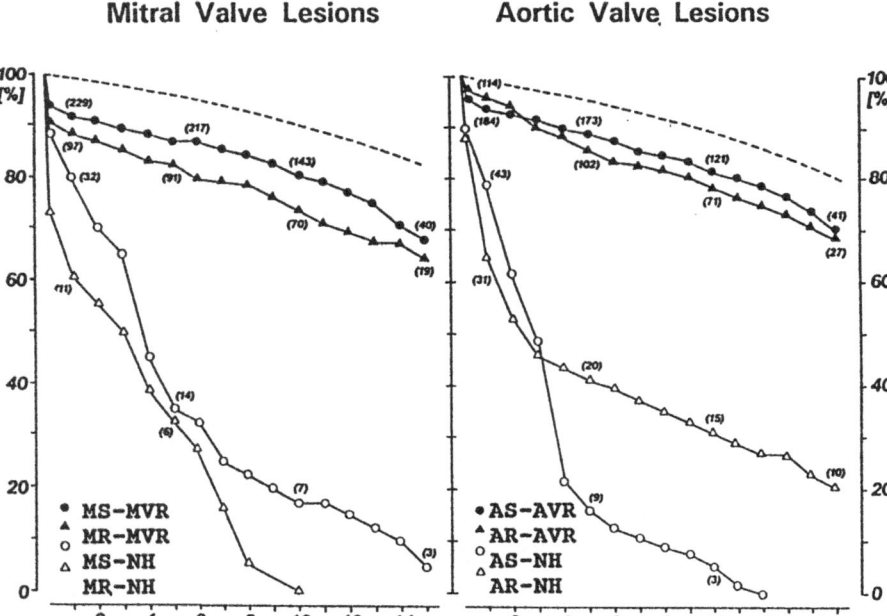

Figure 1. Natural history (NH) of acquired mitral and aortic valve lesions after surgical intervention was indicated. The NH is compared with the prognosis of patient, in whom the indication
for surgical intervention was given and the operation was performed by implantation of a
mechanical prosthesis during the same period. The dotted line represents the prognosis of an
age-related so called normal population. MS = mitral stenosis, MR = mitral regurgitation, AS =
aortic stenosis, AR = aortic regurgitation, MVR = mitral valve replacement, AVR = aortic
valve replacement.

to work is a preoperative employment status of the patient, gives a further
argument not to postpone surgery.

On the other hand, an intervention performed too early does not only
expose the patient to an unnecessary operative risk but also to the specific
late complications of heart valve substitutes.

The timing of surgery is further made difficult because there are no generally agreed criteria how the optimal time for surgical intervention should
be determined [8,9].

2. Surgical intervention and replacement valves

We are still awaiting 15 to 20 year results from randomized studies comparing
mechanical and tissue valves, different mechanical valves or different bioprosthetic devices [10,11].

According to the scientifically so far limited experiences, there are some arguments for homografts at least in children. They are, however, not widely used, as homograft insertion needs a considerable technical skill and prolonged perfusion times.

Considering the inherent advantages and disadvantages of the different prosthetic devices available as well as the lack of consensus regarding superiority of one device over another, an individual approach is preferred when selecting a heart valve prosthesis for the individual patient.

It is generally agreed that valve preserving procedures with a primary satisfactory result are superior to replacement using any type of prosthesis. To be scientifically accurate one has to insist, however, not to compare patients with repair procedures with those who have undergone valve replacement. Such a comparison is strongly biased and results in misleading conclusions, as these two groups of patients are strictly not comparable.

The high percentage (up to 45%) of early postoperative neurophysiological dysfunctions demands a careful perioperative management. The prospective comparison of cognitive function following valve surgery or coronary artery bypass surgery does not support the earlier hypothesis of poorer cognitive function in valvular than in coronary artery bypass patients.

3. Postoperative treatment

Thromboembolic complications and anticoagulant-related hemorrhage are still the major sources for postoperative morbidity and mortality and the thrombogenicity of mechanical prostheses is still their most important disadvantage [12,13], although improved designs and the use of new, more biocompatible materials have reduced the incidence of thromboembolic events [14]. It is questionable whether a further significant reduction of the thrombogenicity of mechanical heart valves is feasible within the near future. A better anticoagulation management, however, could be implemented at once. New therapeutic strategies, for instance low-intensity anticoagulation in combination with home prothrombin estimation may contribute to a significant decrease in thromboembolic and bleeding complications in patients with valvular replacement [15].

With respect to the return to work it would be ideal to allow the patients a maximum flexibility to adjust the working hours to their physical wellbeeing. One has to keep in mind, however, that all prostheses are obstructive to forward blood flow and that there may be a clinically important increase in pulmonary artery pressures with consequent presentation of dyspnea in patients with mitral valve replacement, which may limit the physical capacity significantly more than after aortic valve replacement [16,17]. In the latter case the overall physiological success of the operative intervention is linked to the residual impairment of left ventricular function.

We are entering a new era of managing valvular patients. Some of the prostheses which are currently available have brought us closer to the 'ideal valve replacement' than has been realized by many. The next step in order to improve quality of life following valve replacement surgery, is now to optimise perioperative and late postoperative treatment.

References

1. Harken DE, Saroff HS, Taylor WJ et al. Partial and complete prosthesis in aortic insufficiency. Thorac Cardiovasc Surg 1960;40:744.
2. Starr A, Edwards ML: Mitral replacement: Clinical experience with a ball-valve prosthesis. Ann Surg 1961;154:726.
3. Hylen JC: Mechanical malfunction and thrombosis of prosthetic heart valves. Am J Cardiol 1972;130:396.
4. Santinga JT, Kirsh MM: Hemolytic anemia in series 2300 and 2310 Starr-Edwards prosthetic valves. Ann thorac Surg 1972;14:539.
5. Lefrak EA, Starr A: eds. Cardiac valve prosthesis. New York: Appleton-Century-Crofts, 1979.
6. Horstkotte D, Loogen F: The natural history of aortic valve stenosis. EHJ 1988;9(Suppl.E):57
7. Horstkotte D, Niehues R, Strauer BE: Pathomorphological aspects, aetiology and natural history of acquired mitral valve stenosis. EHJ 1991;2(Suppl.H):55.
8. Horstkotte D: Operationsindikation bei erworbenen Herzklappenfehlern. In: Horstkotte D, Loogen F. eds. Erworbene Herzklappenfehler. München-Wien-Baltimore: Urban & Schwarzenberg 1987.
9. Bonow RO: Asymptomatic patients with significant aortic or mitral incompetence and left ventricular dysfunction should undergo operation. Z Kardiol 1985;75(Suppl.2):124.
10. Horstkotte D: Prosthetic valves or tissue valves – A vote for mechanical prostheses. Z Kardiol 1985;74(Suppl.6):19.
11. Horstkotte D, Trampisch HJ: Long-term follow-up after heart valve replacement. Z Kardiol 1986;75:641.
12. Horstkotte D, Körfer R, Seipel L, Bircks W, Loogen F: Late complications in patients with Björk-Shiley and St. Jude Medical heart valve replacement. Circulation 1983;6:175.
13. Horstkotte D, Körfer R: The influence of prosthetic valve replacement on the natural history of severe acquired heart valve lesions: Comparsion of complications and hemodynamic findings after implantation of Björk–Shiley, St. Jude Medical, and other heart valve prostheses. In: De Bakey ed. Advances in Cardiac Valves. New York: York Medical Book, 47, 1983.
14. Bokros JC, La Grange LD, Schoen FJ: Control of structure of carbon for use in bioengineering. In: Walker PL ed. Chemistry and physics of carbon, Vol 9:103, New York: M. Dekker, 1973.
15. Bernardo A, Halhuber C, Horstkotte D: Home prothrombin estimation. In: Butchart EG, Bodnar E eds. Thrombosis, Thromboembolism and Bleeding London: ICR, 1991.
16. Horstkotte D, Haerten K, Seipel L: Central hemodynamics at rest and during exercise after mitral valve replacement with different prostheses. Circulation 1983;68(Suppl.II):161.
17. Horstkotte D, Loogen F, Bircks W: Is the late outcome of heart valve replacement influenced by the hemodynamics of the heart valve substitute? In: Horstkotte D Loogen F. eds. Update in heart valve replacement. Darmstadt: Steinkopff, 1986.

PART TWO

QUALITY OF LIFE AFTER CORONARY BYPASS SURGERY

A: Physiological State

10. Morbidity and mortality after myocardial revascularization in patients with ischemic heart disease

W.J. KEON and S.C. MENZIES

Introduction

Coronary artery bypass grafting for atherosclerotic heart disease is one of the most common procedures performed in North America; the number of cases doubling between 1979 and 1986 [1]. Over the years, it has been recognized that there are benefits in having comprehensive profiles and outcomes of patients undergoing bypass surgery hence the large number of clinical trials. These trials give a clear view of the performance, provide useful data on characteristics of patients and the long-term impact of treatment.

In 1980 the American College of Cardiology and the American Heart Association established a Task Force on the assessment of diagnostic and therapeutic cardiovascular procedures. Their comprehensive report, spanning ten years of review, was published in March 1991. Part of their mandate was to review the incidence of coronary artery bypass graft surgery and current indications for its use [2]. On reviewing the existing literature and extensive information from the clinical trials, they classified the indications for bypass surgery into three treatment groups; (1) conditions for which the operation is indicated on the basis of a demonstrated advantage over medical treatment in terms of longevity or relief of symptoms or both (Table 1); (2) conditions for which the operation is acceptable treatment but for which the advantages over medical treatment have not yet been fully defined; and (3) conditions for which the operation is not generally considered to be indicated because of lack of demonstrated advantage over medical treatment. Given the current state of knowledge, they developed generally accepted guidelines for the individual presenting for bypass surgery.

Surgical practice is constantly changing. Innovative technology and new knowledge result in new indications for bypass surgery. As the practice of clinical cardiology and surgery have changed, so has the clinical profile of the patient presenting for surgery, surgical management of the patient and the operative outcome. The development of interventional cardiology has changed the type of patient coming to bypass surgery. However, the im-

Paul J. Walter (ed.): *Quality of Life after Open Heart Surgery*, 107–114.
© 1992 Kluwer Academic Publishers.

Table 1. ACC/AHA treatment class I categories for CABG [2].

Asymptomatic and mild, moderate or severe ischemia with non-invasive stress testing.

- Left main disease regardless of L.V. function
- 3–vessel disease with moderate or severe L.V. function

Chronic, stable Class I–II angina and mild ischemia with non-invasive stress testing.

- Left main disease regardless of L.V. functions
- 3–vessel disease with moderate or severe L.V. function

Chronic, stable Class I–II angina with severe ischemia with non-invasive stress testing.

- Left main disease regardless of L.V. function
- 3–vessel disease regardless of L.V. function

Chronic, stable Class III or IV angina with mild, moderate or severe ischemia with non-invasive stress testing.

- Left main disease regardless of L.V. function
- 3–vessel disease regardless of L.V. function

plementation of coronary angioplasty is not the only factor responsible for the change in the profile of the bypass surgical patient. The changing demographics of our populations and the increasing percentage of elderly is a continuing trend. Improvement in operative techniques and methodologies has extended our indications for surgery to the older population. Also, with the increasing age comes the increasing incidence of other chronic diseases such as diabetes and hypertension. The individual now presenting for bypass surgery is sicker, older, is more frequently a repeat surgery, has poorer ventricular function and more diffuse disease (Tables 2 and 3). Consequently, despite improved operative techniques and myocardial protection, the patient in the 1990s is at more risk of operative mortality and morbidity. Conversely, high risk patients are known to benefit most from surgery and because of

Table 2. Two decades of open heart surgery. Ottawa Heart Institute Clinical Profile.

	1970–74	1990
N	600	500
Mean Age	48.9 yrs	60.5 yrs
Male %	91.2	81
Female %	8.8	19
Elective %	84	91
Emergency/Urgent %	16	9
Reoperations	1.6	11.2
Angina Class I %	11.7	0.4
Angina Class II %	31.7	12.6
Angina Class III %	33.5	53
Angina Class IV %	23.1	28
Length of Stay	22.7 days	15.3 days

Table 3. Two decades of open heart surgery. Ottawa Heart Institute Angiographic findings.

	1970–74	1990
# of diseased vessels		
% lDV	8	4.5
% 2DV	28	18.4
% 3DV	64	77.2
Left ventricle function		
% Class IV	11.9	9.9
% Class III	9.5	18.3
% Class II	27.8	24.5
% Class I	14.8	25.5
% Normal	36	21.8
% CHF	9.6	17.8

their acuity of symptoms often have no alternative to surgical intervention [2]. Operative mortality alone is an inappropriate yard stick by which to judge a surgical procedure and the acuity of the patient must always be kept in perspective.

2. Experience at the Ottawa Heart Institute

The Ottawa Heart Institute has been performing coronary artery bypass surgery since 1970 and during that time has surgically treated in excess of 14 000 patients. The first 600 consecutive patients coming to bypass surgery between 1970 and 1974 were compared with a second group, 500 patients undergoing bypass surgery in 1990. The medical records of these groups of patients were retrospectively analyzed. A comparison of their clinical profile is presented in Tables 2 and 3. The mean age increased by 12 years, the percentage of females doubled, the percentage of reoperations increased sevenfold, the number of patients with three-vessel disease increased 13% and the number of individuals with normal ventricular function decreased 15%. This change in patient profile is similar to that seen in other published studies both in Canada and the United States (Table 4) [3–7].

Auxiliary surgical procedures were performed on 102 (20%) of patients as illustrated in Table 5 Intra-aortic balloon was required in 4.8% of the patients and internal mammary arteries were used as grafting in 63% of patients. The mean number of grafts per patient was 2.8. Complete revascularization was achieved, in 100% of patients with double and single vessel disease and in 92.1% of patients with triple vessel disease. The majority of those patients with single vessel disease required surgery, not just for coronary artery disease but for valve disease, left ventricular aneurysm repairs or septal defects and the isolated bypass grafts were performed as a secondary procedure.

Table 4. Recent clinical profile of patients undergoing CABG.

	Royal Victoria Montreal '88 [3]	Toronto Hospital Registry '86 [4]	Ottawa Heart Institute	Emory '87 [6]	SLU '85 [5]	Penn State [7]
N	393	1852	500	1513	185	603
Mean Age	62	59.5	60.5	61	61.4	61
% Female	22	19	19	22	23	20.4
Left Main	20	17	7.2	14.7	19	–
% Emergency	17	19	9	9.7	18	12.8
% Class III/IV Angina	88	–	75	72	–	95.6
Abnormal LV	65	63	78.2	–	30	–
% Reop	9	5.8	11.2	7.7	7	6.3
% IABP	5.6	–	4.8	4.7	–	7.1
# Grafts/pt	3.3	3.2	2.8	3.8	3.6	3.3
% Used IMA	87	54	63	88	–	49.6

The overall mortality was 3.4%. Operative mortality was higher in females, 6.3% versus males at 2.7%; in emergencies 12% versus 2.4% elective; in reoperations 10% versus 2.5%; in patients with additional procedures, 4.9% versus 3%. Mortality was also directly related to preoperative angina class with 0% mortality in individuals presenting with Class I or II, 2.6% mortality with Class III angina and 5.9% mortality with Class IV angina. Ventricle class was also a predictor of operative mortality, being 1% with normal ventricles, 2.6% with Class I, 3.7% with Class II, 6.2% with Class III and

Table 5. Auxiliary procedures 1990.

Manual coronary endarterectomy	50
Laser coronary endarterectomy	2
Endarterectomy and left ventricular aneurysm	1
Left ventricular aneurysm repair	6
Left ventricular repair and VSD	1
Aortic valve replacement	16
Aortic valve replacement and aortic aneurysm	1
Aortic valve replacement and mitral valve replacement	1
AVR, MVR, L.V. aneurysm and pulmonary artery repair	1
Mitral valve replacement	5
Mitral valve replacement and tricuspid valve repair	1
Aortic aneurysm repair	2
ASD closure	2
VSD closure	1
Bental procedure	1
MVR, ASD and L.V. aneurysm	1
Lobectomy	2
Subendocardial resection	2
Implantable defibrillator	6
Total	102

Table 6. Comparison of clinical profile versus hospital mortality.

	Alive (N483)		Died (N17)	
Mean Age	60.2 yrs		67.8 yrs	
	N	%	N	%
Female	89	19	6	35
Male	394	81	11	65
Angina Class III–IV	418	86.5	17	100
LV Class III–IV	133	27	8	47
Emergency/urgent	43	8.9	6	35
Reoperations	55	11	5	29
Left main disease	10	2	7	41
Additional procedures	97	20	5	29

9.1% with Class IV. As expected, operative mortality was also related to the number of complications with 0 mortality in individuals with no complications ranging to 8% mortality with one complication to 66% with five complications. In our hands the following factors increased the risk of operative mortality; increased age, female gender, severity of angina, poor ventricular function, emergency status, reoperation and left main disease (Table 6). The rate of postoperative complications is indicated in Table 7. They range from benign atrial fibrillation to perioperative infarction (of which 7 of 39 were fatal) through to multiple organ failure. The infection rate of 6.6% includes 5 sternal wound infections, 6 pneumonias, 6 urinary tract, 14 leg wound infections and 2 patients with septecemia.

Pulmonary complications included 19 patients with atelectasis, 2 with pneumothorax, 6 with pleural effusion, 1 each with pulmonary edema and pulmon-

Table 7. Postoperative complications 1990.

	N	%
Arrhythmias	53	10.6
Periop MI	39	7.8
Pulmonary	31	6.4
Infection	33	6.6
CHF	31	6.2
LCO	27	5.4
Bleeding	18	3.6
Post pump syndrome	14	2.8
Hematoma	12	2.4
Hypertension	7	1.4
Renal failure/insufficiency	5	1.0
Liver failure	2	0.4
DVT	1	0.2
CVA	1	0.2
Pericarditis	1	0.2
Malunion of sternum	1	0.2

Table 8. Cause of hospital deaths 1990 (*N*500).

Perioperative M.I.		7
*LCO		8
with CHF	2	
with multi-organ failure	1	
with intraoperative bleeding	1	
with incomplete revascularization	1	
LCO Alone	3	
Ventricular fibrillation		1
Pulmonary Emboli		1

* LCO = low cardiac output

ary emboli and 2 with respiratory insufficiency requiring tracheostomy. Of the 18 patients with bleeding complications, 12 required reopening. The cause of death in these 17 patients who had hospital mortality are listed in Table 8.

3. Operative techniques and management

Meticulous surgical technique is the rule for all bypass surgery. Intraoperative hemostasis, particularly at reoperation can be improved with the use of homologous blood, ultrafiltration devices on the pump oxygenator and the cell saver for intraoperative shed blood.

In the case of reoperations where the operative risk is high, management of cardiopulmonary bypass, chest entry, myocardial preservation and handling of previously constructed bypass grafts is very important. Some authors advocate exposure of the femoral artery before sternotomy [8]. Careful sternotomy with division of the anterior table of the sternum and retraction with rakes and the lungs deflated is an acceptable technique. Another approach is to use the routine sternal saw with careful dissection of the right ventricle, by means of the subxyphoid approach, lifting the sternum anteriorly as the saw is directed cephalad. Great care must be taken to protect any internal mammary artery pedicles since these are currently the preferred bypass graft material. Patent grafts that are to be preserved during repeat surgery should have minimal manipulation. If angiography demonstrated that they contain atherosclerotic material, early ligation can prevent atheroemboli from being dislodged and causing perioperative infarction. When patent vein grafts have diffuse atheroma, we use groin cannulation, single right atrial cannulation, isolate the proximal aorta above the grafts, institute cardiopulmonary bypass, arrest with crystalloid cardioplegia and as the last procedure dissect the heart free dividing the vein grafts as soon as they are encountered. In come cases we have used retrograde coronary perfusion but have found this requires extra dissection prior to cardiac arrest.

Myocardial protection using moderate systemic hypothermia and crystalloid potassium cardioplegia at 5%c is our preferred method of protection. This is in agreement with most other authors who advocate short aortic cross clamp times, cardiac decompression and uniform cooling of the heart with cold cardioplegia [9]. Our current incidence of manual coronary endarterectomy in patients presenting with diffuse disease is 10%. With manual endarterectomy, spatulae are spiralled distal to the incision until the core of atheroma is free from the vessel wall. Gentle traction is then applied to remove the specimen, however, the ease with which the core is extracted is totally unpredictable. Complete core removal is essential for successful procedures to ensure distal side and end branches are tapered off naturally and not abruptly. Endarterectomy widens the scope of eligible candidates for coronary revascularization, however, it should not generally be performed if there is a graftable distal vessel of 1.5 mm or greater in diameter. It is associated with higher risks of operative mortality, perioperative infarction and late infarction and lower graft patency [10]. It is imperative to develop a standard process whereby these patients are carefully selected with consideration of the potential risks and benefits involved.

The use of the internal mammary artery as a bypass conduit has increased over the years. It is noted that its patency is considerably higher with 95% patent at 10 years [11]. It provides a potentially large runoff and is preferable to use it to graft the anterior descending artery.

The more complete the revascularization, better the long-term results for the patient. Therefore, complete revascularization must be attempted in all cases. It is recommended that all diseased vessels greater than 1 mm be grafted [2] and it is preferred that sequential grafting is used only if required [12]. The major problem with sequential graft has been the difference between patency rates of end to side and side to side anastomosis. Alternate conduits available other than saphenous vein and internal mammary include the right gastro-epiploic artery, inferior mesenteric and the inferior epigastric artery. If homologous material is not available, one can resort to the use of dacron grafts.

4. Conclusions

Our patient profile is similar to those published by other groups with respect to the characteristics and management of coronary artery disease (Table 4). The mortality rate for bypass grafting remains relatively stable in our hands despite the increased acuity of the patient presenting for surgery. This reflects the improved operative management including myocardial protection. The hospital morbidity appears to be increasing. However, it must be noted that operative mortality and morbidity alone is not indicative of the success of a procedure. It must be analyzed in the context of the individual risk of patients. Parsonnet et al. [13] performed an elegant study on risk stratifi-

Table 9. Mortality and complications (%).

Institution (yr)	Emory 87	SLU 85	Penn State 87	OHI 90
N	1513	185	603	500
Mortality	3.1	–	3.8	3.4
Elective	–	–	1.9	2.4
Emergency	–	–	16.8	12
Hemorrhage			2.6	3.6
Sternal infection	3	–	4.3	1
Respiratory failure	–	–	0.33	0 4
Periop MI	5.5	5	–	7.8
Length of stay	–	–	11.2	15.3 days

cation. Univariant regression analysis was used to classify patients into levels of predicted operative mortality (Table 9) [13]. The experience at our Institute supports the conclusions of Parsonet in terms of high risk patients. Table 6. With the number of high risk patients presenting themselves for surgery increasing, the challenge to the surgeons will be ongoing.

References

1. Feinleib M, Havlik RJ, Gillum R et al: Coronary heart disease and related resources: National hospital discharge survey data. Circulation 1989;79(Suppl. I):13–18.
2. Kirklin JW, Akins CW, Blackstone EH et al: ACC/AHA guidelines and indications for coronary artery bypass graft surgery. Circulation 1991;83:1125–1173.
3. Morin JE, Symes JF, Guerraty AJ et al: Coronary artery bypass profile in Canada and the United States. Can J Cardiol 1990;8:319–322.
4. Christakis GT, Ivano VJ, Weisel RD et al: The changing pattern of coronary artery bypass surgery. Circulation 1989;80:1151–1161.
5. Haunhien KS, Fiore AC, Wadley J et al: The changing mortality of myocardial revascularization: Coronary artery bypass and angioplasty. Ann Thorac Surg 1988;46:666–674.
6. Jones EL, Weitraub WS, Craver JM et al: Coronary bypass surgery: Is the operation different today? J Thorac and Cardiovasc Surg 1991;101:108–115.
7. Davis PK, Parascandola SA, Miller CA et al: Mortality of coronary artery bypass grafting before and after the advent of angioplasty. Ann Thorac Surg 1989;47:493–498.
8. Grunwald RP: A technique for direct-vision sternal re-entry. Ann Thorac Surg 1985;40:521–522.
9. Keon WJ: Reoperation for coronary artery disease. Current Opinion in Cardiology 1986;1:907–910
10. Keon WJ, Bédard P, Brais M et al: Coronary endarterectomy: Improving techniques and results. J Thorac and Cardiovasc Surg 1981;22:503–509.
11. Loop FD, Lytle BW, Cosgrove DM et al: Influence of the internal mammary artery graft on 10 year survival and other cardiac events. N Engl J Med 1986;314:1–6.
12. Keiser TM, FitzGibbon GM and Keon WJ: Sequential coronary bypass grafts: long term follow-up. J Thorac and Cardiovasc Surg 1986;91:5,767–772.
13. Parsonnet V, Dean D and Bernstein AP: A method of uniform stratification of risk for evaluating the results of surgery in acquired adult heart disease. Circulation 1989;79(Suppl 1):3–12.

11. Long-term results of patients after coronary artery bypass surgery

CHARLES J. MULLANY and BERNARD J. GERSH

1. Introduction

Although aorto-coronary artery bypass grafting is a relatively recent innovation, surgery for the ischemic myocardium has been undertaken since the early 1900s. These early procedures included cervical sympathectomy [1], indirect revascularization by promotion of epicardial collaterals (Beck [2] and Vineberg [3] procedures), and coronary sinus arterialization (Beck II procedure [4].) It was not until the 1950s that direct coronary revascularization was first performed, initially by coronary endarterectomy [5] and later by direct aorto-coronary bypass procedures [6,7]. In 1966, Favaloro [8] from the Cleveland Clinic and Johnson [9] from Milwaukee, popularized routine coronary artery bypass grafting. Since then, approximately 300 000 aorto-coronary artery bypass procedures [10], as well as a similar number of coronary angioplasties [11], are performed annually in the United States. The efficacy of these procedures, both in the relief of symptoms and in the prolongation of life, have been the subject of much debate. In this chapter we will address long-term results of coronary revascularization by coronary artery bypass surgery, with emphasis upon survival, symptom relief, and overall quality of life.

2. Role of clinical trials and registry studies

Prior to the widespread application of coronary artery bypass grafting, there had been few attempts to objectively assess the efficacy of coronary revascularization. Although randomized prospective trials would appear to be the most effective means of assessing a therapeutic procedure, they do have particular disadvantages [12] (Table 1). These trials, by having limited entry criteria, necessarily exclude a large number of patients who eventually undergo coronary artery bypass grafting. Moreover, by the time the results of such trials are published, advances in therapy may make the results of a

Paul J. Walter (ed.): *Quality of Life after Open Heart Surgery*, 115–131.
© 1992 Kluwer Academic Publishers.

Table 1. Types of clinical studies*

Type	Control	Strengths	Weakness
Retrospective, matched	Historical or life table	Simplicity Large population	Selection bias Comparability not ensured
Registry	Concurrent, non-randomized	Large population Selection bias can be reduced by statistical adjustment	Unrecorded baseline variables may prevent valid comparison
Prospective randomized	Random assignment	Removes investigator bias Balances groups for all variables	Crossover Low participation rates Changes in therapy with time

* Reproduced, with permission from McGoon *et al.*, Surgical treatment of coronary artery disease. Cardiology: Fundamentals and Practice. Eds. Giuliani, *et al.*, Mosby 1991, p. 1491.

particular trial invalid. Increasing rates of crossover from one therapeutic modality to another also confound the ultimate results. In the Coronary Artery Surgery Study (CASS), at the end of ten years, at least 38% of patients treated medically had crossed over into the surgical arm [13]. It must also be accepted that the major benefits of coronary revascularization upon survival in comparison with medical therapy have been noted among 'sicker' patients considered at higher risk. Moreover, such patients, particularly if they are severely symptomatic, are also less suitable for inclusion into randomized trials. For this and other reasons, observational studies on registry patients are now playing an increasingly important role in the assessment of myocardial revascularization. The major randomized trials which compare surgery to medical therapy are the Veteran's Cooperative Study (VACOOPS, 1972–1974) [14–17], The European Coronary Surgery Study (ECSS, 1973–1976) [18,19], and more recently, the Coronary Artery Surgery Study of North America (CASS, 1975–1979) [13,20–24]. Trials currently in progress compare percutaneous transluminal coronary angioplasty with surgery or medical therapy. Major registry studies include the CASS Registry [25–35], the Duke Data Bank [36], and Seattle Heart Watch [37].

3. Results of coronary artery bypass grafting

3.1. *Symptoms*

For patients with proximal stenosis of the coronary arteries, with good distal vessels, and who are having significant angina pectoris, there is little doubt that coronary artery bypass grafting results in dramatic relief of symptoms. Even in patients with mild preoperative symptoms, there is good evidence that patients treated surgically have better relief of symptoms, require less anti-anginal medication, have fewer activity limitations, and have less evidence of exercise induced ischemia than those patients who have continued on medical therapy alone [21]. In the CASS randomized trial, at 5 years, a large proportion of surgical patients were asymptomatic (63% vs 38%). By the end of 10 years these differences became far less apparent with only 47% of surgical patients being asymptomatic [22]. However, if one excludes the large number (37%) of medical patients who crossed over to surgical therapy, then the differences in symptomatic status between the two groups still remained pronounced (Figure 1) [22]. Clearly the impact of a large number of 'crossovers' on symptom relief is substantial. Nevertheless, the benefits of coronary artery bypass grafting upon symptoms do diminish with time as graft attrition and progression of disease in the native vessels take their toll.

3.2. *Long-term survival*

The bulk of the controversy regarding coronary artery bypass grafting relates to its effect upon long-term survival. Studies comparing *all* patients undergoing either coronary artery bypass grafting or medical therapy have failed to demonstrate significant differences in survival between the two treatment modalities at the end of 5 or 10 years. However, there are clearly subgroups of patients who benefit from surgery with an increase in their life expectancy. The message from all the trials is consistent; i.e. the survival benefit is greatest in those at higher risk.

3.2.a. *Left main coronary artery stenosis*
The impact of coronary artery disease upon survival in patients with severe disease of the left main coronary artery is dramatic. In the Veteran's Study, of those patients with significant disease of the left main coronary artery, 42 month cumulative survival rate in the medical group was 65% compared to 88% in the surgical group [15]. Similar improvement in survival has been demonstrated both in symptomatic [26] and in asymptomatic patients [27] enrolled in the CASS registry. For asymptomatic patients, 5 year survival of medically and surgically treated patients was 57% and 88% respectively. The greater the degree of left main stenosis and/or impairment of the left ventricular function, the poorer is the prognosis of the patient if treated medically and the greater are the surgical benefits [26]. This also applies to the patient with an associated right coronary artery occlusion [38].

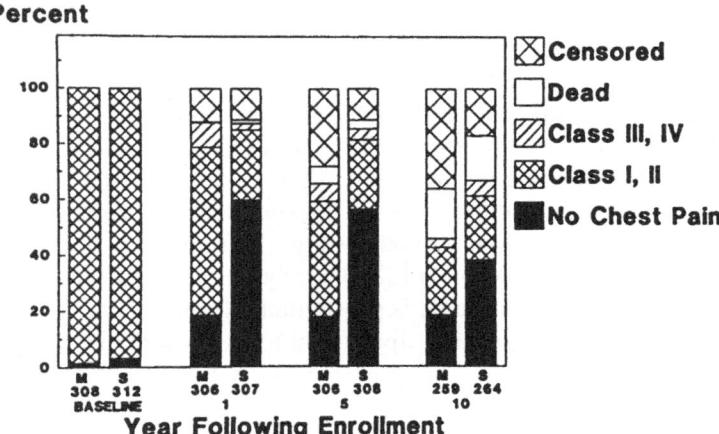

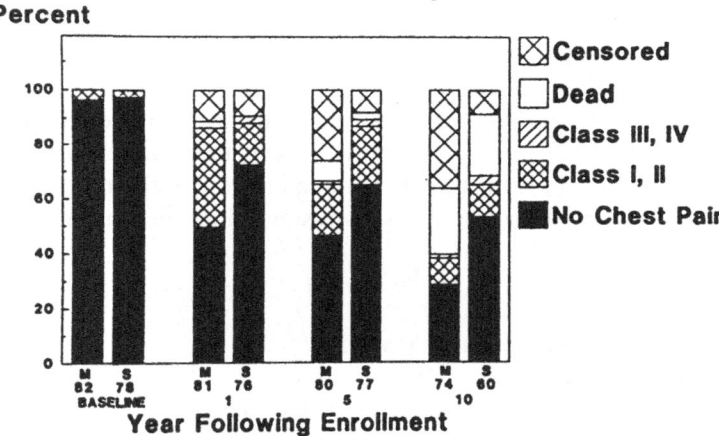

Figure 1A and 1B. Chest pain status in patients randomized to surgical (S) or medical (M) therapy. Data from the medical group were removed from the strata at the time of coronary artery bypass graft surgery, data from the surgical group patients were included only after they actually underwent surgery, and data from the surgical group patients were censored when repeat surgery was performed. Group A: Mild angina and normal left ventricle; Group B: Mild angina and moderately impaired left ventricular function; Group C: Free of angina after myocardial infarction. Reproduced with permission from Rogers *et al.*, Circulation 1990;82:1647–1658.

3.2.b. *Extent of coronary artery disease*

The major determinants of prognosis in coronary artery disease are left ventricular function, the number of vessels diseased, the severity of ischemia, and the electrical stability of the myocardium. It is not surprising, therefore, that the major benefits of coronary bypass surgery are found among patients with multivessel disease and left ventricular dysfunction, particularly in the face of severe symptoms or documented ischemia on stress testing.

3.2.b.1. *Single vessel disease.*

The prognosis of single vessel disease, treated either medically or surgically, is excellent with no studies indicating an advantage of either form of treatment. In CASS, 10 year survival for single vessel disease was 82% (medical) and 85% (surgical) [13]. Twenty-two percent of patients randomized to medical therapy had undergone coronary artery bypass grafting at 10 years [13]. What is yet unresolved is whether symptomatic patients with single vessel disease manifested by a tight proximal left anterior descending stenosis, particularly prior to the origin of the first septal perforator, should be treated medically, by percutaneous transluminal coronary angioplasty, or by internal mammary artery bypass grafting. Although percutaneous transluminal coronary angioplasty is attractive in that it has the potential to avoid surgery, the high incidence of restenosis in the proximal left anterior descending remains a problem. In a nonrandomized study reported from the Cleveland Clinic [39], patients with proximal left anterior descending stenosis who were treated surgically had a better long-term survival with a greater freedom from cardiac events, even when repeat percutaneous transluminal coronary angioplasty is excluded, than those patients who were treated by initial angioplasty (Figure 2).

3.2.b.2. *Two vessel disease.*

The interaction of severity of ischemia, as manifested by angina or noninvasive testing, and left ventricular function, determines whether the patients with two vessel disease have improved longevity with coronary revascularization [40]. In early studies reported from the European Coronary Surgery Study Group [18], a documented benefit of surgery upon survival was noted in patients with two vessel disease, but only when this included stenosis of the proximal left anterior descending coronary artery. In the CASS randomized trial, the presence of a 50- or 70-percent stenosis of the left anterior descending coronary artery as a component of one or two vessel disease was not associated with a survival benefit from surgery compared to medicine [13]. In the CASS randomized trial, unlike the European Coronary Surgery Study, patients with Class III or IV angina were excluded. It is therefore not surprising that in the CASS population confined to patients with mild stable angina or asymptomatic survivors of a prior myocardial infarction a survival benefit with surgery was not seen. Moreover, the CASS surgical and medical mortality and survival rates were better than with equivalent patients in the Veterans and European trials [13].

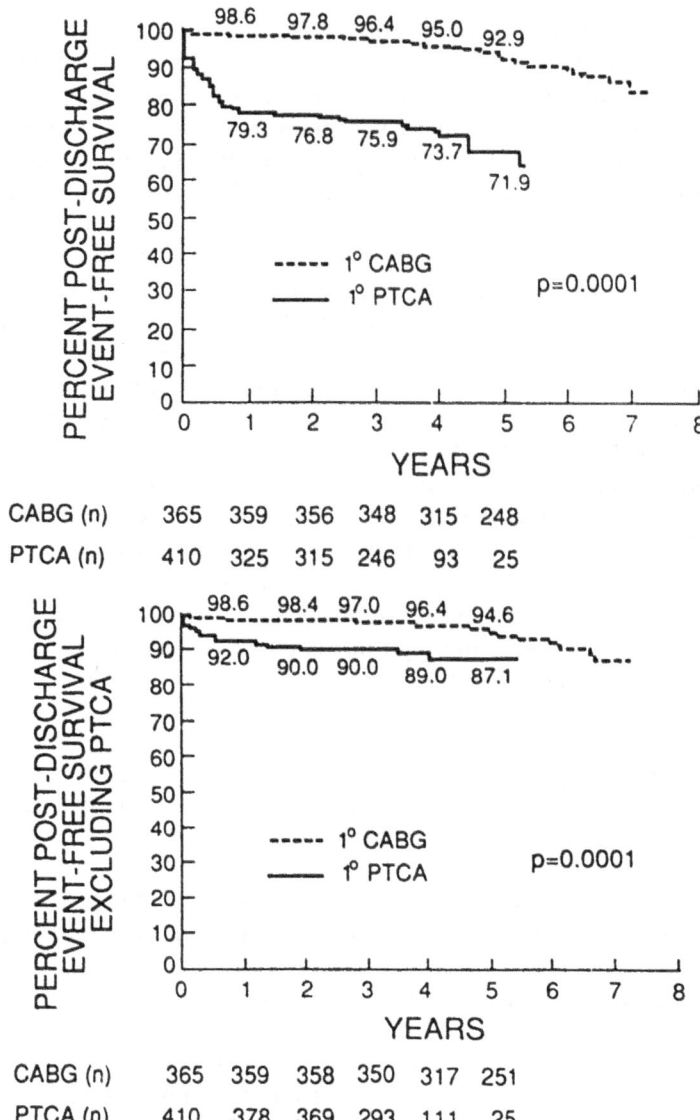

Figure 2A and 2B. Post-discharge event-free survival rates for 775 patients treated with PTCA and CABG for isolated left anterior descending stenosis (A). Event-free survival rates for 775 patients with isolated left anterior descending stenosis by primary treatment group where in-hospital events and PTCA are excluded as events (B). Reproduced with permission from Kramer *et al.*, Am Heart J 1989;261:1144–1153.

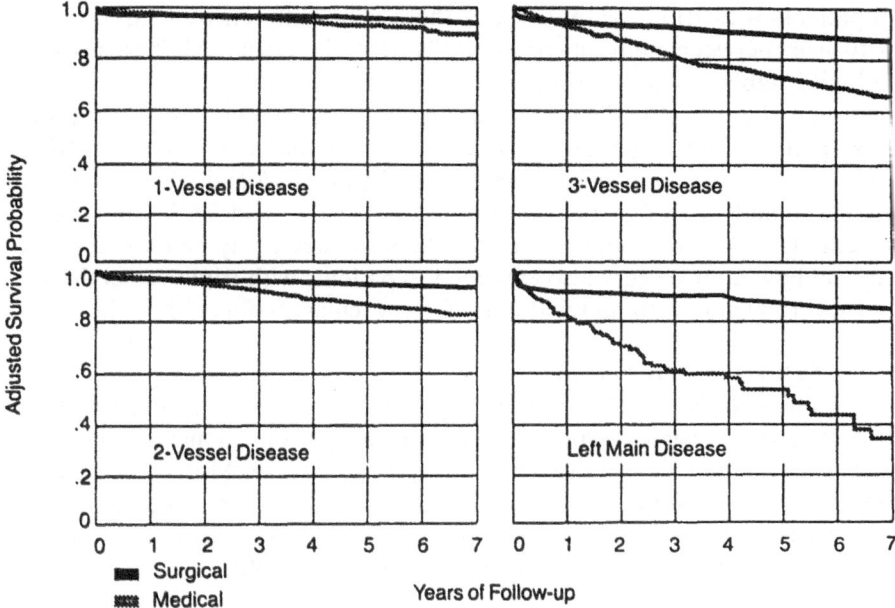

Figure 3. Survival of patients treated medically or surgically in 1984 with one-vessel disease, two-vessel disease, three-vessel disease, and left main coronary artery disease. The survival curves are adjusted for all known important baseline characteristics. Reproduced with permission from Califf *et al.*, JAMA 1989;261:2077–2086.

Most of the data published regarding prognosis of patients according to extent of disease comes from the surgical series commenced in the 1970s. In the CASS randomized study, confined to patients with mild angina or asymptomatic patients following myocardial infarction, patients with two vessel disease and an ejection fraction of <0.50 treated surgically had a 5 year survival of 82% compared to 65% to those treated medically [20]. Although there was a trend to a better survival with surgery, this was not statistically significant. In contrast, in a CASS registry study, which included patients with severe angina, the survival after coronary artery bypass grafting in patients with two vessel disease and diminished left ventricular function was significantly better than those who had been treated medically [30]. With normal left ventricular function there was no difference between medical and surgical treatment.

There is now reasonable evidence of the improving prognosis of patients managed surgically in more recent times [36]. The information from the Duke data bank [36] indicates that by 1984, two vessel disease was associated with a significantly better survival if treated surgically rather than medically (Figure 3).

3.2.b.3. *Triple vessel disease.* In the CASS [13] randomized trial, comparing all patients with triple vessel disease, there is no difference in survival at 5 or 10 years between medically or surgically treated patients. All these patients had mild stable angina or were asymptomatic after a myocardial infarction. However, there is little dispute regarding the beneficial effects of surgery in those patients with impaired left ventricular function. For those with triple vessel disease and an ejection fraction less than 0.50, 5 and 10 year survival was 81% and 58% for medical patients and 90% and 75% for surgical patients [13]. On the other hand, a CASS registry study showed that the survival benefit of surgery also extended to patients with triple vessel disease and severe angina with and without left ventricular dysfunction [33].

3.2.c. *Left ventricular function*
Left ventricular dysfunction, initially regarded as a potential contraindication or deterrent to coronary bypass surgery, has now become a major indication, particularly in patients with two and three vessel disease. Moreover, perhaps the greatest improvement in survival after coronary artery bypass compared to medical therapy is in the subset of patients with left ventricular dysfunction and demonstrable reversible ischemia [13,19,23,30,32,40].

3.2.d. *Elderly patients*
In general, the elderly can be characterized as a higher risk subgroup, primarily on the basis of an increased prevalence of severe symptoms, left ventricular dysfunction, and multivessel and left main coronary artery disease [41]. As such, the potential for coronary bypass surgery to improve survival over medical therapy is enhanced. The potential long-term benefits of coronary bypass surgery do, however, come at a price, since perioperative morbidity and mortality of cardiac surgery in the elderly is increased, particulary among the 'old old', i.e. patients aged 75 years and older [41]. Nonetheless, excellent symptom relief and survival among patients of advanced age who leave the hospital has been documented [41]. Crucial to the early and long-term success of coronary bypass surgery in the elderly is careful patient selection. Comorbid medical conditions must be recognized in advance, since they may have a powerful and deleterious impact not only upon the perioperative period, but also upon late survival. In the CASS study, the number of associated medical diseases was one of the major determinants of late outcome [29]. The older the patient, the more we should focus upon quality of life as an end point and not purely survival. It is mandatory, therefore, that any decision to perform cardiac surgery in this age group takes into account the patient's current quality of life, their aspirations, expectations, motivation, and the presence and the severity of other medical conditions.

3.2.e. *Diabetes*
The influence of diabetes upon long-term survival in patients undergoing coronary artery bypass grafting has been controversial [42–45]. Diabetics

tend to have more extensive coronary artery disease and a greater degree of left ventricular dysfunction when compared to nondiabetics [44,46]. They are also likely to be older, female, and have more unstable symptoms. No adverse effect of diabetes on late survival was reported in either the CASS registry [25], or by Cosgrove [43]. However, both Lawrie [45] and Morris [44] have demonstrated that diabetes mellitus has an adverse effect upon survival independent of the above risk factors. At five years, survival of non-diabetic patients was 91% compared to 80% in diabetics. The increasing proportion of patients who undergo coronary artery bypass grafting and who are also diabetic emphasize the need to further study the influence of diabetes upon all therapeutic modalities for coronary artery disease [44].

3.2.f. *Gender*
Early reports from the CASS registry [25,34] and other series [40,46,48] documented in women a higher perioperative mortality after coronary artery surgery and poorer long-term symptom relief. It was initially felt that the explanation was primarily technical and the consequence of the smaller caliber of coronary arteries in women, as well as a possible association with diabetes [35]. Whereas this may be the case in many patients, it is unlikely to be the sole explanation for the difference in outcome between men and women. In this regard, a recent report [47] implies a gender bias towards the selection of women for coronary artery bypass. It would appear that for a given severity of symptomatology, men are more likely than women to be referred for angiography and coronary revascularization. An additional factor might relate to the practice, during 'routine' physicals in men, of stress testing which could lead to earlier referral. Another potentially infuential factor relates to the perception that chest pain and ST segment changes in women are a manifestation of atypical symptoms or a false positive test. The entire issue of coronary artery disease in women, its etiology, management, and prognosis, merits further investigation.

3.3. *Recurrent disease and symptoms*

Despite the excellent early symptomatic relief that coronary artery bypass grafting provides, recurrence of angina pectoris, particularly after 5 years, becomes increasingly common. In 1801 patients reported by Rowe *et al.* [46], 79% of patients were free of angina pectoris at 5 years. However, by 10 years, only 35% of patients were free of angina. Likewise, freedom from angina in the CASS surgical randomized patients was 63% at 5 years and 47% at 10 years [22]. In many instances the angina pectoris is mild and can be managed medically, with not all patients requiring further invasive treatment such as angioplasty or reoperation.

Causes of recurrent angina pectoris are progression of the patient's own coronary artery disease as well as occlusion or narrowing of grafts due either to technical problems (early) or by graft atherosclerosis (late). It is estimated that 15–20% of vein grafts close during the first postoperative year with a subsequent closure rate of 0.5 to 3.0% over the next 10 years [49]. Very early closure (<1 month) may be due to thrombotic occlusion at the graft anastomosis, possibly related to small distal vessels, a narrowed anastomosis, or endothelial injury at the time of surgery [50]. Occlusions occurring between 1 and 12 months after surgery seem to be related to intimal hyperplasia [50]. Thereafter atherosclerosis is the major pathological finding in occluded or stenosed saphenous vein bypass grafts (Figure 4). At the Montreal Heart Institute [49,51], after 10 years, only 53% of saphenous vein grafts were patent, compared to 84% of internal mammary artery grafts. Likewise, in those patients treated at the Cleveland Clinic, cumulative vein graft patency at a mean follow-up of 88 months was only 45%, compared to internal mammary artery patency of 93% [52].

The overwhelming greater patency of the internal mammary artery compared to saphenous vein has led to its wide acceptance as a preferred conduit, particularly to the left anterior descending coronary artery. Initially, only a few centers routinely used the internal mammary artery as a coronary conduit. However, after realization of the greater patency and better long-term results with this conduit and the increasing experience in harvesting and handling the internal mammary artery, the application of the internal mammary artery, as well as other arterial conduits (bilateral mammary grafts, gastroepiploic, and inferior epigastric arteries) are being expanded rapidly. There are now good data that internal mammary artery grafting leads to a better 10 year survival and possible freedom from cardiac events [53] than in comparable patients who received vein grafts alone. In regard to symptoms, relief differences between the internal mammary artery or saphenous vein are less evident [10], but may favor the former. However, there is no evidence to date that the use of two internal mammary artery grafts is any better than single internal mammary artery grafts [54]. Since the left anterior descending coronary artery is the most important artery in the majority of patients, the role of the internal mammary artery on improved survival may be related to maintenance of blood flow to the anterior surface and septum of the left ventricle [10]. In addition, the use of the internal mammary artery most probably converts patients from triple vessel disease to two vessel disease and that any further improvement in long-term survival with multiple arterial grafts will be very difficult to demonstrate.

The relative immunity of the internal mammary artery from atherosclerosis may be related to both anatomic and biochemical factors. Sims [55] has demonstrated that the internal mammary artery has a particularly prominent internal elastic lamina throughout its whole length, and has postulated that this prevents migration of medial smooth muscle cells into the intima, thickening of the intima, and subsequent development of atherosclerosis. The

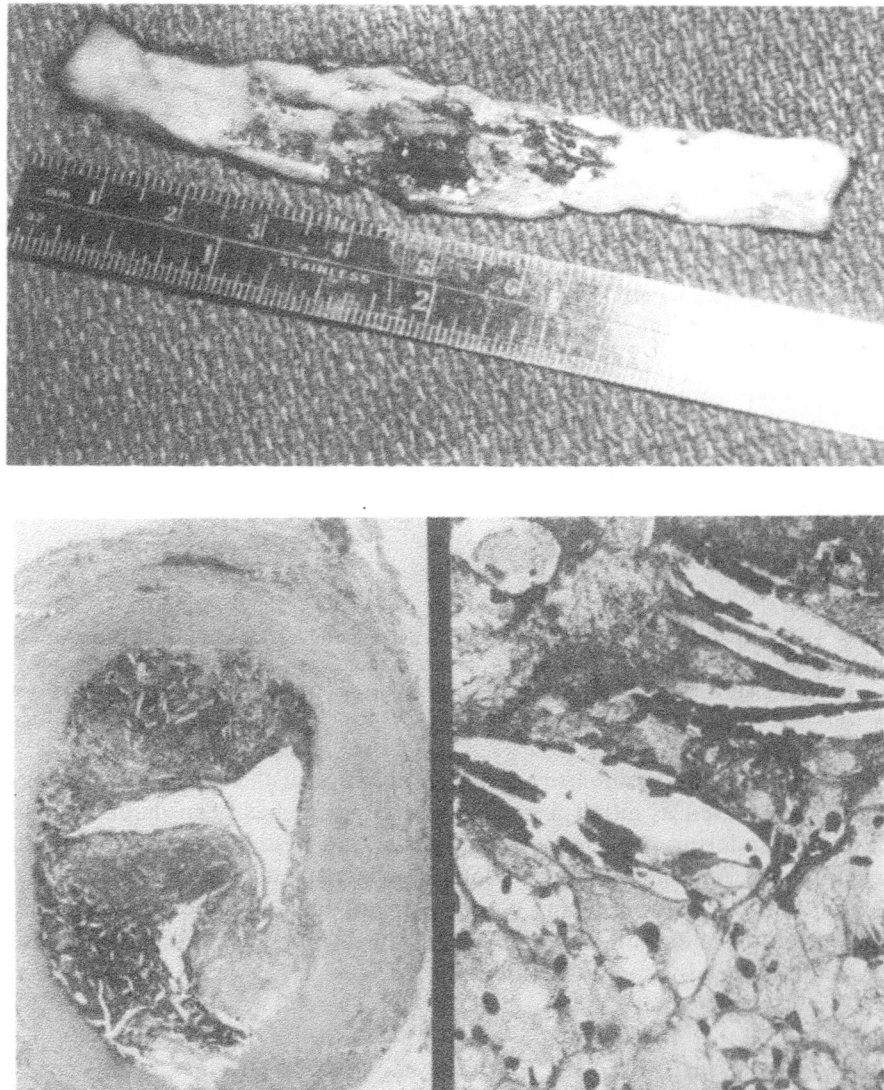

Figure 4A and 4B. Atherosclerotic plaque involving saphenous vein graft (A). Histological section of saphenous vein graft involved with atherosclerosis (B). Reproduced with permission from Mullany, Modern Medicine of Australia, March 1989;62–68.

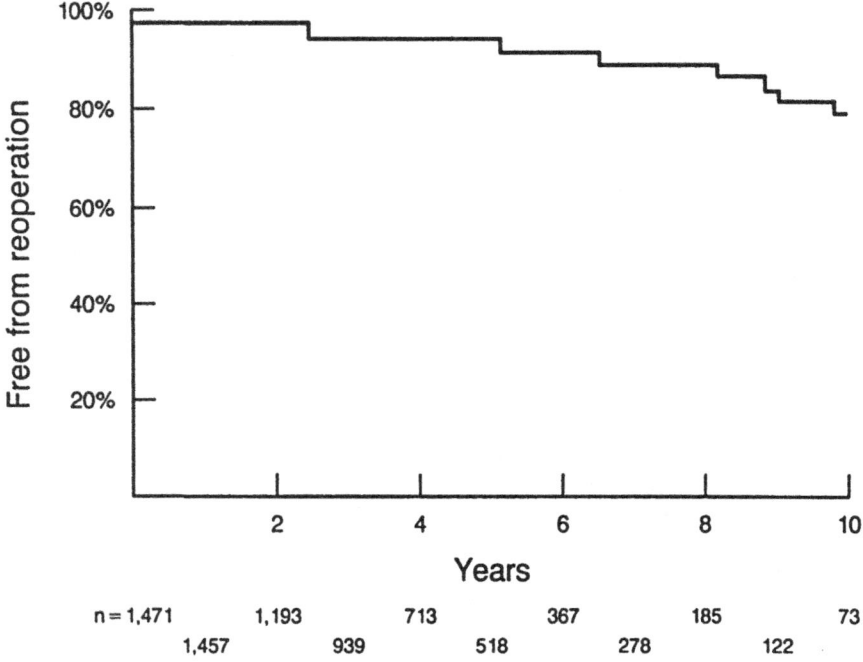

Figure 5. Cumulative freedom from reoperation in patients who survived initial coronary-artery bypass surgery. At 10 years, the freedom from reoperation was 82.8% ± 3.0%. Number of at-risk patients shown by year. Reproduced with permission from Rowe, *et al.*, Med J Aust 1989;150:682–693.

preservation of the vasa vasorum and lymphatics of the internal mammary artery, when used as either a pedicle or free graft, has been demonstrated in animal models to prevent ischemia of the graft vessel and the subsequent development of intimal thickening [56]. The internal mammary artery, when compared to saphenous vein, has also been demonstrated to have high concentrations of endothelial relaxing factor which may inhibit histamine and serotonin induced vasoconstriction [57].

3.4. *Reoperations*

Because of recurrent angina pectoris, a number of patients will need repeat coronary artery bypass grafting. Repeat surgery is not common before five years. However, by 10 years, 10–15% of patients will require repeat surgery (Figure 5) [46]. Risk factors for reoperation are young age at initial surgery, non-use of the internal mammary artery as a conduit, continued smoking, persistent hyperlipidemia, incomplete revascularization, and Class IV symptoms at initial surgery [46,58].

Management of risk factors, such as smoking and hypercholesterolemia, are extremely important for the patient who has had coronary artery surgery. In a multivariate analysis of patients undergoing repeat coronary artery bypass grafting, Solymoss *et al.* [59] found that continued smoking after initial coronary artery bypass grafting was a most significant factor leading to graft thrombosis. In both medically and surgically treated patients enrolled in the CASS registry, smoking cessation lessened the risk of subsequent death or myocardial infarction [31]. Moreover, the benefits of smoking cessation upon subsequent events was noted across *all* age groups. An autopsy study of young males under the age of 35 years demonstrated that smokers had over a twofold increased chance of having raised atherosclerotic lesions in the right coronary artery when compared to nonsmokers [60]. Finally, patients who were randomized to surgery in the CASS study and who continued to smoke had a poorer survival and increased number of late hospitalizations [24]. In view of the above data it is essential that patients who have coronary artery disease, and certainly those who have undergone coronary artery bypass grafting, should abstain from smoking.

An adverse serum lipid profile with an elevated level of LDL cholesterol as well as a low level of HDL cholesterol, has been demonstrated to be associated with the development of saphenous vein graft atherosclerosis and thrombosis [59,61]. Patients who have been treated aggressively with lipid lowering drugs have been found to have less progression of atherosclerotic lesions both in grafted and ungrafted segments of the coronary circulation as well as in venous grafts [62]. A combination of cigarette smoking and high serum cholesterol is particularly deleterious and emphasizes the need for active intervention to improve the effectiveness of coronary artery bypass grafting. Following revascularization, patients should be advised to achieve an ideal body weight, stop smoking, consume a low saturated fat and cholesterol diet, and to participate in regular moderate aerobic exercise. Ideal blood lipid values for postbypass grafting patients include total cholesterol less than 5.2 mOsm/L, LDL cholesterol less than 3.4 mOsm/L, a ratio of total cholesterol to HDL cholesterol less than 4.5, and triglycerides less than 1.5 mOsm/L. Many patients with elevated cholesterol levels can be adequately managed by proper diet and exercise. However, some patients will require drug therapy for lipid levels consistently above the desirable concentrations.

4. Conclusions

Coronary bypass surgery has been a major therapeutic advance, and an extensive body of information, emanating primarily from the 1970s and early 1980s, has identified subsets of patients in whom coronary bypass surgery prolongs survival compared to medical therapy. The issue for the 1990s will be to define the optimal method of revascularization in different subgroups of patients – whether by coronary artery bypass, balloon angioplasty, or other catheter-based interventional devices.

In regard to the late results of coronary artery bypass surgery, the focus has been on survival and symptom relief, but other less tangible manifestations of the quality of life have understandably received less attention. As our population continues to age, the expanding use of invasive cardiovascular procedures in patients of advanced age should direct efforts towards a careful evaluation of our therapies upon quality of life, and not on survival alone.

Aggressive approaches towards the maintenance of graft patency by means of different conduits, drugs (e.g., aspirin), and risk factor modification are crucial if the full benefits of coronary artery bypass surgery upon late outcome and the quality of life are to be realized.

References

1. Jonnesco T: Traitement chirurgical de l'angine de poitrine guerie par la resection du sympathique cervico-thoracique. Bull Acad Med Paris 1920;84:93.
2. Beck CS: The development of a new blood supply to the heart by operation. Ann Surg 1935;102:801–813.
3. Vineberg AM, Niloff PH: The value of surgical treatment of coronary artery occlusion by implantation of the internal mammary artery into the ventricular myocardium. Surg Gynecol Obstet 1950;91:551–561.
4. Beck CS: Revascularization of the heart. Ann Surg 1948;128:854–864.
5. Bailey CP, May A, Lemmon WM: Survival after coronary endarterectomy in man. JAMA 1957;164:641–646.
6. Sabiston DC, Jr: The coronary circulation. Johns Hopkins Med J 1974;134:314–329.
7. Garrett HE, Dennis EW, DeBakey ME: Aortocoronary bypass with saphenous vein graft: Seven year follow-up. JAMA 1973;223:792–794.
8. Favaloro RG. Saphenous vein graft in the surgical treatment of coronary artery disease. J Thorac Cardiovasc Surg 1969;58:178–185.
9. Johnson WD, Flemma RJ, Lepley D, Ellison EH Extended treatment of severe coronary artery disease: A total surgical approach. Ann Surg 1969;170:460–470.
10. ACC/AHA: Guidelines and indications for coronary artery bypass surgery. Circulation 1991;83:1125–1173.
11. King SB, Talley JD: Coronary arteriography and percutaneous transluminal angioplasty: Changing patterns of use and results. Circulation 1989; 79(Suppl I):19–23.
12. McGoon MD, Fuster V, Gersh BJ, Mullany CJ: Surgical treatment of coronary artery disease. B. Revascularization versus medical management of coronary artery disease. In Giuliani E, Fuster V, Gersh B, McGoon M, and McGoon D. (eds.) Cardiology Fundamentals and Practice Volume II, 1991:1490–1502.
13. Alderman EL, Bourassa MG, Cohen LS, Davis KB, Kaiser GC, Killip T, Mock MB, Pettinger M, Robertson TL for the CASS Investigators: Ten year follow-up of survival and myocardial infarction in the randomized coronary artery surgery study. Circulation 1990;82:1629–1646.
14. Peduzzi P, Hultgren HN: Effect of medical vs surgical treatment on symptoms in stable angina pectoris. The Veterans Administration Cooperative Study of Surgery for Coronary Arterial Occlusive Disease. Circulation 1979;60:888–900.
15. Takaro T, Peduzzi P, Detre KM, Hultgren HN, Murphy ML, Vander Bel-Kahn J, Thomsen J: Survival in subgroups of patients with left main coronary artery disease. Veterans Admin-

istration Cooperative Study of Surgery for Coronary Arterial Occlusive Disease. Circulation 1982; 66:14–22.

16. Murphy ML, Hul tgren HN, Detre KM, Thomsen J, Takaro T: Treatment of chronic stable angina: A preliminary report of survival data of the randomized Veterans Administration Cooperative Study. N Engl J Med 1977;297:621–627.

17. Veterans Administration Coronary Artery Bypass Surgery Cooperative Study Group: Eleven-year survival in the Veterans Administration randomized trial of coronary bypass surgery for stable angina. N Engl J Med 1984;311:1333–1339.

18. European Coronary Surgery Study Group: Long-term results of prospective randomized study of coronary artery bypass surgery in stable angina pectoris. Lancet 1982;2:1173–1180.

19. Varnauskas E and The European Coronary Surgery Study Group: Twelve year follow-up of survival in the randomized European Coronary Surgery Study. N Engl J Med 1988;319:332–337.

20. CASS Principal Investigators Coronary artery surgery study (CASS): A randomized trial of coronary artery bypass surgery: Survival data. Circulation 1983;68:939–950.

21. CASS Principal Investigators: Coronary artery surgery study (CASS): A randomized trial of coronary artery bypass surgery: Quality of life in patients randomly assigned to treatment groups. Circulation 1983;68:951–960.

22. Rogers WJ, Loggin CJ, Gersh BJ, Fiske LD, Myers WO, Oberman A, Sheffield LT for the CASS investigators: Ten year follow-up of quality of life in patients randomized to medicine versus coronary bypass graft surgery: The coronary artery surgery study (CASS). Circulation 1990;82:1647–1658.

23. Passamani E, David KB, Gillespie MJ, Killip T, and the CASS principal investigators and their associates: A randomized trial of coronary artery bypass surgery: Survival of patients with low ejection fraction. N Engl J Med 1985;312:1665–1671.

24. Cavender JB, Rogers WJ, Finder LD, Gersh BJ, Coggin CJ, Myers WD For the CASS investigators. Impact of cigarette smoking on quality and duration of life in patients randomized to medicine or coronary artery bypass grafting in the coronary artery surgery study (CASS): 10 year follow-up. Clinical Res 1989;37:2A.

25. Myers WO, Davis K, Foster ED, Maynard C, Kaiser GG: Surgical survival in the coronary artery surgery study (CASS) registry. Ann Thorac Surg 1985;40:245–260.

26. Chaitlan BR, Fisher LD, Bourassa MG, Davis K, Rogers WJ, Maynard C, Tyras DH, Berger RL, Judhins MP, Ringrist I, Mock M, Killip T, and participating CASS medical centers: Effect of coronary bypass surgery on survival patterns in subsets of patients with left main coronary artery disease: Report of the collaborative study in coronary artery surgery (CASS). Am J Cardiol 1981;48:765–777.

27. Taylor HA, Deumite NJ, Chaitman BR, Davis KB, Killip T, Rogers WJ: Asymptomatic left main coronary artery disease in the coronary artery surgery study (CASS) registry. Ciculation 1989;79:1171–1179.

28. Gersh BJ, Kronmal RA, Frye RL, Schaff HV, Ryan TJ, Gosselin AJ, Kaiser GC, Killip T, and participants in the CASS: Coronary arteriography and coronary artery bypass surgery: Morbidity and mortality in patients ages 65 and older. A report from the coronary artery surgery study. Circulation 1983;67:483–491.

29. Gersh BJ, Kronmal RA, Schaff HV, Frye RL, Ryan TJ, Myers WO, Athearm MW, Gosselin AJ, Kaiser GC, Killip T: Long-term 5–year results of coronary bypass surgery in patients 65 years or older: A report from the coronary artery surgery study. Circulation 1983;68(supl II):II-190–199.

30. Mock MB, Fisher LD, Holmes DR Jr., Gersh BJ, Schaff HV, McConney M, Rogers WJ, Kaiser GC, Ryan TJ, Myers WO, Killip TC, and participants in the coronary artery surgery study: Comparison of effects of medical and surgical therapy on survival in severe angina pectoris and two vessel coronary artery disease with and without left ventricular dysfunction: A coronary artery surgery study registry study. Am J Cardiol 1988;61:1198–1203.

31. Hermanson B, Omenn GS, Kronmal RA, Gersh BJ, and participants in the coronary artery surgery study: Beneficial six year outcome of smoking cessation in older men and women

with coronary artery disease: Result from the CASS registry. N Engl J Med 1988;319:1365–1369.

32. Fisher LD, Tristini FE, and the CASS investigators: Comparison of coronary artery bypass surgery and medical therapy in patients with exercised-induced silent myocardial ischemia: A report from the Coronary Artery Surgery Study (CASS) Registry. JACC 1988;12:595–599.

33. Kaiser GC, Davis KB, Fisher LD, Myers WO, Foster ED, Passamani ER, Gillespie MJ: Survival following coronary artery bypass grafting in patients with severe angina pectoris (CASS): An observational study. J Thorac Cardiovasc Surg 1985;89:513–522.

34. Kennedy JW, Kaiser GC, Fisher LD, Maynard C, Fritz JK, Myers W, Mudd JG, Ryan TJ, Coggin J: Multivariant discriminant analysis of the clinical and angiographic predictors of operative mortality from the Collaborative Study in Coronary Artery Surgery (CASS). J Thorac Cardiovasc Surg 1980;80:876–885.

35. Fisher LD, Kennedy JW, David KB, Maynard C, Fritz JK, Kaiser G, Myers WO, and the participating CASS clinics: Association of sex, physical size, and operative mortality after coronary artery bypass in the Coronary Artery Surgery Study (CASS). J Thorac Cardiovasc Surg 1982;84:334–341.

36. Califf RM, Harrell FE, Lee KL, Rankin JS, Hlatky, MA, Mark DB, Jones RH, Muhlbaier LH, Oldham HN, Pryor DB: The evolution of medical and surgical therapy for coronary artery disease: A 15 year prospective. JAMA 1989;261:2077–2086.

37. Hammermeister KE, Derouen TA, Dodge HT: Comparison of survival of medically and surgically treated coronary disease patients in Seattle Heart Watch: A nonrandomized study. Circulation 1982(Suppl II);65:53–59.

38. Rittenhouse EA, Sauvage LR, Mansfield PB, Smith JC, Hall DG, Davis CC, O'Brien MA: Severe left main coronary arterial stenosis with right coronary arterial occlusion: Results of bypass graft surgery. Am J Cardiol 1982;49:645–650.

39. Kramer JR, Proudfit WL, Loop FD, Goormastic M, Zimmerman K, Simpfendorfer C, Horner G: Late follow-up of 781 patients undergoing percutaneous transluminal coronary angioplasty or coronary artery bypass grafting for an isolated obstruction in the left anterior descending coronary artery. Am Heart J 1989;118:1144–1153.

40. Gersh BJ, Califf RM, Loop FD, Akins CW, Pryor DB, Takaro TC: Coronary bypass surgery in chronic stable angina. Circulation 1989;79(Suppl I):46–59.

41. Mullany CJ, Darling GE, Pluth JR, Orszulak TA, Schaff HV, Ilstrup DM, Gersh BJ: Early and late results after isolated coronary artery bypass surgery in 159 patients aged 80 years and older. Circulation Suppl 1990;82:IV-229–236.

42. Saloman NW, Page US, Okis JE, Stephens J, Klause AH, Bigelow JC: Diabetes mellitus and coronary artery bypass: Short-term risk and longterm prognosis. J Thorac Cardiovasc Surg 1983;85:264–271.

43. Cosgrove DM, Loop FD, Lytle BW, Gill CG, Golding L, Gilson C, Stewart RW, Taylor PC, Goormantic M: Determinants of 10 year survival after primary myocardial revascularization. Amm Surg 1986;202:480–490.

44. Morris JJ, Smith LR, Glower DD, Jones RH, Morris PB, Rankin S. Diabetes as an independent risk factor for survival after coronary artery bypass. Abstract, Circulation 1990;82(Suppl III):No. 4, III–360.

45. Lawrie GM, Morris GC, Glaeser DH: Influence of diabetes mellitus on the results of coronary bypass surgery. JAMA 1986;256:2967–2971.

46. Rowe MH, Mullany CJ, White AL, Wilson AC, Clarebrough JK: Early and late survival after coronary artery surgery. Med J Aust 1989;150:682–693.

47. Khan SS, Nessim S, Gray R, Czer LS, Chaux A, Matloff J: Increased mortality of women in coronary artery bypass surgery: Evidence for referral bias. Ann Intern Med 1990;112:561–567.

48. Loop FD, Golding LR, Macmillan JP, Cosgrove DM, Lytle BW, Sheldon WC: Coronary artery surgery in women compared with men: Analyses of risks and long-term results. J Am Coll Cardiol 1983;1:383–390.

49. Grondin CM, Campeau L, Lesperance J, Enjalbert M, Bourassa MG: Comparison of late changes in internal mammary artery and saphenous vein grafts in two consecutive series of patients 10 years after operation. Circulation 1984;70(Suppl I):208–12.

50. Smith S, Greer J: Morphology of saphenous vein coronary artery bypass grafts: 7 to 116 months after surgery. Arch Pathol Lab Med 1983;107:13–18.

51. Bourassa MG, Campeau L, Lesperance J, Grondin CM: Changes in grafts and coronary arteries after saphenous vein aorto-coronary bypass surgery: Results at repeat angiography. Circulation 1982;65(Supple II):90–97.

52. Lytle BW, Loop FD, Cosgrove DM, Easley K, Taylor PC Long-term (512 years) sequential studies of internal mammary artery and saphenous vein coronary bypass grafts. Circulation 1983;68(Suppl III):114.

53. Loop FD, Lytle BW, Cosgrove DM, Stewart RW, Goormastic M, Williams GW, Golding LAR, Gill CC, Taylor PC, Sheldon WC, Proudfit WL: Influence of the internal mammary artery graft on 10-year survival and other cardiac events. N Engl J Med 1986;314:1–6.

54. Morris JJ, Smith LR, Glower DD, Muhlbaier LH, Reves JG, Wechsler AS, Rankin S: Clinical evaluation of single versus multiple mammary artery bypass. Circulation 1990;82(Supple IV):IV-2141223.

55. Sims EH: Discontinuities in the internal elastic lamina: A comparison of coronary and internal mammary arteries. Artery 1985;13:127–143.

56. Daly RC, McCarthy PM, Orszulak TA, Schaff HV, Edwards WD: Histologic comparison of experimental coronary artery bypass grafts – similarity of in situ and free internal mammary artery grafts. J Thorac and Cardiovasc Surg 1988;96:19–29.

57. Yang Z, Diederich D, Schneider K, Siebenmann R, Stulz P, von Segesser L, Turina M, Buhler FR, Luscher TF: Endothelium-derived relaxing factor and protection against contractions induced by histamine and serotonin in the human internal mammary artery and in the saphenous vein. Circulation 1989;80:1041–1048.

58. Cosgrove DM, Loop FD, Lytle BW, Gill CC, Golding LAR, Gibson C, Stewart RW, Taylor PC, Goormastic M: Predictors of reoperation after myocardial revascularization. J Thorac Cardiovasc Surg 1986;92:811–821.

59. Solymoss BC, Nadeau P, Millette D, Campeau L: Late thrombosis of saphenous vein coronary bypass grafts related to risk factors. Circulation 1988;78(Suppl I):I-140–143.

60. Pathological Determinants of Atherosclerosis in Youth (PDAY) Research Group: Relationship of atherosclerosis in young men to serum lipoprotein cholesterol concentrations and smoking. JAMA 1990;264:301813024.

61. Stewart WJ, Goormastic M, Healy BP, Lytle BW, Hoogwerf BJ, Cressman MD, Sheldon WC, Loop FD: Clinical outcome 10 years after coronary bypass: Effects of cholesterol and triglycerides in 4913 patients (abstract). J Am Coll Cardiol 1988;11:7A.

62. Blankenhorn DH, Nessim SA, Johnson RL, SanMarco ME, Azen SP: Beneficial effects of combined colestipol cniacin therapy on coronary atherosclerosis and coronary venous bypass grafts. JAMA 1987;257:3233–3240.

12. Comprehensive cardiac care and quality of life in patients after surgical revascularization

JAN J. KELLERMANN

1. Introduction

In recent years we have learned that patients who underwent coronary aortic bypass grafting (CABG) had not only a diminished rate of return to work, but also a low score in social readjustment. Those findings varied from country to country. In some places the decrease of return to work after surgery and the maintenance of a good quality of survival seemed to be a function of the socio-economic structure of a country and its insurance policies [1].

The question may be raised why return to work should represent a variable of such dominant importance when discussing the patient's perceived quality of life. It is well documented in our studies that the 'biological phenomenon of work' proves to be the 'master key' to other dependent variables such as symptomatology and emotional stability. We have found, that there is a correlation between the reason 'to get up in the morning' and the loss of the urge linked with a basic need for creativity and performance.

2. Comprehensive cardiac care (CCC)

Twenty-nine years ago we introduced a CCC program which is based on physiological, psychological and social aspects and includes a close clinical follow-up of our patients. Our model can be considered a typical model of a comprehensive care program. Of late we have treated 347 patients with documented coronary artery disease (CAD) 42.2% after CABG and 7.5% after PTCA (see Table 1).

An exercise training program is introduced as one of the therapeutic modalities utilized. We have always found a significant rise in physical work performance and a number of cardio-circulatory and respiratory parameters, as a consequence of prolonged-physical training [2]. In some patients such an improvement has not been reached, but in all our patients the emotional

Paul J. Walter (ed.): Quality of Life after Open Heart Surgery, 133–138.
© 1992 Kluwer Academic Publishers.

Table 1. CCC. Mode of intervention ($n = 347$).

Exercise only	4.3%
Exercise + drugs	46.0%
Exercise + CABG + drugs	42.2%
Exercise + PTCA + drugs	7.5%

stability increased while anxiety and fear had already decreased after a 16–week program [3]. Twenty-three years ago we published our first results in Israel concerning the return to work of patients after myocardial infarction. In this report we analysed the working status of a group of 390 patients, past myocardial infarction, who did not undergo an advised or supervised rehabilitation program [4]. We found that 91% of our patients returned to work and only a few had to change their types of work. It was also found that 17% of those patients who returned to work should actually have been disqualified on medical grounds. We assumed that the reason for this remarkably high rate of return to work was the socio-economic structure in Israel, which made it difficult for the patient to manage to live on such national insurance income and other unemployment benefits as they may receive.

Patients participating in our CCC program are accepted at least 12 weeks after an acute coronary event or after surgery. Functional and clinical conditions are repeatedly examined by means of non-invasive testing procedures and nuclear studies. The patients participate twice weekly in an individually-tailored training program. Risk factors are eventually modified; these includes: a complete cessation of smoking, dietary measures, and the control of hypertension and/or diabetes. If hyperlipidemia continues after the implementation of a dietary regimen, lipid reducing compounds are prescribed. Arrhythmia is monitored closely and antiarrhythmic therapy is occasionally initiated.

A complete reassessment of the patient's clinical condition is performed after six months (if there is no reason for an earlier reassessment) which includes subjective maximum exercise testing, echo-Doppler imaging, Holter monitoring and, in selected patients, radionuclide ventriculography. In those patients in whom the symptomatology deteriorates, functional capacity decreases or the frequency of ischemic episodes (silent or overt) increases, coronary angiography is repeated and, naturally, the CCC program is interrupted. This program continues for every patient for many years on an ambulatory basis.

3. Quality of life

It is generally accepted that a number of variables influence the perceived quality of life (see Table 2). In our studies we have found that a 16–32-week program of CCC improves symptomatology, enhances the patients'

Table 2. Patients perceived quality of life dependent variables.

A. Symptoms
B. Emotional stability
C. Social adjustment*

* Dependent on educational and cultural background (cross-culture validations).

self-image, both in the family and socially, reduces absence at work, drug dependency, and anxiety. This has been observed in patients after CABG and without surgery. We have supported the notion that the return to work is one of the crucial factors of the quality of life. On another occasion we have stated that the work site may be hated by some, tolerated by some, loved by others and accepted by few. As a consequence of such a love-hate relationship, the work site may become a nightmare, a shelter or, occasionally a most faithful companion. It is certainly obvious that extreme cross-cultural variabilities exists at the work site around the world and people will have different needs, expectation, demands and environmental stresses, not only according to the various countries and continents, but sometimes even at different places of work within the same country [5].

4. Return to work

Six years ago we examined two groups of patients post-CABG: one group underwent a CCC program, the other did not, and was only follow-up routinely. The age range was similar in both groups. The patients did not suffer from congestive heart failure, unstable angina or other underlying diseases.

Out of the group after CABG without CCC, 65.7% return to work after surgery, 48.6% to the same job. Out of the group which participated in our CCC program, 88.4% return to work, 84.6% to same job. One fascinating finding was that 22.9% retired in the group without CCC in comparison to 7.7% in the CCC group.

5. Follow-up study

The effects on patients of a long-term comprehensive rehabilitation program after CABG were studied by means of comparison between 51 participants and 45 non-participating control patients. Preoperational comparison of the two groups showed no significant difference in age, body weight, resting systolic and diastolic blood pressure, heart rate, percentage of patients with one myocardial infarction or one or two vessel disease, or number of grafts

Table 3. Work status at one year and 4.8 ± 1.9 years after CABG. Comparison between trained and untrained patients.

	One year			4.8 ± 1.9 years		
	Trained (N = 51)	Untrained (N = 45)	P <	Trained (N = 51)	Untrained (N = 45)	P <
Stopped working (%)	1.9	26.6	0.01	3.9	34.0	0.001
Working at same job and regular hours (%)	58.8	20.0	0.0001	47.0	7.0	0.0001
Decreased working hours (%)	39.2	53.3	0.03	49.0	59.0	0.05

performed. No significant group difference was found in the level of education, annual income, or type of employment. In both groups all patients continued to work regularly until two weeks before the operation. Postoperatively, compared with the untrained group, the trained group showed significantly ($p < 0.05$) higher functional capacity and percentage or patients resuming work ($p < 0.001$) after one year, as well as after 4.8 ± 1.9 years. The increased rate of return to work in the trainees may be a function of the fact that they are volunteers and thus may be better motivated to return to work in any case [6] (Table 3).

6. Present study

As mentioned in our introduction, there are 347 coronary patients in our CCC program at present. Out of these patients 174 (50.2%) are patients who underwent CABG, while 173 (49.8%) patients have not undergone surgery, all of them with documented CAD.

Table 4 shows the work status of the two groups of patients. It can be seen that, while 80.3% are working in the group without surgery, 76.3% return to work after coronary surgery. In both groups a similar percentage – namely 16.1% and 16.7%, respectively – are retired. In the group after CABG, 6.1% have a physical occupation and 46.9% a sedentary profession.

Table 4. Work status of patients with and without CABG (N = 347).

Status	Post CABG	No surgery
Full time	81 (46.5%	96 (55.5%)
Part time	52 (29.8%)	43 (24.8%)
Retired	28 (16.1%)	29 (16.7%)
Unemployed	13 (7.5%)	5 (2.9%)
Total N	174	173

23.1% are working in occupations demanding a moderate caloric expenditure (2.5–3.5 kcal.)

Physical work capacity was established by means of a subjective maximum exercise test. Physical work capacity, heart rate (HR) and rate pressure products (RPPs) in patients with and without CABG have been tested. A statistically significantly higher PWC was obtained in patients past surgery than in patients without surgery.

The physical work capacity was significantly higher both in patients with part-time jobs or full time occupation when compared to the retired patients. In the patients past CABG no change in threshold HR (THR) and threshold RPP (TRPP) has been found, either in the groups with full time employment, part-time or those who were retired. In the patients without surgery a significantly higher THR was found when the patients were fully employed as compared to those who were retired. It must also be noted, as mentioned earlier, that almost all the patients past CABG were under drug therapy in addition to exercise training. 33.3% were on beta blockers, 32.1% on calcium antagonists and 15.4% on antiarrhythmic therapy.

7. Discussion

It is our opinion that CCC represents the best available comprehensive management for coronary patients after and without CABG. we have learned that a medically misguided patient will often be confused and helpless after surgery, the reason being that, unfortunately, some surgeons give the impression that all the patient's problems are solved by the operation. Patients are not aware of the fact that they are suffering from coronary atherosclerosis. Secondary preventive measures such as risk modification and life style control should be followed for many years.

We have observed an enhanced quality of survival in patients who underwent a CCC program after CABG.

The present study demonstrate a high percentage of patients who returned to work after surgery. When we compare our results obtained in CCC patients to those without CCC, the return to work is significantly higher for the intervention group. While there are various factors which can influence the return to work (see Table 5) it seems that a supervised comprehensive rehabilitation program can improve the psychosocial and economic status, and beneficially influence the patient's clinical condition.

We have learned that, in Israel, as in other countries, there can be marked intercenter variabilities and one should be cautious when comparing the results from different hospitals because of the possible different composition of the patient's material. An effective patient education is mandatory and may eventually further enhance the complete rehabilitation of patients past CABG.

Table 5. Possible factors influencing the return to work after CABG.

---

* Age
* Premature retirement
* Severity of symptoms
* Prior working status
* Education
* Medical misguidance
* Time of absence from work prior to surgery

---

8. Summary

From our study, which involved patients who underwent supervised rehabilitation, it may be concluded that patients after CABG should undergo a comprehensive coronary care program. It is generally thought that the quality of survival is closely linked to severity of symptoms, the emotional stability and functional capacity. With CCC you can obviously beneficially influence these variables and, therefore, the effect on the emotional and occupational status of patients undergoing such a program is not surprising.

References

1. Walter PJ (ed.): Return to work after coronary artery bypass surgery. Berlin, Heidelberg: Springer Verlag, 1985.
2. Kellermann JJ, Modan B, Feldman S, Kariv I: Return to work after myocardial infarction. Geriatrics 1968;23:151–156.
3. Wintner I, Kellermann JJ: Psychological factors in cardiac rehabilitation. In: Stockmeier R, Halhuber MJ (eds.), Psychological approach to the rehabilitation of coronary patients. Berlin, New York: Springer Verlag, 1976:156–172.
4. Kellerman JJ: Cardiac rehabilitation – The Israeli experience. In: Pollock M, Schmidt DH (eds.), Heart disease and rehabilitation. 2nd ed. New York: John Wiley & Sons Inc, 1985:517–534.
5. Weinberg SD, Kellermann JJ, McIntosh HD: Work site-based education of the cardiac patient. In: Wenger NK (ed.), The education of the patient with cardiac disease in the twenty-first century. Le Jacq Publishing Inc, 1986;400–404.
6. Ben Ari E, Kellermann JJ, Fisman EZ, Pines A, Peled B, Drory Y: Benefits of long-term physical training in patients after coronary artery bypass grafting – a 58-month follow-up and comparison with a nontrained group. J Cardiopulm Rehab 1986;5:165–170.

B: Intellectual Functioning

13. The intellectual function of patients after coronary bypass surgery

PAMELA J. SHAW

1. Introduction

Neuropsychological testing has been used to assess changes in intellectual function after heart surgery since the report of Priest *et al*. in 1957 [1]. This is the best method available at present for obtaining a quantitative assessment of cognitive change following surgery. Changes in neuropsychological scores after heart surgery have been shown to correlate with cerebrospinal fluid biochemical indices of cerebral damage such as adenylate kinase [2].

Virtually all studies in which neuropsychological tests have been used to measure the impact of cardiac operations on brain function, have found evidence of deterioration in the early postoperative period. However, controversy exists regarding the degree and duration of impairment, on factors that predispose to its development, and on whether intellectual deterioration is a specific complication of cardiopulmonary bypass (CPB) operations.

In this chapter I will review data on the neuropsychological sequelae of coronary artery bypass graft (CABG) surgery published by other workers, and then present the neuropsychological results obtained in the Newcastle prospective study of neurological and neuropsychological complications of CABG surgery carried out in the mid 1980s.

2. Review of published data on intellectual dysfunction following CABG surgery

2.1. *Incidence*

The incidence of postoperative cognitive dysfunction following CABG surgery is difficult to define precisely because it depends on such factors as the detail with which patients have been assessed, the particular psychometric tests used, the timing of postoperative assessment and the definition used for significant abnormality. The earlier after surgery and the more extensively

Paul J. Walter (ed.): Quality of Life after Open Heart Surgery, 141–153.
© 1992 Kluwer Academic Publishers.

the patients have been tested, the greater the frequency and severity of the observed intellectual deterioration.

Savageau and her colleagues, using a small battery of psychometric tests and postoperative testing at 9 days and 6 months, showed that 30% of patients had significant intellectual impairment early after cardiac surgery, but only 5% were still abnormal at 6 months [3,4]. Seventy-six per cent of the 227 subjects in this study had undergone CABG operations. Ellis and associates found that 75% of 30 CABG patients had deterioration in some aspect of intellectual function 7 days after surgery. At 4 weeks 17% were still impaired but all had returned to normal by the end of 6 months [5].

2.2. *Type of cognitive changes observed*

Those aspects of cognitive function observed most commonly to deteriorate after cardiac surgery include short-term memory, new learning ability, attention span and psychomotor speed [6–8].

2.3. *Functional impact of cognitive changes after CABG surgery*

There has previously been little detailed information on the functional impact of intellectual deterioration after CABG surgery, but in general it appears that many of the observed cognitive changes do not give rise to major symptomatic complaints. Some authors have emphasised that the domestic and employment activities of many individuals may not require the level of intellectual performance required to complete a psychometric test battery [6,9].

2.4. *Long-term prognosis*

Detailed studies of the long-term prognosis for CABG patients with postoperative intellectual impairment have been few. Several authors have found that much of the early deterioration resolved within 6 months [4,5]. Indeed Ellis *et al.* considered that the lack of long-term cognitive dysfunction indicated that low flow-rates and low arterial pressures could safely be used during CPB. Late postoperative psychometric results may show improvement over those obtained before operation. This observation has generally been considered indicative of practice effects rather than genuine cognitive improvement [10]. Other authors have demonstrated persistent intellectual impairment following heart surgery. Aberg and Kihlgren in 1974 found that 11 to 23% of patients showed intellectual deficit 12 months after surgery [10].

Savageau *et al.* found that 20% of patients with early neuropsychological deterioration after cardiac operations were still impaired at 6 months [4]. This group also found that in some patients neuropsychological decrements could develop as a late finding, when there had been no impairment in the early postoperative period. This late deterioration cannot automatically be attributed to the cardiac surgery, though it is interesting to note that delayed deterioration can occur following a cerebral hypoxic-ischaemic insult [11]. Two studies have considered neuropsychological performance as late as several years after cardiac surgery, but both of these referred to patients undergoing heart valve replacement operations [12,13]. The study of Sotaniemi showed several interesting findings: firstly, after an initial improvement, some patients showed a late deterioration between one year and five years; secondly the group of patients who had shown early neurological complications displayed significantly poorer neuropsychological functioning at 5 years, compared to the group who had not shown early complications [13]. It will be interesting to determine whether similar long-term neuropsychological changes will be found in patients undergoing CABG surgery.

2.5. *Association between post-operative neuropsychological deterioration and clinical neurological disorders*

The association between postoperative neuropsychological dysfunction and clinical neuropsychological disorders has received the attention of several authors and the conclusions have been conflicting. Some authors have found good correlation between the two sets of findings [10,14], but others have observed the contrary [6,15,16].

2.6. *Neuropsychological testing to predict post-operative outcome*

Several studies have attempted to use neuropsychological testing to predict outcome after operation and to assess possible improvements in CPB technology. Willner and colleagues showed that a test of analogical reasoning, the conceptual level analogy test (CLAT), had some ability to predict immediate as well as late postoperative outcome in terms of psychiatric symptoms and mortality [17,18]. Patients whose postoperative CLAT scores indicated severe cognitive dysfunction were at significantly increased risk of death and psychiatric complications, both in hospital and at follow-up 18 months and 5 years later.

3. Is neurophyschological deterioration specific to cardiac operations?

There are methodological problems associated with the use of psychometric tests to evaluate patients on repeated occasions. The tests do not have perfect test–retest reliability coefficients and it is possible that some of the observed neuropsychological deterioration could be due to fatigue, depression or lack of motivation after a major operation, rather than a specific deleterious influence of CPB on cerebral function. Many of the early studies which reported on intellectual deterioration after CABG surgery failed to include a control group who were not exposed to CPB [3,4,19]. There is some evidence that general surgical operations and conventional anaesthesia produce very few changes in intellectual function. Gruvstad *et al.* showed that patients developed little impairment of neuropsychological function 7 days after surgery for lumbar disc prolapse [20], and Aberg and Kihlgren concluded that patients undergoing thoracotomy without CPB did not show significant postoperative intellectual deterioration [10]. More recently Raymond *et al.* performed psychometric testing on 31 patients undergoing CABG surgery and a small group of 16 patients undergoing general surgical procedures [21]. The CABG group showed significant postoperative deterioration in several psychometric tests, but these abnormalities were not present in the control group. Other studies however, have failed to show important differences in postoperative neuropsychological deficit between CABG and surgical control patients. Smith and associates studied 53 CABG patients and 19 controls having thoracic or major vascular surgery [22]. They found that 65% of CABG patients had neuropsychological impairment after surgery, but unexpectedly, comparable deterioration was present in the surgical control group. It is noteworthy that the numbers in this surgical comparison group were relatively small and the authors subsequently stated that, in comparison to the CABG group, they were older and appeared 'sicker' in terms of metabolic status and requirement for perioperative pharmacological support [16]. A further study of 46 CABG patients and 14 controls undergoing peripheral vascular surgery also concluded that non-specific effects of surgery rather than specific effects of CPB substantially contributed to postoperative intellectual deterioration [8].

It therefore seems that changes in intellectual function can occur after major general surgical procedures as well as CPB operations. Controversy exists as to whether all the intellectual changes seen after CABG surgery, are simply a non-specific effect of general surgery, or whether there is a superimposed specific risk of cerebral damage related to the use of CPB.

4. Risk factors for neuropsychological deterioration after CABG surgery

Preoperative factors which have been identified as risk factors for neuropsychological deterioration following CABG surgery include age [3,23] (older patients being at greater risk of cerebral injury), and the type, severity and duration of preoperative heart disease [3]. Several authors have also found that the duration of extra-corporeal perfusion was a determinant of postoperative cerebral outcome [3,16]. It has been suggested that the cumulative effect of cerebral microembolism during bypass might account for this observed phenomenon.

The literature contains conflicting evidence regarding the importance of low intra-operative levels of mean arterial blood pressure (MAP) in the pathogenesis of cerebral injury. Several studies have shown that sustained MAP levels of less than 50 mm Hg are significantly correlated with postoperative cerebral dysfunction [14,15,22,24,25]. Kolkka and Hilberman, however, have argued that MAP during bypass is not a major determinant of neuropsychological dysfunction [26]. Similarly Ellis and colleagues put forward the view that low flow rates and arterial pressures could be employed safely during bypass because they found no evidence of long-term cerebral dysfunction after operations in which these methods had been employed [5]. Both of these groups emphasised the potential advantages of low flow rates and pressures in terms of myocardial preservation during surgery.

Nevin and coworkers provided evidence for involvement of hypocapnia and hypoperfusion in the aetiology of neuropsychological deficit after CABG [27]. They observed that accidental hyperventilation leading to hypocapnia was common prior to bypass. The group of patients with pre-bypass hypocapnia showed swings in arterial PCO_2, increases in cerebral venous pressure and lower cerebral perfusion pressures in the first 10 minutes of bypass. A reduction in postoperative neuropsychological morbidity was observed in the patient group in whom strict normocapnia was maintained.

Some authors have reported that CABG surgery produces less cerebral injury than surgery for cardiac valvular disease [26]. This may result from a reduced potential for cardiogenic cerebral embolism during CABG procedures where the heart chambers are not usually opened. Other authors, however, have not found that valve replacement surgery imposes a greater threat to the brain than CABG surgery [23].

Unexpected catastrophes during CABG surgery such as air embolism, aortic dissection, profound hypotension or hypoxia are occasional hazards and are often accompanied by cerebral and intellectual deterioration [28,29].

Postoperative factors have received scant attention because neurological complications of heart surgery have been so closely attributed to intraoperative factors. Breuer *et al.*, however, found that postoperative use of inotropic agents or an intra-aortic balloon pump (both markers for hypotensive and severely ill patients) correlated with the development of prolonged postoperative encephalopathy a [30].

5. Prediction of neuropsychological deficit

It is at present difficult to continuously monitor cerebral wellbeing during cardiac operations, as there is no available method for direct measurement of cerebral oxygenation. There are practical difficulties associated with conventional EEG recording and interpretation in the operating theatre. The cerebral function analysing monitor (CFAM) which provides simplified and compressed information from the raw EEG is probably the best practical apparatus currently available for cerebral surveillance. Nevin *et al.* reported that significant changes on the CFAM recording during surgery correlated with the development of postoperative neuropsychological deficit [31]. Most of the abnormalities on the CFAM trace were observed to occur at the onset of bypass though some were observed at other times during the operation.

6. Newcastle study of neuropsychological complications of coronary artery bypass (CABG) surgery

As part of a major prospective study of neurological and neuropsychological complications of CABG surgery, involving 312 patients, detailed psychometric testing was carried out before and 7 days after operation on 298 patients. Six months after operation 259 patients underwent psychometric reassessment.

The psychometric tests employed included the Halstead-Reitan trail making test Part B, all 7 subtests from the Wechsler memory scale (WMS), and the block design and vocabulary subtests from the Wechsler Adult Intelligence Scale (WAIS). These tests were chosen to assess a wide range of cognitive abilities (psychomotor speed, attention and concentration, audioverbal and visual short-term memory, visuo-spatial abilities, new learning ability and verbal comprehension) within a time scale (35–50 minutes) which would not be too demanding for the patients.

Our major objectives in undertaking this study were to assess:

1. The incidence and severity of neuropsychological complications occurring after CABG surgery.
2. The functional impact of these complications in terms of the patients everyday activities.
3. Whether neuropsychological complications are a specific feature of cardiac operations using CPB, or a non-specific effect of major surgery.
4. The long-term prognosis and recovery of the early postoperative neuropsychological complications of the CABG group.
5. Preoperative, intraoperative and postoperative factors which predispose to the development of neuropsychological complications.

6.1. *Patients and operative methods*

The CABG group consisted of 276 (88.5%) males and 36 (11.5%) females, with an age range of 33–70 years (mean 53.4 ± 7.4 years). The anaesthetic regime used was based on a modified form of neuroleptanalgesia. CPB was instituted using moderate haemodilution and hypothermia (28°C). Membrane oxygenators were used in 66% and bubble oxygenators in 34%. Cardiotomy reservoirs with integral microaggregate filtration were employed, but arterial line filters were not included in the circuit. Non-pulsatile perfusion was employed in 57% of operations and pulsatile perfusion in 43%.

A comparison group of 50 patients undergoing major surgery for peripheral vascular disease (PVD) was also studied. They were similar to the CABG group from the point of view of age, duration of operation, anaesthetic methods, time spent in ITU after surgery, and the fact that they suffered from atherosclerotic vascular disease. The major difference between the two groups related to the use of CPB [32].

6.2. *Early neuropsychological dysfunction following CABG surgery*

For each of the 10 psychometric tests employed, the differences between the preoperative and postoperative scores were the variables used in the statistical analysis of the data. A patient was considered to show significant deterioration on a particular test if his postoperative scores dropped by more than SD below his preoperative score. The non-parametric Wilcoxon signed rank test was used to assess whether significant deterioration occurred for the group of 298 patients as a whole.

At the end of the seventh postoperative day significant deterioration was observed for the group of patients as a whole in 7 of the 10 psychometric tests (Table 1). Table 2 shows the percentage of patients deteriorating by more than 1 SD on each test. This ranges from 35.6% for the WMS associate learning to as low as 1% on the WAIS vocabulary test.

Seventy-nine per cent (235/298) deteriorated on at least one subtest. Twenty-four per cent (71/298) deteriorated on 3 or more subtests and were considered to show moderate cognitive deterioration, 5% (14/298) deteriorated on 5 or more subtests and were considered to show severe cognitive deterioration.

The cognitive abilities which deteriorated most were those of psychomotor speed, attention and concentration, new learning ability and auditory short-term memory.

In terms of the functional impact of the observed neuropsychological deterioration, 123 of the 235 patients (52%) whose scores deteriorated had no significant symptoms while in hospital, 89 (38%) complained of cognitive

Table 1. Mean changes in neuropsychological test scores in CABG patients and PVD control group.

Test	CABG group preoperative → 7 days postoperative		CABG group preoperative → 6 months postoperative		PVD group preoperative → 7 days postoperative	
	Mean change in score	p	Mean change in score	p	Mean change in score	p
Trail making	−23.4 ± 70	<0.002*	+15.61 ± 38.03	<0.0001	+4.74 ± 25.56	0.29
WMS information	+0.07 ± 0.61	0.066	+0.08 ± 0.70	0.098	+0.19 ± 0.39	0.0077
WMS orientation	−0.08 ± 0.45	0.0035*	+0.01 ± 0.38	0.64	+0.10 ± 0.31	0.043
WMS mental control	−0.78 ± 1.83	<0.002*	−0.05 ± 1.61	0.79	+0.21 ± 1.37	0.35
WMS memory passages	−0.55 ± 2.68	<0.002*	−0.13 ± 2.48	0.28	+1.34 ± 2.29	0.0004
WMS digits total	−0.63 ± 1.74	<0.002*	−0.22 ± 1.66	0.079	+0.29 ± 1.69	0.22
WMS visual reproduction	+0.43 ± 2.42	0.002	+0.35 ± 1.98	0.005	+1.77 ± 1.79	<0.0001
WMS associate learning	−2.48 ± 3.61	<0.002*	+0.54 ± 3.23	0.012	−0.10 ± 2.88	0.81
WAIS block design	−0.18 ± 2.03	0.3	+0.49 ± 1.94	0.0001	+0.69 ± 1.52	0.005
WAIS vocabulary	−0.29 ± 0.88	<0.002*	−0.19 ± 0.90	0.0014*	+0.10 ± 0.63	0.30

* Indicates the tests in which significant deterioration of the whole group occurred.

Table 2. Percentage of CABG and PVD patients showing deterioration by >1 SD in neuropsychological scores after operation.

Test	CABG group at 7 days after operation	CABG group at 6 months after operation	PVD group at 7 days after operation
Trail making	21.5%	3.1%	4.2%
WMS information	10.7%	17.4%	0%
WMS orientation	10.4%	3.9%	0%
WMS mental control	32.6%	16.2%	10.4%
WMS memory passages	17.1%	10.4%	2.1%
WMS digits total	23.8%	16.6%	12.5%.
WMS visual reproduction	7.1%	5.4%	0%
WMS associate learning	35.6%	12.4%	6.3%
WAIS block design	8.4%	5.8%	0%
WAIS vocabulary	1.0%	0.4%	0%

impairment and 23 (10%) were considered to be overtly disabled by their intellectual dysfunction [33].

6.3. *Long-term intellectual dysfunction following CABG surgery*

Using the same battery of psychometric tests, 259 patients underwent repeat psychometric assessment at 6 months after CABG surgery [34]. The mean neuropsychological scores for the whole group remained unchanged or improved compared to preoperative scores for the majority of the 10 tests (Table 1). The percentage of patients showing deterioration by more than 1 SD on each subtest at 6 months ranges from 0.4 to 17.4% as shown in Table 2. Analysis of the test scores for individuals showed that 147/259 (57%) patients showed deterioration on at least one test score at 6 months. The degree of impairment was usually mild: 130/147 (88%) showed mild cognitive dysfunction (score deterioration on 1 or 2 tests), and only 17/147 (12%) had moderate or severe impairment (score deterioration on ≥3 tests). It was also apparent that detectable neuropsychological deterioration at 6 months often did not matter to the patient in functional terms. Seventy-one per cent of the patients whose scores were impaired had no significant symptoms; 27% had minor symptoms and only 2% were seriously disabled. Of the patients unemployed at 6 months in only one case was intellectual deterioration the factor preventing return to work.

6.4. *Early postoperative neuropsychological outcome in the peripheral vascular disease (PVD) control group*

The same neuropsychological methods were used to evaluate the surgical control group before and 7 days after operation [35]. The results for this group can be considered in the same 3 ways outlined above for the CABG patients. The test score changes are shown in Table 1. In none of the 10 tests did significant worsening of the PVD group as a whole occur after surgery. In 5 tests significant improvement was observed and in the other 5 no significant change was seen. This is in marked contrast to the early findings in the CABG group, where significant score deterioration occurred in 7 of the 10 tests. The percentage of control patients whose score deteriorated by greater than 1 SD for each test is shown in Table 2. The percentage of PVD patients deteriorating on individual subtests ranged from 0–12.5%. For each test the PVD group showed less impairment than the CABG group. Fifteen of the 48 (31%) PVD patients showed deterioration on one or more test scores, compared with 79% of the CABG group. Of these 15, 13 were impaired on one test only and 2 patients on 2 subtests. No patient in the surgical control group showed moderate or severe degrees of neuropsychological dysfunction (defined as impairment on 3 or more subtests). This is in contrast to the CABG group where 71/298 (24%) deteriorated on 3 or more tests. None of the 15 PVD patients with psychometric score deterioration had significant symptoms or disability.

6.5. *Risk factors associated with the development of neuropsychological complications in the CABG group*

We analysed 50 preoperative, intraoperative and postoperative factors with the aim of identifying predisposing factors for perioperative neuropsychological morbidity [36]. The data were analysed using the SPSSX package of the University of Newcastle Multiple Access computer. The 50 variables were analysed for significant association with neuropsychological outcome initially employing univariate analysis with the chi-square test (with Yates' correction where appropriate) for discrete variables and the Wilcoxon signed rank test for continuous variables. A multivariate analysis was then performed on those univariate factors found to be significant at the level of $p < 0.05$.

Table 3 shows those factors found to show an association with moderate and severe degrees of neuropsychological impairment. Several factors implying the presence of cerebrovascular or other extra-coronary vascular disease (history of cerebrovascular accident (CVA), history of transient ischaemic attack (TIA), peripheral vascular disease) showed significant correlation with the development of neuropsychological impairment. Postoperative hypotensive events and large decreases in haemoglobin level during

Table 3. Factors correlating with neuropsychological deterioration in CABG patients.

Neuropsychological impairment on ⩾3 tests (moderate)		Neuropsychological impairment on ⩾5 tests (severe)	
1. History of CVA	$p = 0.004$	1. Peripheral vascular disease	$p = 0.009$
2. History of TIA	$p = 0.01$	2. Haemoglobin drop during operation	$p = 0.004$
3. Diabetes	$p = 0.04$	3. Time in ITU after operation	$p = 0.004$
4. Significant postoperative hypotension (systolic BP <80 mm Hg for >5 min)	$p = 0.02$		

surgery, both of which may cause cerebral ischaemia, also appeared to be important predisposing factors. Diabetic patients were at greater risk of intellectual dysfunction. The increased time spent after surgery in the Intensive Therapy Unit by patients with severe neuropsychological impairment, is likely simply to reflect the fact that these patients had more complicated postoperative courses.

6.6. *Conclusions from the neuropsychological results of the Newcastle CABG study*

1. CABG surgery is associated with a high incidence of postoperative neuropsychological dysfunction. Seventy-nine per cent (235/298) of our patients showed deterioration in some aspect of cognitive function in the early postoperative period.
2. A high proportion of the early neuropsychological deterioration is asymptomatic. Only 30% of our patients with score deterioration had significant symptoms and 8% were overtly disabled by intellectual impairment in the early postoperative period.
3. Minor neuropsychological score impairment may persist at 6 months, but only 27% of patients with score deterioration are symptomatic and only 2% are seriously disabled by intellectual dysfunction.
4. Some deterioration in neuropsychological scores may occur as a nonspecific effect of major surgery. It would, however, seem reasonable to postulate that the greater frequency and severity of cognitive impairment in CABG compared to the PVD control patients, reflects a superimposed cerebral injury resulting specifically from cardiopulmonary bypass.
5. Several factors show an association with, and may predispose to, moderate and severe degrees of neuropsychological impairment including: extracoronary vascular disease, diabetes, a large decrease in haemoglobin level during surgery and postoperative hypotensive events.

Acknowledgements

I warmly thank Consultant Cardiothoracic Surgeons: Mr Blesovsky, Mr Hedley-Brown, Mr Hilton, Mr Holden and Mr Morritt; and Consultant Vascular Surgeons: Mr Chamberlain, Mr Dickinson, Mr McNeill, Mr Proud and Mr Taylor of the Royal Victoria Infirmary and Freeman Hospital, Newcastle upon Tyne, for kindly allowing me to study the patients under their care. Thanks are also due to Mr John Welch for advice on the neuropsychological test battery and Mrs Joyce French for help with statistics and computing.

References

1. Priest WS, Zaks MS, Yacorzynski GK, Boshes B: The neurologic, psychiatric and psychologic aspects of cardiac surgery. Med Clin North Am 1957;41:155-169.
2. Aberg T, Ronquist G, Tyden H, Ahlund P, Bergstrom K: Release of adenylate kinase into cerebrospinal fluid during open-heart surgery and its relation to postoperative intellectual function. Lancet 1982;1:1139-1142.
3. Savageau JA, Stanton BA, Jenkins CD, Klein MD: Neuropsychological dysfunction following elective cardiac operation. I Early assessment. J Thorac Cardiovasc Surg 1982;84:585-594.
4. Savageau JA, Stanton BA, Jenkins CD, Frater RWM: Neuropsychological dysfunction following elective cardiac operation. II A six-month reassessment. J Thorac Cardiovasc Surg 1982;84:595-600.
5. Ellis RJ, Wisniewski A, Potts R, Calhoun C, Loucks P, Wells MR: Reduction of flow rate and arterial pressure at moderate hypothermia does not result in cerebral dysfunction. J Thorac Cardiovasc Surg 1980;79:173-180.
6. Juolasmaa A, Outakoski J, Hirvenoja R, Tienari P, Sotamiemi K, Takkunen J: Effect of open-heart surgery on intellectual performance. J Clin Neuropsychol 1981;3:181-197.
7. Sotamiemi KA, Juolasmaa A, Hokkanen ET: Neuropsychologic outcome after open heart surgery. Arch Neurol 1981;38:2-8.
8. Hammeke TA, Hastings JE: Neuropsychological alterations after cardiac operation. J Thorac Cardiovasc Surg 1988;96:326-331.
9. Gilberstadt H, Sako Y: Intellectual and personality changes following open heart surgery. Arch Gen Psychiatry 1967;16:210-214.
10. Aberg T, Kihlgren M: Effect of open heart surgery on intellectual function. Scand J Thorac Cardiovasc Surg 1974;Suppl 15:1-63.
11. Plum F, Posner JB, Hain RF: Delayed neurological deterioration after anoxia. Arch Intern Med 1962;110:18-25.
12. Aberg T, Ahlund P, Kihlgren M: Intellectual function late after open heart operation. Ann Thorac Surg 1983;36:680-683.
13. Sotaniemi KA, Mononen H, Hokkanen TE: Long-term cerebral outcome after open heart surgery. A five-year neuropsychological follow-up study. Stroke 1986;17:410-416.
14. Tufo HM, Ostfeld AM, Shekelle R: Central nervous system dysfunction following open heart surgery. JAMA 1970;212:1333-1340.
15. Lee WH, Miller W, Rowe J, Hairston P, Brady MP: Effects of extracorporeal circulation on personality and cerebration. Ann Thorac Surg 1969;7:562-570.
16. Smith PL: The cerebral complications of coronary artery bypass surgery. Ann Roy Coll Surg Eng 1988;70:212-216.

17. Willner AE, Rabiner CJ, Wisoff BG, Hartstein M, Struve FA, Klein DF: Analogical reasoning and postoperative outcome. Arch Gen Psychiatry 1976;33:255–259.
18. Willner AE, Rabiner CJ, Wisoff BG *et al*: Analogy tests and psychopathology at follow-up after open heart surgery. Biol Psychiatry 1976;11:687–696.
19. Freeman AM, Folks DG, Sokol RS *et al.*: Cognitive function after coronary bypass surgery: effect of decreased cerebral blood flow. Am J Psychiatry 1985;142:110–112.
20. Gruvstad M, Kebbon L, Lof B: Changes in mental functions after induced hypotension. Acta Psychiatr Scand 1962;37:Suppl 163.
21. Raymond M, Conklin C, Schaeffer J, Newstadt G, Matloff JM, Gray RJ: Coping with transient intellectual dysfunction after coronary bypass surgery. Heart Lung 1984;13:531–539.
22. Smith PLC, Treasure T, Newman SP *et al.*: Cerebral consequences of cardiopulmonary bypass. Lancet 1986;i:823–825.
23. Townes BP, Bashein G, Hombein TF *et al*: Neurobehavioral outcomes in cardiac operations. J Thorac Cardiovasc Surg 1989;98:774–782.
24. Henriksen L.: Evidence suggestive of diffuse brain damage following cardiac operations. Lancet 1984;1:816–820.
25. Stockard JJ, Bickford RG, Schauble JF: Pressure-dependent cerebral ischemia during cardiopulmonary bypass. Neurology 1973;23:521–529.
26. Kolkka R, Hilberman M: Neurologic dysfunction following cardiac operation with low-flow, low-pressure cardiopulmonary bypass. J Thorac Cardiovasc Surg 1980;79:432–437.
27. Nevin M, Adams S, Colchester ACF, Pepper JR: Evidence for involvement of hypocapnia and hypoperfusion in aetiology of neurological deficit after cardiopulmonary bypass. Lancet 1987;ii:1493–1495.
28. Coffey CE, Massey W, Roberts KB, Curtis S, Jones RH, Pryor DB: Natural history of cerebral complications of coronary bypass graft surgery. Neurology 1983;33:1416–1421.
29. Folks DG, Freeman AM, Sokol RS, Govier AV, Reves JG, Baker DM: Cognitive dysfunction after coronary artery bypass surgery: A case-controlled study. South Med J 1988;81:202–206.
30. Breuer AC, Furlan AJ, Hanson MR *et al*: Central nervous system complications of coronary artery bypass graft surgery: prospective analysis of 421 patients. Stroke 1983;14:682–687.
31. Nevin M, Colchester ACF, Adams S, Pepper JR: Prediction of neurological damage after cardiopulmonary bypass surgery. Anaesthesia 1989;44:725–729.
32. Shaw PJ: Neurological and neuropsychological complications of coronary artery bypass graft surgery. MD Thesis, University of Newcastle upon Tyne 1987.
33. Shaw PJ, Bates D, Cartlidge NEF *et al.*: Early intellectual dysfunction following coronary bypass surgery. Quart J Med 1986;225:59–68.
34. Shaw PJ, Bates D, Cartlidge NEF *et al*: Long-term intellectual dysfunction following coronary artery bypass graft surgery: a six month follow-up study. Quart J Med 1987;239:259–268.
35. Shaw PJ, Bates D, Cartlidge NEF *et al*: Neurological and neuropsychological morbidity following major surgery: a comparison between coronary artery bypass and peripheral vascular surgery. Stroke 1987;18:700–707.
36. Shaw PJ, Bates D, Cartlidge NEF *et al*: An analysis of factors predisposing to neurological injury in patients undergoing coronary bypass operations. Quart J Med 1989;267:633–646.

14. Perceived and assessed cognitive function following coronary artery bypass surgery – mechanisms and intervention

STANTON NEWMAN

1. Introduction

Coronary artery bypass surgery has shown a dramatic increase in frequency in most industrialised societies. The reduction in mortality has led to an increased interest in morbidity. One area of morbidity is that of changes in cognition following surgery which are taken to reflect changes in brain function. This area of research utilises neuropsychological tests and has been performed for some time in cardiac surgery. Evaluation of this research over time is complicated by changes in surgical practice, different numbers and types of neuropsychological tests administered and the mode of analysis performed on the data [1]. Surgical practise has altered in a number of ways and is now further evolving in the light of data from neuropsychological studies. One index which reflects these changes is the duration of time on extracorporeal circulation (bypass time). In early studies long bypass times were recorded while in our own work a mean bypass time of approximately 85 minutes is common. The number of neuropsychological tests performed has varied considerable. Some studies report using one or two tests [2,3] while in our studies we have used ten tests which are described elsewhere [4–6]. It is important also, to place the form of neuropsychological assessment performed in the context of cardiac surgery into perspective. The design of all studies require adjustments to be made to accommodate the clinical environment. The resultant neuropsychological assessment involve a selection of tests and in no way represent a comprehensive assessment of neuropsychological functioning which would be difficult to perform without a considerable increase in the time required. As a result these do not offer a comprehensive understanding of the areas of cognition that will show changes but offer only limited information regarding the areas of deterioration and areas of preservation of function.

The manner in which data from these studies has been analysed has also varied. One technique has been to compare mean performance of groups (See for example Ref. [7]). As we have stated elsewhere this approach is

Paul J. Walter (ed.): *Quality of Life after Open Heart Surgery*, 155–165.

limited as it assumes deficits in all patients and denies the possibility of learning on neuropsychological tests. To take a hypothetical example, if approximately 20% of patients show some deterioration and approximately 60% show some learning effects with the remaining showing no change, then the overall trend will be towards some improvement. Group data analysis consequently fails to detect those patients with deficits and it is only by considering individual performance that the deficits may be detected. The analysis of the data of individual patients may take many forms. We have tended to approach the data analysis for incidence studies in a different manner from intervention studies. With incidence studies we wish to establish a figure of the percentage of patients showing deficits. This is arrived at by determining an index of deterioration in performance not seen in control subjects undergoing repeated testing. The amount of deterioration and the number of tests that are considered to reflect a deficit is essentially a conventional decision much like arriving at a figure of blood pressure that reflects hypertension or weight to height ratio as reflecting obesity. In our data we have defined a patient's performance on a test as showing a significant deterioration if a drop in performance greater than the standard deviation of all preoperative performances occurs. A subject is only considered to have a *neuropsychological deficit* if two or more tests show such a deterioration. We feel this is sufficiently conservative definition of deficit but it is important that the percentages ascribed to incidence studies are seen in the light of this being conventional in nature. With intervention studies one is not establishing the frequency of deficits but contrasting two forms of treatment. We have, in our intervention studies, compared change scores across the two or more conditions of the study in a variety of manners.

2. Incidence

We have performed a number of incidence studies, using the definition of neuropsychological deficit as outlined above, and have established the incidence of neuropsychological deficits in a group of patients who have undergone coronary artery bypass grafts over twelve months. This group consisted of 121 patients undergoing routine elective Coronary Anery Bypass Grafting.

Our data shows that 24% of patients show neuropsychological deficits 12 months after surgery and that these deficits are related to age and and the duration of bypass.

In order to establish that our incidence studies are in not peculiar to the environments where our studies are performed, we have conducted a collaborative study in the USA which has yielded a similar level of incidence with a similar battery of tests [8].

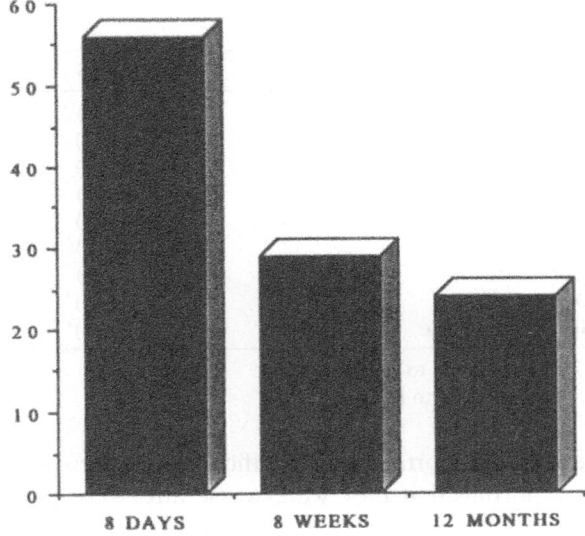

Figure 1. Percentage of patients with neuropsychological deficit after CABG.

3. Relationship to subjective complaints

Some surgeons became sensitised to the possibility of cognitive changes occurring in their patients when they heard patients complaining about cognitive changes following surgery. One question which this provokes is whether the patients that have been identified as demonstrating cognitive changes on neuropsychological tests are the same patients that report these changes. If this were the case the need for neuropsychological assessment as a technique of identifying patients with deficits would be unnecessary. In order to examine this we assessed a sample consisting of 62 coronary artery bypass surgery (CABS) patients (57 male and 5 female). The mean age for the male group was 55.2 (sd = 7.8) and the mean age for the female group was 54.4 (sd = 8.8) with a range of between 44 and 65.

The neuropsychological tests previously described were administered as well as two mood state measures. State anxiety was assessed by the Spielberger state 40 item inventory (STAI) [9] and depression was assessed by the Beck Depression Inventory (BDI) [10]. In addition to these measures patients were also given a semi-structured interview which included nine questions on perceived cognitive changes to which patients indicated whether the particular aspect of cognitive functioning had improved, deteriorated or shown no change from before surgery.

The patients' responses to the nine item questionnaire on perceived cognitive functioning are shown in Table 1. The data from the self reported changes have been collapsed into 'improved' and 'no change' versus 'worse'.

Table 1. Number of patients reporting reduced cognitive abilities
following CABS

	%	(No.)
1. Memory	27.4	(17)
2. Problem solving	17.7	(11)
3. Clarity of thinking	16.1	(10)
4. Concentration	16.1	(10)
5. Making mistakes	14.5	(9)
6. Attention	12.9	(8)[+]
7. Clumsiness	9.7	(6)
8. Decision making	8.1	(5)[+]
9. Speed of response	6.5	(4)*

* = 2 patients failed to respond.
[+] = 1 patient failed to respond.

The most frequently reported area of difficulty with these patients is memory, with 28% reporting that they were worse after surgery (see Table 1). Problem solving (18%) is the next most common cognitive complaint followed by clarity of thinking (16%) and concentration (16%).

The relationship between the subjective reports and neuropsychological assessment were examined by analysing whether the group who perceived a deterioration in an area of cognition showed a greater deterioration in tests measuring that function. For example complaints of a deterioration in memory were examined on the Rey AVLT and the two Non-Verbal memory Tests. The group reporting a deterioration in performance produced scores that were no different on any of the assessed cognitive measures to those reporting no change or an improvement in cognition. To ensure that reports did not reflect an absolute performance a comparison between those reporting a deterioration and those not reporting a deterioration was made on the absolute performance on the neuropsychological tests at twelve months. No differences were found between the groups on this measure. We conclude that subjective reports are unrelated to changes in cognition after CABS or the absolute performance at the time of reporting on cognition.

To investigate what factors determine the subjective complaints reported by some individuals we examined the relationship between subjective complaints and mood state. The relationship between the areas of cognition assessed by the questionnaire and depression as measured on the Beck Depression Inventory is shown in Figures 2 and 3.

In all cases the score on the Beck Depression Inventory was higher for those who considered their cognition had deteriorated. In all but three cases the differences were highly significant. The differences between the groups were similar for measures of anxiety with the group reporting a deterioration in cognition tending to have higher scores on the Spielberger State Anxiety measure [11,12]

These data suggest that complaints regarding cognition after cardiac surg-

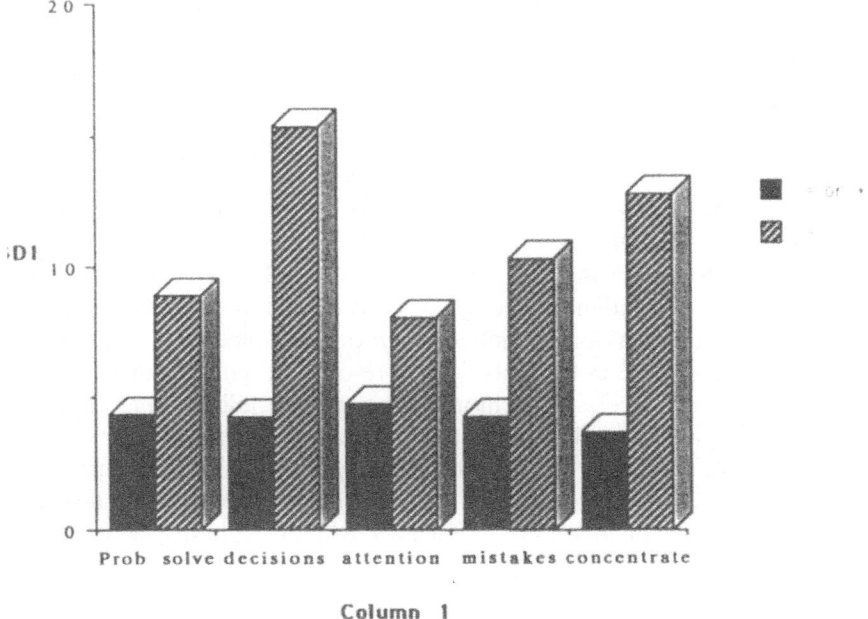

Figure 2. Levels of depression and self reports of cognition after CABS–1.

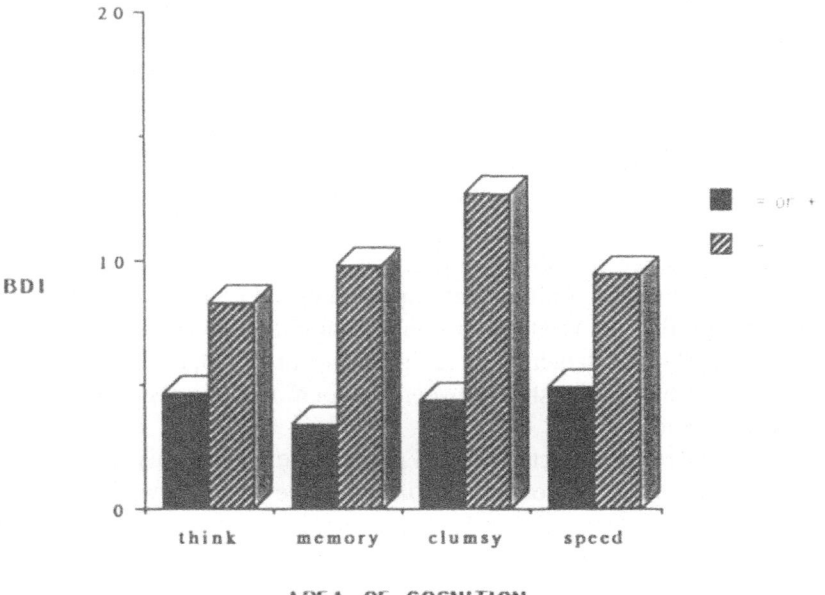

Figure 3. Levels of depression and self reports of cognition after CABS–2.

ery are not an accurate reflection of actual cognitive performance and appear to be influenced by mood state. The mechanism by which patients with low mood report cognitive deficits after surgery in the absence of assessed deterioration in cognition may be related to other research on the influence of mood on memory and judgment [13]. Studies that have examined judgments of health status, which involve both memory (saliency of symptoms) and a judgment (appraisal of health status), and experimental manipulations have shown that an induced mood leads to perceptions of health status concurrent with mood state [14]. In the case of CABS the patients who had low mood may have had increased accessibility to their memories of everyday normal failures of cognition and judged their performance as having deteriorated. In contrast those individuals who were of more positive mood did not have any increase access to memories of cognitive failures and thus considered their cognition to be adequate. The magnification of minor events is consistent with cognitive theories of depression where the evaluation of reality is distorted by the individual [10,15]. Thus the more depressed individual may also have magnified the importance of their cognitive failures.

4. Mechanism of damage

The main contenders as the mechanism causing the neuropsychological deficits observed in patients undergoing CABS are microemboli (particulate and/or air) and/or perfusion related damage as a result of extracorporeal circulation. To give an example of the nature of our studies that have attempted to determine whether a relationship exists between a particular measure and neuropsychology I report on our study investigating microemboli below. We have reported elsewhere on our studies that have investigated rCBF, EEG changes and investigations of the microvasculature by means of retinal fluorescein angiography in relation to neuropsychological changes [16–18].

The study had two main aims. Firstly to investigate whether a 40 micron filter on the arterial line reduced neuropsychological deficits and secondly to attempt to quantify and relate the frequency of microemboli to the incidence of neuropsychological deficits. For the purposes of this chapter the emphasis is placed upon the relationship between microembolic events and neuropsychological outcome.

One hundred routine elective CABS patients were randomised to the filter or non filter condition. Following evaluation in the laboratory a Transcranial Doppler (TC2-64 EME) was used during surgery to detect high amplitude flow disturbances during the course of surgery [19]. As we were unable to discriminate between 30 and 200 microns in the laboratory, we defined a microembolic event as each flow disturbance. Microembolic events were

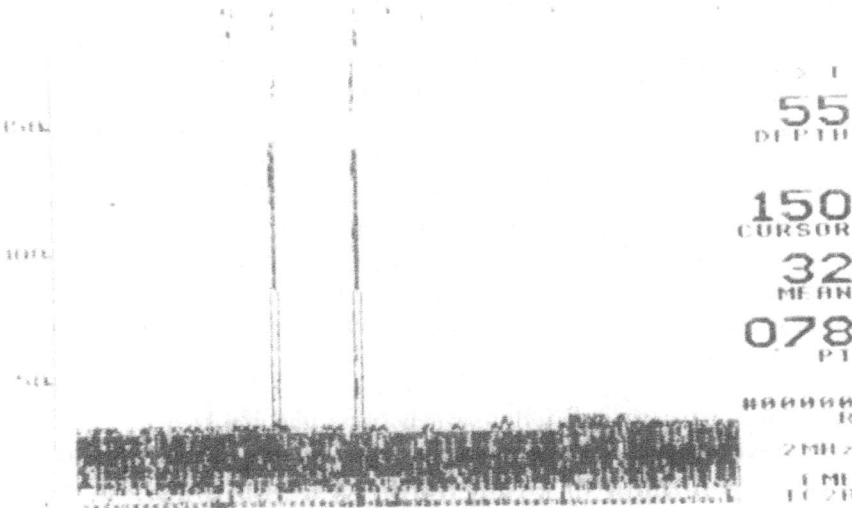

Figure 4. Transcranial Doppler output indicating microemboli during cardiac surgery.

particularly in evidence at the time of cannnulation and at the inception of bypass and were also signficantly more frequent in non filtered patients [20–22]. An example of the output on the transcranial doppler showing microemboli in surgery is shown in Figure 4.

An examination of the frequency of microembolic events in relation to neuropsychological outcome can be seen in Table 2. This table demonstrates that the deficits on the neuropsychological battery used in our studies are related to the frequency of microembolic events occurring in surgery as detected by assessing flow disturbances in the transcranial doppler.

Table 2. The relationship between neuropsychological outcome 8 weeks after surgery and the number of microembolic events in surgery

MEE count during cardiopulmonary bypass	No patients	No with deficit	% deficit
<200	58	5	9%
201–500	13	3	23%
501–1000	16	5	31%
>1000	7	3	43%

5. Interventions

We have performed a number of intervention studies including comparisons between arterial line filter and non-filter groups as mentioned above [21,22]. In a recent study performed by the brain research groups of University College & Middlesex School of Medicine and the Royal Postgraduate Medical School, Hammersmith Hospital we investigated the impact on neuropsychology of different forms of oxygenation. One hundred routine elective CABS patients were entered into the the study and randomly assigned to two conditions. One group had surgery performed using a Harvey H 1700 bubble oxygenator while the other group received a Cobe CML flat sheet membrane oxygenator. As in all our studies, the anaesthetic technique and surgical techniques were conducted in as standard a manner as possible. In this study all patients had a 40 micron arterial line filter. The mean age of the patients was 56 years and the mean bypass time was 88.2 minutes. There were no age or bypass time differences between the groups

Neuropsychological assessment was performed preoperatively and at 8 days and 8 weeks postoperatively. In addition all patients received a number retinal fluorescein angiograms during surgery.

I report here some selective preliminary results of this research to illustrate the findings and the nature of the intervention studies that we perform. The retinal angiograms performed 5 minutes prior to the discontinuation of bypass were compared to the measures performed prior to bypass by both a semiautomatic and an automatic analysis to detect the number and area of microvascular changes [23]. Both of these techniques indicated a larger area of involvement in patients who had surgery with the bubble oxygenator [18,24].

On the neuropsychological assessment, an analysis was performed on the number of patients producing a deficit, as defined above, on each of the tests. The 8 days assessments indicated no differences between the two conditions. At the time of the 8 week assessments the bubble oxygenator group had more subjects with deficits in 80% of the tests. Not all of these were statistically significant, due largely to small numbers. An illustration of these findings is shown in Figure 5. This indicates the performance of the two groups on the tests of memory.

We conclude from this study that flat sheet membrane oxygentors afford better protection to the brain that do bubble oxygenators.

6. General conclusions

Our research has indicated that neuropsychological deficits are apparent and do persist following CABS. We feel that the neuropsychological battery, we

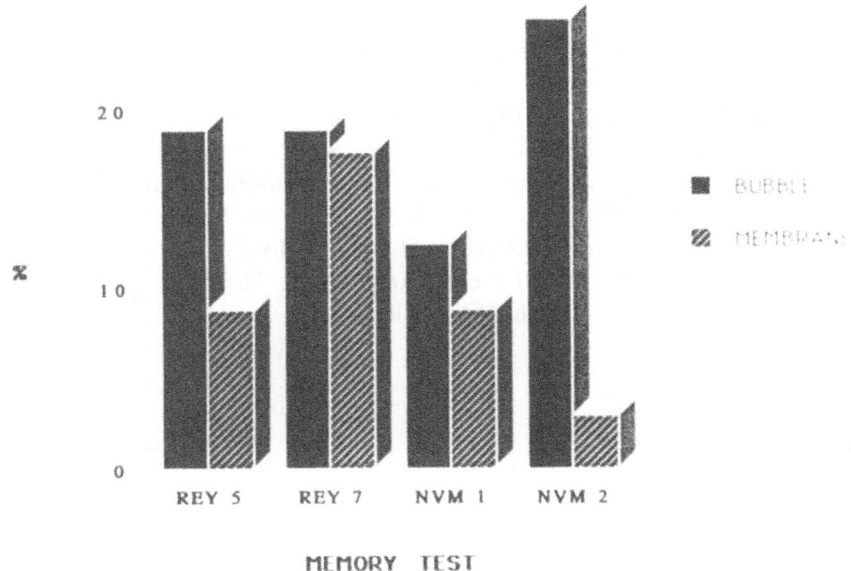

Figure 5. Percentage of patients with deficits on memory tests 8 weeks after CABS – bubble vs membrane oxygenators.

specifically designed to assess changes in cognition following cardiac surgery, is a sensitive tool for assessing these changes. Care needs to be taken in the mode of statistical analysis applied to the data as well as the design of the studies. Furthermore the neuropsychological changes that are detected by formal assessment are not accurately reported by patients and complaints of changes in cognition following CABS appear to be underpinned by levels of depressed mood and anxiety.

Our current attention, which has been illustrated by two studies above, has focussed on two issues. Firstly we are attempting to determine the relationship between mechanisms which may bring about the neuropsychological changes observed. Secondly we are examining modes of intervention to reduce the frequency of neuropsychological disturbance following CABS. The neuropsychological tests we have performed appear to be directly related to the number of microembolic events in CABS. Furthermore, the use of a 40 micron filter on the arterial line reduces the incidence of neuropsychological deficits as does the use of a membrane as opposed to a bubble oxygenator. We are currently investigating other forms of intervention in order to suggest further techniques to reduce the incidence of neuropsychological deficits in CABS.

Acknowledgements

The work reported in this chapter involved the combined efforts of the Brain Research Groups of University College & Middlesex School of Medicine and the Royal Postgraduate Medical School, Hammersmith Hospital. Individuals particularly involved in the studies above are Mr Peter Smith, Mr Graham Venn, Mr Wilf Pugsley, Mr Tom Treasure, Mr Chistopher Blauth, Prof Ken Taylor, Prof Michael Harrison, Mr John Amold, Ms Louise Klinger, Ms Istra Toner & Ms Frances Siddons. I would also like to acknowledge the financial support of the British Heart Foundation, The Medical Research Council and the Sir Jules Thorn Charitable Trust.

References

1. Newman S: The incidence and nature of neuropsychological morbidity following cardiac surgery. Perfusion 1989;4:93–100.
2. Savageau JA, Stanton B, Jenkins CD, Klein MD: Neuropsychological dysfunction following elective cardiac operation. 1 Early assessment. J Thorac Cardiovasc Surg 1982a;84:585–594.
3. Savageau JA, Stanton B, Jenkins CD, Fraser RWM: Neuropsychological dysfunction following elective cardiac operation. 11 A six month reassessment. J Thorac Cardiovasc Surg 1982b;84:595–600.
4. Smith P, Treasure T, Newman S, Joseph P, Ell P, Harrison M: Cerebral consequences of cardiopulmonary bypass. Lancet 1986;1:823–825.
5. Newman SP, Smith P, Treasure T, Joseph P, Ell P, Harrison M: Acute neuropsychological consequences of coronary artery bypass surgery. Curr Psych Res Rev 1987;6:115–124.
6. Newman S, Klinger, L, Venn G, Smith P, Harrison M, Treasure T: The persistance of neuropyschological deficits 12 months after coronary artery bypass surgery. In: Wilner A, Rodewald G (eds) Impact of Cardiac Surgery on the Quality of Life: Neurological and Psychological Aspects. Plenum Press, 1991.
7. Klonoff H, Clark C, Kavanagh-Grey D, Mizgala H, Munro I: Two-year follow-up study of coronary bypass surgery. J Thorac Cardiovasc Surg 1989;97:77–85.
8. Stump D, Newman S, Coker L, Phipps J, Miller C: Persistence of Neuropsychological Deficits following CABG. Anaesthesiology 1990;73:A113.
9. Spielberger C: Test Anxiety Inventory. Palo Alto: Consulting Psychologists Press, 1980.
10. Beck AT: Depression: Clinical, Experimental and Theoretical Aspects. New York: Harper, 1967.
11. Newman S, Klinger L, Venn G, Smith P, Harrison M, Treasure T: Subjective reports of cognition in relation to assessed cognitive performance following coronary artery bypass surgery. J Psychosomatic Res 1989;33:227–233.
12. Newman S, Klinger L, Venn G, Smith P, Harrison M, Treasure T: Reports of cognitive change, mood state and assessed cognition following coronary artery bypass surgery. In: Wilner A, Rodewald G (eds.) Impact of Cardiac Surgery on the Quality of Life: Neurological and Psychological Aspects. Plenum Press, 1991.
13. Isen AM: Toward understanding the role of affect in cognition. In: Wyer RS, Scrull TK (eds) Handbook of Social Cognition, Vol. 3. New Jersey: Lawrence Erlbaum, 1984:179–236.

14. Croyle RT, Uretsky MB: Effects of mood on self-appraisal of health status. Health Psychol 1987;6:239–253.
15. Ingram RE, Hollon SD: Cognitive therapy of depression from an information processing perspective. In: Ingram RE (ed.) Information Processing Approaches to Clinical Psychology. New York: Academic Press, 1986:259–281.
16. Venn G, Sherry K, Treasure T, Newman S, Harrison M, Klinger L: Cerebral blood flow during cardiopulmonary bypass. Eur J Cardiothoracic Surg 1988;2:360–363,
17. Venn G, Sherry K, Treasure T, Newman S, Harrison M, Klinger L: Clinical implications of cerebral blood flow changes during cardiopulmonary bypass. Perfusion 1988;3:271–280.
18. Blauth C, Smith P, Newman S, et al: Retinal microembolisation and neuropsychological deficit following clinical cardiopulmonary bypass: comparison of a membrane and a bubble oxygenator. Eur J Cardiothoracic Surg 1989;3:135–139.
19. Padayachee TS, Parsons S, Theobald et al: Computerised techniques for detecting gaseous microemboli in blood using pulsed Doppler ultrasound. Perfusion 1987;2:213–218.
20. Pugsley W: The use of Doppler ultrasound in the assessment of microemboli during cardiac surgery. Perfusion 1989;4:115–122.
21. Pugsley W, Treasure T, Klinger L, Newman S, Pascalis C, Harrison M: Microemboli and cerebral impairment during cardiac surgery. Vasc Surg 1990;24:34–43.
22. Treasure T, Pugsley W, Klinger L, Paschalis C, Aspey B, Harrison M, Newman S: Arterial Line Filtration reduces microembolism and significantly improves neuropsychological outcome in coronary artery surgery. In: Wilner A, Rodewald G (eds) Impact of Cardiac Surgery on the Quality of Life: Neurological and Psychological Aspects. Plenum Press, 1991.
23. Jagoe JR, Blauth CI, Smith PL, Arnold JV, Taylor KM, Wooten R: Quantification of retinal damage during cardiopulmonary bypass: Comparison of computer and human assessment. Proc IEE 1990;137 Part 1(3):170–175.
24. Smith P, Blauth C, Newman S, Arnold J, Siddons F, Taylor K: Cerebral microembolism and neuropsychological outcome following coronary artery bypass surgery (CABS) with either a membrane or bubble oxygenator. In: Wilner A, Rodewald G (eds) Impact of Cardiac Surgery on the Quality of Life: Neurological and Psychological Aspects. Plenum Press, 1991.

C: Emotional State

15. Psychological status of patients before and after coronary bypass surgery

H. BOUDREZ, J. DENOLLET, B.J. AMSEL, G. DE BACKER, P.J. WALTER, J. DE BEULE and R. MOHAN

1. Introduction

During the past two decades coronary artery bypass surgery (CABG) has become a widespread therapeutic tool in the management of coronary artery disease. Extensive scientific research has been performed leading to considerable technical mastery of the procedure and refinement of the selection criteria. As a result the number of patients undergoing CABG has gradually increased. A few controlled trials have been undertaken to evaluate the results of CABG [1–4]. In these studies the overall survival rates improved in favour of surgical patients, provided they responded to a specific range of criteria. The level of angina decreased markedly after surgery. However, chest pain recurred in a large number of patients within seven years. The main end-points in these trials were mortality and morbidity. However, undergoing cardiac surgery implies a life-threatening situation for most patients and their families. Some patients fail to adapt and do not function well psychologically. Increased presurgical anxiety and depression have already been noted by several authors [5,6] even beyond the level of clinical psychological dysfunction.

Although psychological and psychosocial aspects of CABG play an important role in the interpretation of the effects of the intervention, these elements (with the exception of resumption of work) have been studied in less detail than somatic functioning and survival. Moreover, such data have not been available for Belgium. Therefore a joint research project was set up in the University Hospital in Antwerp (Department of Cardiac Surgery) and in the University Hospital in Ghent (Department of Cardiac Rehabilitation). The main objectives of the project were to measure the presurgical psychological situation, the evolution of psychological and other quality-of-life-parameters and to detect and isolate factors that could predict postsurgical well-being.

This article reports on the methods and the initial results concerning the presurgical psychological situation compared with the situation 4 months after surgery.

Paul J. Walter (ed.): Quality of Life after Open Heart Surgery, 169–176.
© 1992 Kluwer Academic Publishers.

2. Methods

Patients were asked to answer several questionnaires at four points in time. The first moment was scheduled several days before surgery, at hospital admission; the second moment was scheduled 3–5 weeks after surgery; the third 4 months after surgery and the last, one year after surgery.

Different questionnaires were used

- SCL-90 (Symptom Check List) [7] measures anxiety, agoraphobia, depression, somatic complaints, cognitive insufficiency, sensitivity, hostility, sleep disturbances. All answers lead to a concluding total score, indicating psychoneuticism.
- The ZBV (Zelf Beoordelings Vragenlijst) [8] is a translation and adaptation of the state-trait anxiety scale, developed by Spielberger (STAI).
- The MPVH (Medisch Psychologische Vragenlijst voor Hartpatienten) [9] is a Dutch scale, measuring subjective well-being, incapacitation, dysphoria, and social inhibition.
- The Marlowe–Crowne Scale measures social desirability as a trait variable. It offers relevant opportunities in combination with anxiety-scores [10].
- A Dutch version of the JAS (Jenkins Activity Survey) was used to measure type-A behaviour.
- The MV (Maastrichtse Vragenlijst) [12,13] provides a measure of vital exhaustion. In prospective epidemiologic research the scale has proven to predict myocardial infarction in a significant way.
- The MBHI (Millon Behavioral Health Inventory) [14] is a rather extensive scale measuring eight coping styles, six psychogenic attitudes, three psychosomatic correlates and three prognostic indices.
- Self-composed questions measured patients' surgical expectations (by means of a visual analogue scale), his social situation (job, civil state, education), his degree of social participation in cultural activities or in leisure time activities and the frequency of contacts with friends and family members.
- Medical data were collected by studying the medical records.

All variables can be categorized as state-variables on the one hand and as trait-variables on the other. Computation of statistical significance was executed by means of the chi-square test, and the paired t-test. Factor analysis and multiple regression analysis were also used.

3. Results

3.1. *Socio-demographic variables*

A group of 330 patients, 284 men and 46 women, 185 German and 145

Table 1. Presurgical psychological data (mean values and sd).

		Men	Women	Total	p
Wellbeing	m	21.7	18.2	21.2	0.003
	sd	7.2	5.8	7.1	
Dysphoria	m	18.0	18.9	18.1	0.24
	sd	4.7	5.3	4.8	
Psychoneur.	m	132.9	150.2	135.4	0.001
	sd	32.2	40.4	33.9	
Depression	m	24.0	28.7	24.7	0.000
	sd	6.5	10.0	7.3	
Anxiety	m	15.5	18.7	15.9	0.000
	sd	4.9	7.3	5.4	
Vit. Exh.	m	7.1	9.6	7.4	0.001
	sd	3.5	2.8	3.5	

Belgian patients undergoing a first CABG, were selected, with a mean age of 59.1 years. Women were significantly older then men, 62.9 versus 59.1 years, respectively. More than 80% (276/330) were married. Most patients were on sick leave (116/330) or retired (156/330). Only 32/330 patients were still working before surgery. The majority of patients (231/330) had only lower education (to the age of 15), only 31/330 had a higher degree (university or higher education). The remainder of the patients followed education to the age of 18.

3.2. *Preoperative data* (Table 1)

A factor analysis of all presurgical psychological state-variables resulted in a data reduction. The single variables with high loadings on each factor were then chosen.

Compared to a group of patients after myocardial infarction [9], subjective well-being and dysphoria reach a moderate mean score. However, some 10–20 percent of all patients score in a clinically dysfunctional way. Results for psychoneuroticism, anxiety and vital exhaustion must be categorised as high, related to a normal population and as low, related to a psychiatric population [7]. Furthermore, 25% of the patients exhibit anxiety scores that, on a clinical-psychological basis, must be interpreted as deficient, based on the same reference groups. Remarkably, statistically and clinically significant differences between men and women can be noted in all variables, excepted dysphoria. These differences are not only statistically significant, they also have clinical relevance. Women feel subjectively worse than men, and score worse on psychoneuroticism, depression, anxiety and vital exhaustion.

Table 2. Psychological evolution pre-CABG – 4 months post-CABG.

	Pre		Post		
	m	sd	m	sd	p
Subj. well-being	21.3	7.3	28.6	7.3	0.000
Dysphoria	18.2	4.8	15.6	4.8	0.000
Psychoneurot.	136.2	35.5	130.1	31.9	0.04
Depression	24.9	7.8	23.2	7.1	0.01
Anxiety	15.9	5.5	14.3	4.5	0.001
Vital exhaustion	7.5	3.5	6.6	3.8	0.009

3.3. *Psychological evolution pre-CABG – 4 months post-CABG* (Table 2)

All variables listed in Table 2 show a significant amelioration for the study group as a whole. In most instances this amelioration is extremely pronounced, as this is the case with subjective well-being, dysphoria, anxiety and vital exhaustion.

The remarkable presurgical differences between male and female patients have completely disappeared 4 months after surgery (Table 3). Moreover women tend to exhibit more favourable scores on all variables than men. The difference even reaches statistical significance for psychoneuroticism, men exhibiting more psychoneuroticism than women at 4 months postoperatively. This means that the female psychological evolution to a more favourable pattern in that time interval is much more pronounced than the evolution of male patients. The evolution of all listed variables in women reach statist-

Table 3. Psychological evolution pre – post-CABG.

		Men			Women			
		pre	post	p	pre	post	p	p*
Well-being	m	21.7	28.4	0.00	18.7	30.1	0.00	0.17
	sd	7.5	7.6		5.8	4.4		
Dysphoria	m	18.0	15.8	0.01	19.1	15.0	0.00	0.37
	sd	4.8	4.9		5.2	4.1		
Psychoneur.	m	133.5	131.8	0.62	153.1	119.8	0.00	0.04
	sd	33.2	33.0		44.2	21.5		
Depression	m	24.1	23.6	0.43	29.9	21.2	0.00	0.07
	sd	6.8	7.3		10.9	5.0		
Anxiety	m	15.4	14.5	0.69	19.3	13.1	0.00	0.10
	sd	4.7	4.6		8.1	3.9		
Vital Exh.	m	7.1	6.7	0.74	9.7	6.0	0.00	0.20
	sd	3.6	3.9		3.0	3.3		

p* = the p-value concerning the score-differences of men and women 4 months after CABG ("post").

Table 4. Multiple regression analysis.

Dependent variable	Predictive variables
Psycho-neuroticism (SCL-90) R^2 0.26	– postsurgical pain during sex and during emotions – MBHI-cardiovascular tendency.
Subjective Well-being (MPVH-W scale) R^2 0.17	– postsurgical activity (biking) – postsurgical pain in cold temperature
Anxiety (SCL-90) R^2 0.24	– performance of postsurgical activity (biking) – cardiac pain during biking – MBHI-gastro-intestinal susceptibility

ical and clinical significance, while in male patients only the evolution for subjective well-being and dysphoria is statistically significant (Table 3).

However, although a considerable positive psychological evolution can be observed, some 10–20% of all patients, four months after surgery, exhibit psychological states that must be interpreted as clinically dysfunctional.

3.4. *Prediction of the postsurgical psychological situation*

A multiple regression analysis was set up in order to detect variables that could predict the postsurgical psychological state. In order to choose the dependent variables in that multiple regression analysis a factor analysis was first executed, resulting in three separate factors. The single variables with the highest factor loading were finally selected. These variables were: psychoneuroticism (SCL-90), subjective well-being (MPVH) and anxiety (SCL-90). A multiple regression analysis was executed in stages, composed of several groups of variables that were entered into the analysis: socioeconomic variables, medical variables, psychological state-variables, psychological trait variables, presurgical activities, presurgical pain during these activities, expected postsurgical activities, expected postsurgical pain during these activities, postsurgical activities performed and postsurgical pain experienced.

All significant variables on each of these stages were then entered in a final analysis with a stepwise selection of the variables. The results of this method resulted in the findings, summarized in Table 4. that indicates the independent variables with predictive power.

The variable psychoneuroticism was significantly predicted by postsurgical pain during sexual activities and emotions and by the cardiovascular tendency variable of the Millon Behavioral Health Inventory. All correlations were positive. Subjective well-being was positively predicted by the capability to perform postsurgical activities like cycling and negatively by experiencing pain in cold temperatures. Postsurgical anxiety was positively predicted by the performance of postsurgical activities like cycling, negatively by cardiac pain during cycling and also negatively by the gastrotintestinal susceptibility variable of the MBHI.

No other presurgical variables, whether medical, social or psychological, could predict the psychological status four months after the surgical intervention.

4. Discussion

The results of a presurgical inquiry were analysed and compared with those four months after the operation. The study group consisted of 284 males and 46 females, selected before a first CABG surgery. The mean age was 59 years. The pre-surgical mean scores on psychological variables must be considered as moderate, compared to a reference group of patients after myocardial infarction, as high compared to a group of normal people, and as low compared to a psychiatric population. Although the mean scores on presurgical psychological state-variables are to be considered as moderate, some 10–20% of patients (or even 25% in the case of anxiety) exhibit scores that go beyond the level of normal psychological functioning.

This finding is comparable to the results of other research [5,15,16], that also observed clinically relevant psychological reactions before surgical intervention. Considerable presurgical differences in most psychological state-variables can be noted between male and female patients, the latter scoring in a much more dysfunctional way. These differences do not only reach statistical but also clinical significance.

All psychological state-scores ameliorate over the time interval studied (pre-operatively vs four months after surgery): patients' subjective well-being increases while depression, anxiety, dysphoria, and psychoneuroticism decrease. However, 10–20% of patients still exhibit dysfunctional psychological states postoperatively. These findings confirm the results from other research [15–18].

The observed presurgical differences between men and women have all disappeared after four months. Moreover, women tend to score in a more favourable way than male patients, contradicting the findings of Zyzanski [19], who observed postsurgically more negative emotions in women than in men. For psychoneuroticism this trend even reaches statistical significance.

Multiple regression analysis revealed only two presurgical variables, cardiovascular tendency (MBHI), and gastro-intestinal susceptibility (MBHI), that can partly explain the variance in three postsurgical factors.

Other presurgical variables, neither medical, social nor psychological could predict the psychological status four months after the surgical intervention. On the contrary, postsurgical performance of activities without cardiac pain explains a great deal of the variance in the regression analysis.

It seems appropriate to stress a few consequences in order to optimize the guidance of CABG patients:

- 10–20% or even more (in the case of anxiety) score presurgically in a psychological dysfunctional way. Identification of those patients can possibly elicit intervention towards them.
- The same remark can be applied to the female subgroup.
- Predictive power can partly be observed in presurgical variables (cardiovascular tendency and trait anxiety), that easily can be screened in a presurgical contact.
- It also seems appropriate to remain alert in order to identify postoperatively those patients (also 10–20%) with a dysfunctional psychological status.

5. Summary

A prospective study has been executed in two University Hospitals in order to evaluate the evolution of some psychosocial aspects in patientes undergoing coronary artery bypass surgery (CABG). For this reason 330 patients (185 German and 145 Belgian patients; 284 men and 46 women) were selected for participation. Several existing measurement scales were used, completed by questionnaires that were composed in light of this inquiry.

Measurement took place at four points in time, ranging from the presurgical situation till one year postoperatively. This article reports results comparing the presurgical situation with that four months after surgery.

Important improvement in psychological well-being can be noted in most patients. However a minority of them still show unfavourable psychological reactions. Furthermore, initial differences between male and female patients have all disappeared after four months. It seems appropriate to identify those patients with unfavourable psychological reactions, as well presurgically as postsurgically, in order to increase psychological well-being and quality of life aspects.

Acknowledgement

This study was supported by Grant No. 3.0007.86N from the National Fund for Scientific Research.

References

1. CASS Principal Investigators and their associates: Coronary-artery surgery study (CASS):A randomized trial of coronary artery bypass surgery. Quality of life in patients randomly assigned to treatment groups. Circulation 1983;5:951–960.
2. CASS Principal Investigators and their associates: Myocardial infarction and mortality in the coronary artery surgery study (CASS) Randomized trial. New Engl J Med 1984;12:750–758.
3. Veterans Administration: Eleven-year survival in the Veterans Administration randomized trial of coronary bypass surgery for stable angina. New Engl J Med 1984;21:1333–1339.
4. European CSSG: Long-term results of prospective-randomised study of coronary artery bypass surgery in stable-angina. Lancet 1982;1174–1180.
5. Klonoff H, Campbell C, Kavanagh-Gray D, Mizgala H, Munro I: Two-year follow-up study of coronary bypass surgery. J Thorac Cardiovasc Surg 1989;97:78–85.
6. Matthews A, Ridgeway V: Personality and surgical recovery: a review. Brit J Clin Psych 1981;20:243–260.
7. Arrindell WA, Ettema JHM: Handleiding bij een multidimensionele psychopathologieindicator. Swets and Zeitlinger 1986;40 pp.
8. Van Der Ploeg HM, Defares PB, Spielberger CD: Handleiding bij de zelf-beoordelings vragenlijst. Swets and Zeitlinger 1980;35 pp.
9. Erdman RAM: Medisch-psychologische vragenlijst voor hartpatienten. Swets and Zeitlinger 1982;16 pp.
10. Shaw RE, Cohen F, Fishman-Rosen J, Murphy MC, Stertzer SH: Psychological predictors of psychological and medical outcomes in patients undergoing coronary angioplasty. Psychosom Med 1986;8:582–597.
11. Appels A: Jenkins activity survey. Swets and Zeitlinger 1985;47 pp.
12. Appels A, Hoppener P, Mulder P: A questionnaire to assess premonitory symptoms of myocardial infarction. Int J Cardiology 1987;17:15–24.
13. Appels A, Mulder P: Excess fatigue as a precursor of myocardial infarction. Eur Soc Cardiology 1988;9:758–764.
14. Green CJ, Millon TH, Meacher RB: The MBHI: Its utilization in assessment and management of the coronary bypass surgery patient. Psychother Psychosom 1983;39:112–121.
15. Jenkins CD, Stanton BA: Quality of life assessed in the recovery study. in: Assessment of qualilty of life in clinical trials of cardiovascular therapies, Le Jacq Publishing Inc., USA, 1984;266–280.
16. Langeluddecke P, Fulcher G, Hughes C, Tennant C: A prospective evaluation of the psychosocial effects of coronary artery bypass surgery. J Psychosom Res 1989;1:37–45.
17. Magni G, Unger HP, Valfre C, Polesel E, Cesari F: Psychosocial outcome one year after heart surgery. Arch Intern Med 1987;147:473–477.
18. Mayou R, Bryant B: Quality of life after coronary artery surgery. Q J Med, New Series 1987;239:239–248
19. Zyzanski St J, Stanton BA, Jenkins CD, Klein MD: Medical and psychosocial outcomes in survivors of major heart surgery. J Psychosom Res 1981;3:213–221.

16. The emotional state of patients after coronary bypass surgery

ELIZABETH LORNA CAY and AINE O'ROURKE

Introduction

For more than a decade coronary artery bypass graft surgery has increasingly become an accepted method of treatment of the patient with intractable angina. More recently early revascularisation has been used to prevent damage to the threatened myocardium. Early on, it became obvious that the physical results were excellent but unexpectedly there was little or no functional improvement in many patients following an apparently successful operation. Studies have demonstrated that the quality of life remains poor in 25–40% of patients [1–3]. Many psychological, social, economic and personality factors have been shown to contribute to a poor outcome; important among these non-cardiac causes is the emotional state of the patient.

2. Emotional reaction after surgery

There are strong emotional reactions after surgery. Two-thirds of a surgically treated group reported symptoms of anxiety, depression, confusion and feelings of irritability in the early weeks after operation [4]. Subsequently there is considerable psychological adjustment with the majority of studies reporting a decrease in levels of anxiety and depression though these symptoms, if untreated, persist in one third [2] and are severe in 14–18% of patients [5,6]. Little is known of the emotional reactions of women to their operations but what evidence there is suggests that they are more disturbed than men [3]. Denial of illness and the operation are frequent in patients with a short history of angina who have emergency surgery as a preventive measure; like the patient after myocardial infarction they have little time to adjust and during early convalescence may react aggressively or become depressed, as they become aware of the implications of the disease. There is no correlation between the success of the operation as assessed by the surgeon and the patient's emotional distress or the quality of life [7].

Paul J. Walter (ed.): Quality of Life after Open Heart Surgery, 177–183.

Table 1. Emotional response and level of exercise at end of programme ($n = 28$).

SAD category	Mean watts attained*
Normal	149.5
Depressed	90.5
Anxious	110.9
Anxious and depressed	90.8

* F ratio = 5.1; $p < 0.01$.

3. The effect of emotional factors on outcome

Patients who remain anxious or depressed have a poor outcome of surgery. They cope poorly and do not go back to work or to their previous social activities. They lack self confidence, sleep badly, complain of numerous physical symptoms and are afraid to resume an active sexual life [3]. Men do better than women, they lead more active lives after operation [8,9]. They perceive themselves as more functionally rehabilitated than women possibly because they are less depressed. Women feel that they cope less well overall than their male counterparts [3].

The response to a rehabilitation programme depends on the emotional state of the patient [10]. When the level of exercise attained by 28 physically comparable patients attending a cardiac rehabilitation class was reviewed at the end of the programme, it appeared that anxious patients did not do so well as those who had no psychological symptoms. Depressed patients and those who presented a mixed picture of anxiety and depression had the worst outcome (Table 1).

4. Factors influencing emotional reaction after surgery

The strongest predictor of emotional distress after operation is pre-existing anxiety or depression [3,7,11], though patients themselves relate emotional distress to their lack of knowledge of what to expect of surgery. When 249 patients were asked whether they felt they had been adequately informed, the topic they felt had been best covered was mobilisation after their operation, but even here only 55% felt they had been very well prepared. Emotional reactions had received scant attention; only 24% felt they had had sufficient advice and guidance. About one third felt that they knew enough about going back to work, resuming sexual activity and the possible physical symptoms that might be expected [9]. Obviously, there is much uncertainty in this group of patients.

Lack of knowledge, anxiety, depression and cardiac invalidism are correlated. They form a vicious circle, resulting in a frightened person who knows little about the illness, makes his or her own interpretations of little understood advice and is fearful of indulging in any physical activity that might further damage the heart or dislodge the grafts.

Understanding the needs of the family, particularly the wife, is vital because the patient's optimal level of function may be influenced by his interaction with the spouse [12]. If she is unaware of a reasonable rate of mobilisation after surgery she can prevent progressive return to activity by becoming overprotective. Though early convalescence was reported to be an anxious, stressful time by the majority of wives there was an increasing sense of well being and optimism as their husband's physical state improved and they became less dependent. The shared experience of the uncertainty of surgery seemed to foster more openness and appreciation of each other [13] especially in a previously stable marriage.

Emotional reactions following surgery are influenced by other individuals who are perceived by the patient as being an important part of his life, his relations, employer, workmates, friends with whom he shares his leisure activities and acquaintances who themselves have undergone surgery. If they are uncertain of what to expect of surgery or if they are aware of those in whom operation has failed they, too, react by becoming overprotective.

To combat anxiety, patients and their families rely heavily on their physician in the period after discharge from hospital. The majority saw him as the most important source of information, most of which was obtained preoperatively. Patients would have welcomed more advice after surgery [13]. An overcautious physician results in an anxious patient who lacks the confidence to return to work and an active life [14]. The converse is equally true; physicians with positive encouraging attitudes can promote recovery. In a series of 413 patients, twice as many returned to work after coronary artery bypass grafting compared to the number working before their operation. This encouraging result was ascribed to careful psychological preparation pre-operatively of patient and family by their doctors so that they understood that return to an active life was to be expected [15].

5. Emotional reactions during rehabilitation

There is general agreement on the components of a comprehensive rehabilitation programme; graded increasing physical activity, education (about the disease, its treatment and secondary prevention), promotion of psychological adjustment and help with social problems. The practical application of these basic principles can vary widely and many different types of programme have been described. Though in the short term graft patency was improved in patients undergoing a physical training programme [16] there is, as yet, unlike patients after myocardial infarction [17], no evidence of a secondary preventive effect in a post-operative group. However, there is no doubt

Table 2. Psychological benefits of cardiac rehabilitation.

Increased energy, enthusiasm, well-being
Decreased depression
Decreased anxiety
Improved self image
Improved ability to deal with stress
Better relaxation, sleep
Improved sexual activity
Fewer tranquillizers, hypnotics

that the quality of their life is improved as the psychological benefits of rehabilitation programmes have been well documented (Table 2).

This is true of male patients undergoing rehabilitation after surgery. There is scant knowledge of the emotional reactions of women, understandable when it is considered that at least three quarters of those undergoing surgery are men. Moreover, women are infrequently referred to a rehabilitation programme and are often excluded from randomised trials [18].

5.1. *Emotional reactions during rehabilitation: the Edinburgh experience*

The Cardio-Thoracic Unit in the Royal Infirmary of Edinburgh carries out some 700 bypass operations per year, 76% of the patients being male. Patients come from a wide geographical area and those from a distance are transferred directly from the surgical unit to their local district general hospital. Of the Edinburgh population, all are offered inpatient treatment at a nearby rehabilitation hospital and are transferred on the 5th–7th post-operative day; about 300 patients are admitted per year. Women take up this offer as readily as men as they comprise 24% of those admitted. Patients stay in the rehabilitation unit for a week during which time they undergo a comprehensive rehabilitation programme. Their spouses attend for educational sessions. They are invited to join an outpatient programme which starts the week after discharge from hospital. Fewer women than men attend as outpatients (Table 3) though there may be a trend in the last year or so for more women to come.

Levels of anxiety and depression were assessed in 169 consecutive outpatients at defined intervals using the Hospital Anxiety and Depression Scale

Table 3. Outpatient rehabilitation after coronary artery bypass surgery.

	Eligible to attend		Patients attending		Total
	males	females	males	females	number
1986	76%	24%	81%	19%	98
1989	72%	28%	85%	15%	210
1990	72%	28%	78%	22%	193

Table 4. Anxiety in post-CABG patients attending a rehabilitation programme.

	Number anxious		
	Males	Females	
On entry	30%	48%	$p < 0.01$
6 weeks	26%	33%	$p < 0.05$
12 weeks	19%	26%	ns
6 months	19%	19%	ns
12 months	20%	26%	ns

(HAD) [19]. As a group, women were initially more anxious than men (Table 4) and they took longer to adjust.

Much the same picture emerged when the depressed patients were examined (Table 5) and in the long term it appeared that the depressed women had not derived much benefit from this programme.

It may be that women who are anxious or depressed tend to attend the programme while those who have adjusted quickly feel they need not come. A proportion of patients, both male and female, are still emotionally upset a year later which suggests that a different type of programme is necessary for those patients. This may be particularly true for women if they are to achieve an optimal quality of life after cardiac surgery.

6. Treatment of adverse emotional reactions

For the majority of patients, short educational programmes before operation have been shown to reduce emotional upset in the immediate post operative phase. They result in improved self confidence, more realistic expectations of surgery and increased compliance with medical advice on mobilisation and resumption of work, leisure activities and sex. Educated patients have fewer physical symptoms. In the long term, these programmes have not been of benefit in areas that require lifelong behavioural changes such as stress

Table 5. Depression in post-CABG patients attending a rehabilitation programme.

	Number depressed		
	Males	Females	
On entry	13%	22%	$p < 0.001$
6 weeks	6%	19%	$p < 0.01$
12 weeks	8%	11%	ns
6 months	6%	19%	$p < 0.01$
12 months	6%	18%	ns

modification and eating habits [20]. Obviously patients only pay heed to the events surrounding the immediate crisis.

After surgery, comprehensive rehabilitation programmes have demonstrable psychological benefits (Table 2). These need not be sophisticated and many patients improve with simple measures which can be carried out by the general practitioner or nurse counsellor using booklets, video tapes or self-help manuals. Only a proportion of patients with severe disturbance require specialist rehabilitation.

Any rehabilitation effort is enhanced if the family is involved. Patients whose wives received instructions before surgery on how to support their husbands in the immediate post operative phase were better orientated, less confused, had fewer delusions and slept longer than controls [21]. At a later stage of recovery, male patients taking part in a rehabilitation programme whose wives joined in educational group discussions adjusted more successfully than did other groups of male patients who either did not participate in the programme or, if they did participate, their wives did not [22].

7. The future

It is essential to disseminate awareness in all those involved in the care of patients after coronary bypass surgery that emotional upset exists and that it can, and should, be treated if their patients are to achieve an optimal quality of life.

Rehabilitation programmes will have to become more flexible and tailored to individual needs. This will require experimentation with different types of programme and may be particularly important in women.

The majority of patients are not severely disturbed and simple interventions by their own doctors can enhance their quality of life. Only a proportion need sophisticated techniques. This is an important message as, when understood, rehabilitation will become widely accepted, not as often at present, a luxury for the selected few.

References

1. Jenkins CD, Stanton BA, Savageau JA, Denlinger P, Klein MD: Coronary bypass surgery. Physical, psychological, social and economic outcomes six months later. J Am Med Ass 1983;250:782–788.
2. Horgan D, Davies B, Hunt D et al: Psychiatric aspects of coronary artery surgery: a prospective study. Med J Aust 1984;141:587–590.
3. Kos-Munson BA, Alexander LD, Culbert Hinthorn PA, Lloyd Gallagher E, Gretze CM: Psychosocial predictors of optimal rehabilitation post-coronary artery bypass surgery. Scholarly Inquiry for Nursing Practice: An International Journal 1988;2:171–193.

4. Soloff PH: Medically and surgically treated coronary patients in cardiovascular rehabilitation – A comparative study. Int Psychol Med 1979;9:93–106.

5. Langeluddecke P, Fulcher G, Baird D et al: A prospective evaluation of the psychosocial effects of coronary artery bypass surgery. J. Psychosom Res 1989;33:37–45.

6. Mayou R. Bryant B: Quality of life after coronary artery surgery. Quart J Med 1987;234:239–248.

7. Magni G, Unger HP, Valfre C et al: Psychosocial outcome one year after cardiac surgery. A prospective study. Arch Intern Med 1987;147:473–477.

8. Douglas JS, Spencer BK, Jones EL: Reduced efficacy of coronary bypass surgery in women. Circulation 1981

9. Stanton BA, Jenkins CD, Savageau JA, Thurer RL: Functional benefits following coronary artery bypass graft surgery. Ann Thor Surg 1984;37:286–290.

10. Cay EL: Psychological adjustments in the coronary patient: anxiety. Quality of Life and Cardiovascular Care 1989;5:54–59.

11. Heller S, Frank K, Kornfeld D: Psychological outcomes following open heart surgery. Arch Intern Med 1974;135:908–913.

12. Dracup K: Psychosocial aspects of coronary heart disease: implications for nursing research. West J Nurs Res 1982;4:257–279.

13. Sikorski JM Knowledge concerns and questions of wives of convalescent coronary bypass graft surgery patients. J Cardiac Rehabil 1985; 5:74–85.

14. Almeida D, Bradford JM, Wenger NK, King SB, Hurst JW: Return to work after coronary bypass surgery. Circulation 1983;68 Suppl II:205–213.

15. Oberman AL, Wayne JB, Kouchoukos NT, Charles ED, Russell RO Jr, Rogers WJ: Employment status after coronary artery bypass surgery. Circulation 1982;65 Suppl II:115–119.

16. Nakai YN, Hiasa Y, Maeda T: Effects of physical exercise training on cardiac function and graft patency after coronary artery bypass grafting. J Thorac Cardiovasc Surg 1987;93:65–72.

17. Oberman A: Does cardiac rehabilitation increase long-term survival after myocardial infarction? Circulation 1989;80:416–418.

18. Wenger NK, Alpert JS: Rehabilitation of the coronary patient in 1989. Arch Intern Med 1989;149:1504–1506.

19. Zigmond AS, Snaith RP: The hospital anxiety and depression scale. Acta Psychiatr Scand 1983;67:361–370.

20. Steele LE, Ruzicki D: An evaluation of the effectiveness of cardiac teaching during hospitalization Heart Lung 1987;16:306–311.

21. Chatham MA: The effect of family involvement in patient's manifestations of post cardiotomy psychosis. Heart Lung 1987;7:995–1001.

22. Dracup KA: The effect of a role supplementation program for cardiac patients and spouses of the at-risk role. (Doctoral Dissertation, University of California, San Francisco, 1982.) Dissertation Abstracts International 43:3534B-3535B.

17. Clinical significance of research on quality of life after coronary artery surgery

RICHARD MAYOU

1. Introduction

In the last decade there has been a substantial body of research describing the impact of coronary artery surgery on quality of life. Concepts and methods have become increasingly sophisticated and, as this book shows, general patterns are now clearly delineated. However, the research findings have yet to be fully applied to clinical practice. General discussion of the significance of psychological and social factors, and of the need for rehabilitation is no substitute for precise testable guidelines. This paper reviews possible applications of research and with reviewing their present status taking illustrations from our own research on coronary artery disease [1,2]. A substantial literature has been reviewed elsewhere [3].

There can be no doubt that the overall benefits for quality of life of successful surgery are very considerable, having significant advantages, as compared with medical treatment [3]. However, we also need to be concerned with those patients for whom the outcome is less satisfactory. Sometimes, the explanation is unsuccessful surgery or cardiac or other complications. For others, it is unrelated social or medical events, but for most, it seems to be a psychologically determined failure to achieve the benefits that might be expected from successful surgery. Since outcome for quality of life must be viewed as multi-dimensional, this minority of patients is not easily categorised. There is no set pattern of quality of life outcome and all aspects must be considered separately. Research workers and clinicians must take account of outcome for work, leisure, social life, family life, mood and subjective satisfaction. The following implications for clinical practice will be considered in turn:

- selection for surgery;
- management of post-operative care and rehabilitation;
- identification of those with psychological or social problems or at risk of them:

Paul J. Walter (ed.): Quality of Life after Open Heart Surgery, 185–192.

– provision of the individual treatment for specific problems.

In each case, we should distinguish between straightforward routine measures for everyone and selective extra care for those who need it and would benefit.

2. Selection for surgery

Although, research has increasingly defined the indications for coronary artery surgery, there remain wide divergences of opinion and practice between experts. It has been suggested that surgery is frequently 'inappropriate' [4]. Discussion has focused on disagreements about physical indications and the role of psychological factors has received far too little attention.

There are few psychiatric contra-indications to surgery when the medical indications are clear. However, it is apparent that disability and emotional distress in patients with angina are not closely related to the more objective measures of symptom severity or frequency [1,3,5]. Many patients with severe angina are able to plan their lives carefully so as to minimise limitations. Others, more cautious and passive, describe considerable problems even though angina itself may be infrequent and not greatly limiting. These cautious patients have less need of surgery and it is known that they have a poor outcome from successful surgery. At present, they often also do badly with routine medical therapy, but this should not deter us from trying to devise more effective medical treatment as an alternative to surgery. Despite encouraging clinical experience and case reports, rather little use has been made of individually planned behavioural and other psychological treatments.

3. Preparation for surgery

Explanation and advice should be routine for all those undergoing surgery, and should cover the nature of the operation, postoperative recovery and convalescence. We need to place more emphasis on an active treatment whilst awaiting surgery. Time on a waiting list should not be regarded as lost time, but as an opportunity for continuing medical treatment and encouraging patients to take positive approach which will serve them well following surgery. Waiting lists are often lengthy and many patients find this upsetting, especially as it often results in social difficulties, particularly for employment. Indeed, a major threat to employment is an indication for early surgery.

The period before surgery is also a time for discussion of any unrealistic expectations. It is clear that some of the dissatisfaction with the outcome of surgery is often due to unjustified expectations that symptomatic relief will transform employment and other prospects. For many people, this is unlikely.

4. Postoperative recovery and rehabilitation

The increasingly large literature on rehabilitation emphasises education and exercise. Both are valuable. However, there has been an over-preoccupation with standard programmes, and neglect of the individual needs of the minority of those who are at risk of a poor outcome and require extra and more individually planned help. There has also been a failure to use modern psychological treatments. We have found that following myocardial infarction, most patients do well without special rehabilitation programmes, even though they enjoy and appreciate taking part in exercise training [6]. Those patients most at risk of medically unnecessary problems are often poor attenders at rehabilitation and find it inappropriate and unhelpful for their particular problems. Those patients should be identified and offered more than the routine information and advice which concentrates on the common, even universal, problems.

5. Identification of those with problems or at risk

It is essential to be aware the predictors of outcome are different for the various aspects of quality of life outcome. Thus work factors are most important in relation to employment, but pre-operative mood and history of psychological problems are overwhelmingly the most important factors for outcome for mood. Some patients at risk of a poor quality of life outcome and therefore in need of extra attention, can be identified before surgery [2].

The main predictors are listed in Table 1. It is difficult to make accurate predictions before surgery, and more satisfactory to place greater emphasis on the early identification of problems during convalescence. Research has shown that those who have difficulties within the first few weeks are very likely to suffer continuing problems [2].

Systematic assessment of quality of life must be part of routine follow-up. It can be simple and should be combined with medical assessment (Table 2). It is in fact particularly easy with patients who have had coronary artery surgery since the usual pattern is of a very positive outcome.

Table 1. Predictors of poor quality of life outcome.

Before surgery
  History of previous psychological problems
  Current emotional distress
  Poor social adjustment
  Over-cautious approach to angina
  Over-cautious and unrealistic expectations
  Over-protective family

Early convalescence
  Persistent cardiac symptoms
  Atypical physical complaints
  Neuropsychiatric complications
  Emotional distress
  Over-cautious mobilisation
  Over-protective family

Table 2. Clinical review of quality of life at follow-up.

1. Coping with physical symptoms
2. Atypical physical symptoms
3. Mood:
     – depression
     – anxiety
     – concentration
     – irritability
     – fatigue
     – insomnia
4. Current physical activity
5. Social, marital and leisure satisfaction
6. Plans for work and social activities
7. Information from relative
8. Any questions?

6. Individual treatment of specific problems

Most standard programmes of rehabilitation are unable to offer treatment of specific problems, medical, social and psychological (Table 3). A few that are more flexible may be able to provide extra help for those who need them, but very few have to the psychological expertise to offer precisely planned individual treatment. Mere advice and exhortation is inadequate.

In some cases, recognition, individual explanation and discussion are all that is required. Awareness of the patient's fears and beliefs may enable the doctor or other therapist to provide an acceptable convincing advice. Other patients require more.

Table 3. Specific problems and their treatment.

1. *Persistent cardiac symptoms*
   Exercise testing and prescription
   Co-ordinate medical care and supportive rehabilitation

2. *Neuropsychiatric symptoms*
   Assess cognitive state
   Assess mood to detect depression
   Psychosocial and practical advice

3. *Excessive caution*
   Explanation and discussion with patient and spouse
   Exercise training
   Behavioural programme (graded practice, diary, etc)

4. *Depression*
   Explanation and discussion
   Consider anti-depressant medication
   Psychosocial advice

5. *Anxiety*
   Explanation and discussion
   Cognitive/behavioural programme

6. *Atypical physical symptoms*
   Explanation and discussion
   Cognitive/behavioural programme

7. *Sexual problems*
   Advice, reassurance

8. *Non-compliance*
   Identify problem with patients and spouse
   Try to agree individual rehabilitation programme

6.1. *Cardiac complications*

Patients with cardiac complications, such as continuing angina or heart failure need extra rehabilitation, not only because of their physical impairment, but because they are especially liable to extra psychologically determined handicaps. Small improvements in physical state from medical treatment and improved morale from well-organised and supportive care can make a substantial difference to the quality of life. For example, in a recent trial of drug treatment of moderately severe heart failure, considerable improvements in quality of life were reported by the placebo group, presumably due to being treated in a special clinic run by a sympathetic and encouraging doctor [7].

6.2. *Neuropsychiatric complications*

Individual plans are necessary, not least for those for whom clinically minor neurological and intellectual impairment pose particular problems. It is essential to be aware that depression is the commonest cause of complaints of poor concentration and memory following surgery.

6.2.1. *Depression*
Depression is common, especially in the early weeks of convalescence and at the time of any complications or set backs, is usually of moderate severity with a good prognosis. Resolution of associated social difficulties is important. An important minority of patients, probably less than five per cent, require anti-depressant medication. Doctors need to be more aware of both the psychological and somatic symptoms of depression and the extent to which it may be responsible for malaise, fatigue, atypical somatic symptoms, and other common complaints following surgery.

6.2.2. *Anxiety and caution*
Anxiety symptoms, even panic, are often associated with worry about returning to normal life and with excessive caution about physical activity. Again, simple encouragement and advice can be effective. There is also substantial scope for applying methods well proven in the psychiatric treatment of anxiety disorders. The importance of behavioural techniques (such as diary keeping, anxiety management and graded practice) and of cognitive methods (eliciting and modifying inappropriate beliefs) has been substantially underestimated in rehabilitation.

6.2.3. *Atypical physical symptoms*
Atypical physical symptoms (atypical non-cardiac chest pain, palpitations and breathlessness) are very frequent following surgery and in our own study, were a cause of distress closely associated with poor social and psychiatric outcome [1,3]. Their occurrence after heart surgery is easily understood. Patients are naturally aware of angina and of the significance of chest pain and find it difficult to interpret minor physiological and physical symptoms which may be attributable to the incision, chest wall pain or other minor medical problems. Sometimes such symptoms are attributable to the autonomic symptoms of panic or generalised anxiety.

I believe that psychological treatment methods (cognitive and behavioural) that we have found to be effective with non-cardiac chest pain in patients without evidence of ischaemic heart disease [8], are also useful in patients recovering from surgery. Patients find a combination of discussion of their beliefs about the causes of symptoms, anxiety management and graded practice is helpful in the treatment of the pain and also in encouraging a return to full activities.

6.2.4. *Sexual problems*
Many patients describe sex as being relatively infrequent following surgery, but they do not necessarily see this as a problem. It is often a long-standing

choice by middle-aged couples. With a minority of patients, sexual difficulties arise from anxiety about implications of heart disease (or indeed from other unrelated reasons) may benefit from advice to couples and simple behavioural treatment. A few patients require specialist referral.

6.2.5. *Vocational guidance*
some patients have unrealistic expectations about return to work, others are uncertain about when to return and whether it is appropriate to make changes in hours or on the nature of their job. Patients and families uncertainties are often made worse by employers over-concern or their eagerness to use illness and surgery as an excuse for medical retirement. Some patients, especially those in manual work and without the security of employment, do require expert advice. They may also benefit from exercise testing as a guide to their capacity and from exercise training.

7. Conclusion

We are already in a position to apply research to clinical practice. Even so, there is a need for much more research to evaluate:

(1) more systematic assessment procedures before and after surgery;
(2) psychosocial measures to improve medical treatment of angina;
(3) more specific rehabilitation techniques for sub-groups of patients following surgery.

Psychological treatments already proven and in routine use in other areas of medicine and psychiatry need to be adapted for patients undergoing coronary artery surgery, and indeed with other cardiac disorders and treatments.

A small proportion of these selective extra interventions will require specialist referral to clinical psychologists and psychiatrists, but I would expect that most could be undertaken by members of cardiac and rehabilitation teams. They will require further training, some continuing supervision and access to specialist referral. It is essential that the newer, more sophisticated programmes are carefully co-ordinated with cardiological care, and that they are shown to be both therapeutic and cost effective.

References

1. Mayou RA, Bryant B: Quality of life after coronary surgery. Qu J Med 1986;239:239–248.
2. Bryant B, Mayou RA: Prediction of outcome after coronary artery surgery. J Psychosom Res 1989;4:419–427.
3. Mayou RA: Invited review: the psychiatric and social consequences of coronary artery surgery. J Psychosom Res 1985;30:225–271.
4. Wennberg J (Ed): The paradox of appropriate care. JAMA 1987;258:2568–2569.

5. Mayou RA: Chest pain, angina pectoris and disability. J Psychosom Res 1973;17:287–291.
6. Mayou RA, MacMahon D, Sleight P, Florencio MJ: Early rehabilitation after myocardial infarction. Lancet 1981;2:1399–1401.
7. Blackwood R, Mayou RA, Garnham JC, Armstrong C, Bryant B: Exercise capacity and quality of life in the treatment of heart failure. Clin Pharmacol Ther 1990;48:325–332.
8. Klimes I, Mayou RA, Pearce MJ, Coles L, Fagg JR: Psychological treatment for atypical non-cardiac chest pain: a controlled evaluation. Psych Med 1990;20:605–611.

18. Psychological reactions to open heart surgery: results of a quantitative and qualitative analysis of the recovery process

W. LANGOSCH and H.-P. SCHMOLL-FLOCKERZIE

1. Introduction

In 1990, approximately 39000 open heart surgeries have been performed in Germany. It seems that, nowadays, open heart surgery has become a well established way of treatment. In earlier studies a high rate of psychiatric disturbances has been documented in the postoperative time [1,2], but in a recent study a much lower incidence of disorders like disorientation, paranoid-hallucinatory symptoms, loss of control, given up has been reported (unpublished manuscript by H. Speidel). In addition, it has been found that patients with valvular disease are more inclined to develop psychiatric disorders than coronary patients [1,2]. Such results makes it necessary not to calculate frequencies of psychiatric disturbances across both groups of patients. In this study, the following questions should be answered:

(a) Are there significant differences between psychological data collected preoperatively, postoperatively and at discharge?
(b) Does the same symptom always predominate, i.e. preoperatively, postoperatively and at discharge?
(c) Can a global score of postoperative psychopathology be predicted by preoperatively collected data?

2. Methods

2.1. *Patients*

The sample consists of 75 male patients who had to undergo bypass surgery between 1985 and 1989. Subjects ages ranged from 37 to 67 years, with a mean of 53.2 years (SD = 6.3 years). Most patients (84%) were married or remarried. Eighty-four percent of subjects were still working; 52% reported that they had worked 46 hours or more per week and even 25% reported of

Paul J. Walter (ed.): Quality of Life after Open Heart Surgery, 193–200.
© 1992 Kluwer Academic Publishers.

having spent at least 56 hours per week on the job. A skilled or unskilled job was held by 39% of subjects, 33% of subjects were managers and 17% of subjects held a clerical job. Only 4% of patients reported not having suffered from cardiac symptoms. Their general attitude towards outcome was described by 77% as good and by 21% as excellent. Nevertheless, 78% of patients spontaneously brought up concerns about their heart condition and 31% mentioned concerns about death.

2.2. *Measures*

Semi-standardized interviews were perfomed with the patients admitted into the study one to two days before surgery, two to three days after surgery, when the patients had been transferred to a semi-intensive care ward, and one to two days before discharge from the hospital, i.e. nearly three weeks after surgery. The Hamburg Rating Scale for Psychic Disturbances (HRPD) has been designed to assess psychological changes after open-heart surgery. Each of 36 symptoms is rated on a four-point scale, ranging from absent to severe. By using factor analysis eight mutually independent syndromes or scales have been constructed: general disorientation, impaired thinking/concentration, paranoid-hallucinatory syndrome, worry/anxiety, sullen inadequacy, hostility, loss of control, given up [3,4]. The Hamilton Psychiatric Rating Scale for Depression (HAM-D) consists of 22 items, which have to be rated immediately after completing the interview with the patient [5]. To increase inter-rater reliability the raters are urged to adhere to well-developed scoring guidelines. The Hamilton Anxiety Scale (HAM-A) comprises 14 items, which are defined by descriptors [6]. Each item has to be rated by the interviewer on a five point rating scale according to the extent the patient is bothered or disturbed by the symptom.

Preoperatively, patients were administered the Spielberger State-Trait Anxiety Scale [7], but at discharge patients had only to complete the state anxiety scale. In addition patients completed preoperatively also the Psychological Screening Inventory for Myocardial Infarction Patients (PSM) which consists of 15 scales covering five aspects of well-being, depressive mood, emotional lability, four aspects of type A behavior, achievement behavior, social desirability, social anxiety, non-assertiveness [8].

2.3. *Statistics*

The two-tailed Student's *t*-test for dependent samples was used for comparison between means of the same scale obtained at each of the three measurement points.

For each measurement, factor analysis (principal component analysis with

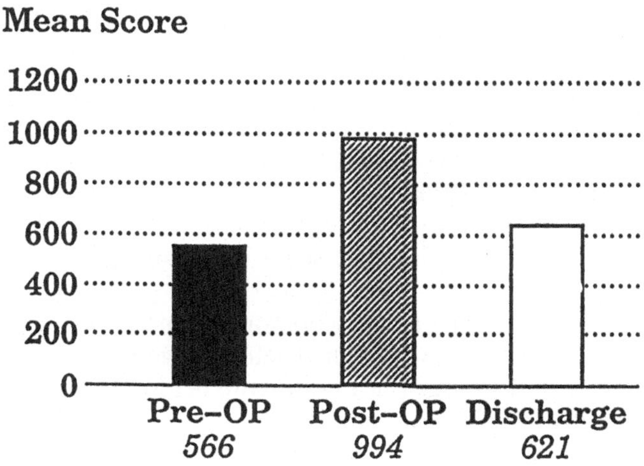

Mean Score

Figure 1. Total score of HRPD before surgery, after surgery and at discharge.

Varimax rotation) was done with the items of the HRPD, HAM-D and HAM-A, provided their mean was >0 and the variance >6%.

After splitting the sample into two groups, using the median of total scores based upon the postoperatively collected HRPD, HAM-D and HAM-A items, step-wise multiple regression analysis was used to determine those preoperative data, allowing us to predict the group of patients with or without psychopathological disturbances, respectively.

3. Results

Postoperatively the total score of the HRPD has increased significantly when compared with the preoperative score ($t = -4.05$, $p < 0.001$) and the total score at discharge ($t = 3.72$, $p < 0.001$) (Figure 1).

The total HRPD-scores obtained before surgery and at discharge were not significantly different ($t = 0.42$, $p = 0.67$).

The score of the HRPD-scale, 'worry/anxiety', changed in quite a similiar way: postoperatively, there was a significant increase in comparison with the score before surgery ($t = 3.40$, $p = 0.001$), but the reduction at discharge was not so clear ($t = 1.82$, $p = 0.73$). Compared with the preoperative value, the discharge score was still somewhat higher ($t = -1.79$, $p = 0.78$). Feelings of sullen inadequacy were significantly higher some days after surgery than before surgery ($t = -6.95$, $p < 0.001$) or at discharge ($t = 6.29$, $p < 0.001$), while there was no significant difference between the scores obtained preoperatively and at discharge ($t = -1.33$, $p = 0.189$).

For the other six HRPD scales a statistical analysis of time-dependent changes was not advisable since these symptoms occurred only very rarely at the different times. Depression – as measured by the HAM-D – was significantly higher postoperatively ($t = -9.59$, $p < 0.001$), but at discharge patients' depression score already was much lower ($t = 8.55$, $p < 0.001$) and no longer different from their preoperative score ($t = 0.89$, $p = 375$).

The HAM-A score changed in nearly the same way: postoperatively, anxiety has significantly increased ($t = 6.50$, $p < 0.001$) and at discharge the anxiety score has returned to the preoperative level ($t = 6.30$, $p < 0.001$), i.e. preoperative score and discharge score were not significantly different ($t = 0.89$, $p = 0.375$).

Patients' preoperative trait anxiety score was within the average range ($T = 48$) and their state anxiety score obtained before surgery was not significantly different from that at discharge (mean raw score before surgery: 32.12; mean raw score at discharge: 32.25).

The following items had to be excluded from the preoperative itempool: 24 symptoms of the HRPD (including all items of the scales paranoid-hallucinatory syndrome, impaired thinking/concentration, given up) five symptoms of the HAM-D (including suicide, depersonalization, paranoid symptoms, obsessional-compulsive symptoms, gastro-intestinal symptoms), one item of the HAM-A (sensory symptoms); postoperatively, the following items could not be considered: 21 symptoms of the HRPD, seven symptoms of the HAM-D (in addition to the first four above mentioned symptoms, the items feeling of guilt, genital symptoms, diurnal variation) and two items of the HAM-A (fears, genitourinary symptoms). At discharge, the following items had to be eliminated: 20 symptoms of the HRPD, six symptoms of the HAM-D (retardation and genital symptoms, in addition to those four symptoms already excluded from the preoperative as well as the postoperative itempool), and one symptom of the HAM-A (fears). The factor analysis with the 41 preoperative items resulted in an eight-factor solution, which accounted for 59.3% of the total variance. Four factors were obtained, when

Table 1. Results of factor analyses with selected items of HRPD, HAM-D and HAM-A.

Pre-op	Post-op.	At discharge
1. Anxious mood	Hypochondriasis, Anxious mood	Depressed mood
2. Hypochondriasis	Somatic symptoms, Fatigue	Hypochondriasis, Anxious mood
3. Restlessness, Nervousness	Insomnia	Insomnia
4. Somatic symptoms, Retardation	Restlessness, Nervousness	Restlessness, Nervousness
5. Depressed mood		Feelings of inadequacy
6. Insomnia		
7. Cognitive difficulties		
8. Sexual problems		
s^2_{cum}: 59.3%	50.7%	49.8%

Table 2. Prediction of high postoperative psychopathology.

Variable	Beta coefficient	t	p
Social desirability	−0.48	−2.78	0.01
Concern about well-being	0.04	2.33	0.03
(Constant)		10.72	0.00
$R = 0.54$		$R^2 = 0.29$	
	adjusted	$R^2 = 0.24$	
$F_{2,25} = 5.20$,		$p = 0.01$	

factor analysis was conducted with the 41 postoperative items. This solution accounted for 50.7% of the total variance. When the 44 discharge items were used, four factors were identified which accounted for 49.8% of the total variance.

Stepwise multiple regression analysis was used to discover those preoperative data allowing for predicting a high or low score of postoperative psychopathology, respectively. This analysis resulted in an equation for predicting high postoperative psychopathology from a low score for social desirability and a high score for concern about well-being. The adjusted $R^2 = 0.24$ indicates that 24% of the variance of high postoperative psychopathology is predictable by these two preoperatively obtained scores.

In contrast, a significant multiple-correlation coefficient was not found for low postoperative psychopathology.

4. Discussion

Serious psychic disturbances like disorientation in time, place or situation, reduced vigilance, visual or auditory hallucinations, derealization and depersonalization, suicidal ideas or behavior, tendencies towards self harm, paranoid ideas, mood or delusions, have not been observed at any of the three interviews. This result confirms that nowadays only a very low incidence of serious psychic disturbances has to be expected, and that the findings of earlier studies can no longer be regarded as valid.

Nevertheless, open heart surgery is still a very stressful procedure for patients, since anxiety, depression and global psychopathology increase significantly immediately after surgery. At discharge, these scores are reduced only to the preoperative level, indicating that even three weeks after surgery, patients' mood, self-confidence, concentration, thinking and memory are disturbed.

Examining the items loading on the factor 'anxiety' at the different times, it becomes clear that the content of anxiety has changed from time to time. Preoperatively, the patient appears tense and mentally troubled, he expresses anxiety in his mood and behavior, his thinking is narrowed to the impending surgery and his disease. The threat to his life, which he is feeling at this time, also manifests itself in the finding that 80% of patients spontaneously express concern with their disease and 30% of subjects spontaneously report concern with death associated with surgery. Nevertheless, nearly all patients emphasize at the same time, that they expect a good or excellent outcome of surgery. It seems that subjects' preferred way of coping with the stress of surgery and their associated upsetting feelings is to maintain hope by minimizing the seriousness of the immediate and intermediate adverse consequences of surgery.

Postoperatively, the subjects suffer from a lot of somatic symptoms, they feel exhausted and they worry about the seriousness of the symptoms which they before surgery had tried to minimize or even to deny. At discharge, patients are concerned with the success of surgery. They observe very carefully their bodily functioning, are preoccupied with their bodily health and are suspicious of their well-being in future.

Subjects' apprehensive concentration on their body is maintained by symptoms like insomnia, fatiguability, reduced appetite, loss of libido, pain, tendencies to sweat. These manifold symptoms are interpreted as signs of clearly reduced strength and capacity, thus eliciting fears of continuing reduction in quality of life. According to the results of the different factor analyses, anxiety is the main symptom before and immediately after surgery, but at discharge depression becomes the predominant syndrome. Inspecting the items which comprise this syndrome reveals that complaints of lack of energy, feelings of worry, pessimistic ideas, blaming their physical condition for being nervous, and narrowed thinking, have the highest loadings. It becomes obvious that depressive mood is the result of being disappointed about suffering from a variety of symptoms three weeks after surgery. At this time, many patients have to give up the illusion that they would regain by surgery nearly the same strength they had had before their disease became worse. Probably this disillusion is more intense the more the patients had coped with their preoperative anxiety by using minimalization or denial. It is assumed that this way of coping is – at least in part – supported by the information which the patients had received before surgery emphasizing the benefits of open-heart surgery, specially the increase in physical fitness that can be expected.

It has been observed that patients who had preferred to cope preoperatively with their surgery by emotional withdrawal were more disappointed with their postoperative course one year after surgery. These subjects had expected a greater improvement and assessed their health as worse compared with their preoperative time [9]. In addition, the authors found that those patients who preoperatively conceived the operation as only a technical event, thus avoiding any emotional involvement, were more depressed, more restless and mentally less stable one year later.

Taking these findings into account, psychological counselling or supportive psychotherapy should be offered to those patients who are depressive three weeks after surgery to help them to accept their physical restrictions as well as to appraise the various symptoms in a more realistic way. Multiple regression analysis shows that patients who, preoperatively, are very concerned about their health and who care less for social rules are at a higher risk of developing psychopathological symptoms in the first two days after surgery. It has been reported that those patients who, in the preoperative period, have been assessed as symptomatic, have a higher incidence of some type of postoperative psychopathology [2], but in this study only self-report data have been included in multiple regression analysis.

The findings of this study point to the importance of emotion – focused forms of coping [10] in the context of surgery, emphasizing the necessity of providing psychological support in the preoperative period for those patients who are disposed to focus their attention on their body.

5. Summary

In this study it has been found that the incidence of serious psychiatric symptoms after bypass surgery is low. In the preoperative and in the postoperative period anxiety is the main symptom, although the content of anxiety is not the same at both periods. Preoperatively, the patient is concerned with the threat to his life: postoperatively, he worries about the meaning of the various somatic symptoms he is suffering from. At discharge, depression predominates, and it is assumed that the main reasons are disappointment with the state of physical health and fears of reduced quality of future life. Patients prone to higher psychopathology in the postoperative period are those who, in general, are apprehensive about their health and who feel less bound by social rules.

It is recommended that those patients who are in general anxious about their health and those who are in a depressed mood two to three weeks after surgery should be offered supportive psychotherapy.

References

1. Rabiner CJ, Willner AE: Differential psychopathological and organic mental disorder at follow-up, five years after coronary bypass and cardiac valvular surgery. In: Speidel H, Rodewald G (eds.) Psychic and neurological dysfunctions after open-heart surgery. Stuttgart, New York: Georg Thieme, 1980:237–249.
2. Götze P, Flemming B, Huse-Kleinstoll G, Meffert HJ, Reimer Ch, Speidel H: Relationship between psychopathological syndromes before and after open-heart surgery. In: Becker R, Katz J, Polonius MJ, Speidel H (eds.) Psychopathological and neurological dysfunctions following open-heart surgery. Berlin Heidelberg: Springer, 1982:84–90.
3. Dahme B, Götze P, Wessel M: Brief psychiatric inventory for assessment of psychopatholog-

ical disorders after open-heart surgery. In: Becker R, Katz J, Polonius MJ, Speidel H (eds.) Psychopathological and neurological dysfunctions following open-heart surgery. Berlin Heidelberg: Springer, 1982:68–76.

4. Götze P, Dahme B, Flemming B, et al: Hamburg Rating Scale for Psychiatric Disturbances – HRPD. In: Becker R, Katz J, Polonius MJ, Speidel H (eds.) Psychopathological and neurological dysfunctions following open-heart surgery. Heidelberg: Springer, 1982:77–83.

5. Hamilton M: Hamilton Depression Scale HAMD. In: Guy W (ed.) ECDEU assessment manual for psychopharmacology. Rev. ed. Rockville: National Institute of Mental Health, 1976:179–192.

6. Hamilton M: Hamilton Anxiety Scale HAMA. In: Guy W (ed.) ECDEU assessment manual for psychopharmacology. Rev. ed. Rockville: National Institute of Mental Health, 1976:193–198.

7. Spielberger C, Gorsuch R, Lushene R: Manual for the State-Trait Anxiety Inventory. Palo Alto, Calif.: Consulting Psychologist, 1970.

8. Langosch W: Psychosomatik der koronaren Herzkrankheiten. Weinheim: VCH edition medizin, 1989.

9. Möhlen K, Davies-Osterkamp S, Müller H, Scheld HH, Siefen G: Relationship between preoperative coping styles, immediate postoperative reactions and some aspects of the psychosocial situation of open-heart surgery patients one year after the operation. In: Becker R, Katz J, Polonius MJ, Speidel H (eds.) Psychopathological and neurological dysfunctions following open-heart surgery. Berlin Heidelberg: Springer, 1982:232–237.

10. Lazarus R, Folkman S: Stress, appraisal and coping. New York: Springer, 1984.

D: Performance of Social Roles

19. Is employment after coronary bypass surgery a measure of the patient's quality of life?

PAUL J. WALTER and B.J. AMSEL

1. Introduction

Return to work after coronary artery bypass surgery may be an important indicator of the overall outcome of the patient and of the social benefit for the community in return for resources spent.

Many adults regard their ability to fulfil a socially useful occupational role as a demonstration of their personal worth. Employment after bypass surgery may therefore currently be regarded as an unstated social goal. The fact that the incidence of return to work after heart surgery is not as high as could be expected from the excellent functional improvement to which one has become accustomed, may be explained by the concept that employment is not the main goal in the individual quality of life assessment. The purpose of this study is to analyse the recent literature on return to work after coronary artery bypass surgery. Integrating the available data, the following hypothesis may be formulated: is the subjective decision of the individual patient for postoperative employment influenced by his feeling that return to work also leads to an improved quality of life?

2. There is a clear discrepancy between objectively measured functional improvement, subjectively stated ability to work and the definitive employment rate

Hacker et al., for example, have shown that, among patients not working after coronary bypass surgery, only 11% felt they would be able to work without limitation in spite of the fact that 39% were in functional class I [1] (Figure 1). Hammermeister et al. also found that subjective clinical improvement may not necessarily lead to increased postoperative employment. They found similar rates of reemployment for medically versus surgically treated patients in spite of better subjective clinical improvement in the surgical patients [2].

Paul J. Walter (ed.): Quality of Life after Open Heart Surgery, 203–213.
© 1992 Kluwer Academic Publishers.

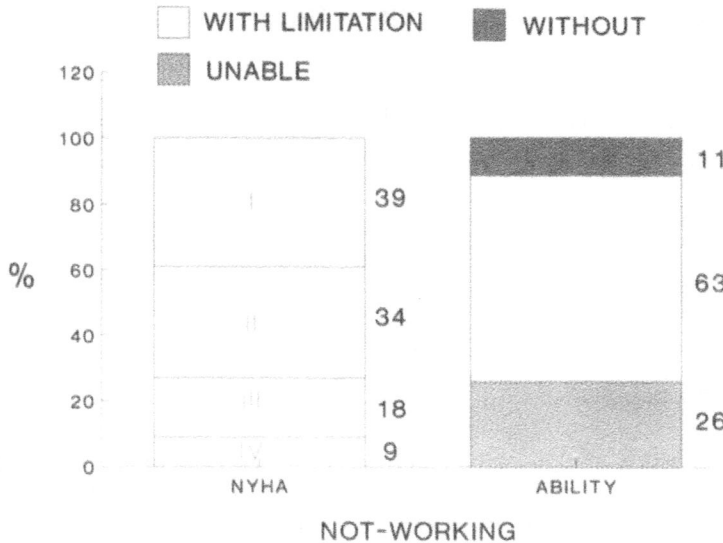

Figure 1. Discrepancy between functional class (NYHA) Subjective ability to work and work status after coronary bypass surgery (from Hacker *et al.* [1]).

Gundle *et al.*, took this a step further when they demonstrated a discrepancy between good physical outcome and poor psychological outcome. They reported on 30 patients of whom only five were employed 12–24 months after surgery. Of them, 69% reached their predicted exercise tolerance while a full 57% had sexual dysfunction, and a significant number of patients had a constricted social life, lack of pleasure from close relationships, serious distortions of body image, and symptomatic depression. This study demonstrates that a very low postoperative employment rate can appear in a group of patients with a reduced quality of life who continue to think of themselves as 'damaged' [13].

The impact of coronary bypass surgery on the quality of life was studied in 95 patients by La Mendola and Pellegrini. Preoperatively 13% were retired in comparison with 38% postoperatively. A clear correlation was shown to exist between the desire to work and actual employment status. Of patients wanting to work, 79% actually worked, whereas 97% of those who did not want to work retired. The desire to work was closely correlated to perceived physical limits. Of patients subjectively without any physical limits and wanting to work, 88% were employed. The fact that almost half of those patients with no desire to work did not feel any physical limits demonstrates once again that other factors than functional ones may play an important role in the patient's decision not to return to work [4]. Thus functional improvement and increased potential for productivity may be used not only on the job but also for enjoying increased leisure time. If, therefore, in spite of an improved functional result of the operation, work resumption is not as high as could be expected, cognitive problems or psychosocial factors may be responsible for this unexpected suboptimal result.

3. The effect of subjective cognitive function on the decision to return to work

Increasing attention has been paid to the role of illness perceptions in the coping process after cardiac surgery. The coping process consists of a complex interplay of cognitive, affective, and behavioral responses. Realistic information and comprehension of the disease and of the surgical procedure are essential for successful coping and may produce a positive affective reaction. This seems to be prerequisite for postoperative employment.

Interestingly, Newman et al. have shown that depression was related more closely to self-reported cognitive dysfunction than to objectively-determined cognitive dysfunction. There was little relation between patients' complaints and their performance on tests of problem solving, clarity of thinking, and concentration. In a study on 62 patients who had undergone coronary bypass surgery, 28% reported a decrease in memory, 18% in the ability to solve problems, 16% in the clarity of thinking, and 16% in concentration. There were no differences in objectively determined memory, concentration, attention, clumsiness, and slowing scores between patients who had subjective complaints in these areas and those who did not. These findings emphasize the importance of subjective perception of physical and mental condition after coronary bypass surgery which may or may not encourage patients to return to work [5].

Positive motivation towards a return to work after coronary bypass surgery is best reached by a coping style comprising four aspects of illness perception: a sufficient knowledge of the disease and the surgical procedure (knowledge), a subjective interpretation of the illness (beliefs), the evaluation of future functioning (expectations), and self perception of health status [6–9]. As indicated above, perception of physical disability may be predictive of postoperative work status. In fact, independent of its clinical severity, a patient's own health perception after a cardiac event has been found to be the most important factor for returning the work [10,11].

The formation of illness cognitions about disease processes may determine the patient's coping strategies and evaluation of treatment. Cardiac patients who initially attribute their symptoms to non-cardiac causes, for example, not only delayed longer before visiting their physicians but also reported more psychosocial problems after surgery [12].

Personal beliefs about the causes of coronary artery disease greatly influence the decision to return to work. In patients who attribute their disease to the stress of work, the rate of return to work is understandably low [13].

4. Emotional changes due to the disease and the operation and their influence on postoperative employment

When there are high levels of hypochondriasis, hysteria and depression, the rate of return to work is low. In their study of 51 patients assigned to medical or surgical therapy only 10 patients were working at least part time after treatment. There were no differences between the medical or surgical group. In spite of potential economic problems, unemployed patients in both groups seemed to be satisfied with their social and family life and with their overall quality of life. It may be assumed that these symptomatic patients adapted to the level of life quality available to them. Many factors would have to improve if general quality of life and the rate of return to work were to increase [14].

Patients' levels of anxiety and depression during hospitalization and the level of cardiac lifestyle knowledge influence expectations of working capacity. These factors are independent of work-related or medical factors. This means that it is not only a patient's perception of his illness during hospitalization, it is also the affective reaction which will have a great influence on his returning to work [15]. The chronic illness suffered by the patient and his subjective experience of the operation influence his state of mind, which in turn influences his expectation of future perspectives of returning to work, among other things.

In a multiple regression analysis of preoperative factors, a patient's expectation concerning postoperative return to work has been found to be the strongest predictor of actual return to work. An affirmative answer to the simple question, 'Do you feel that you will be able to go back to work after surgery?' predicted return to work in 82% while only 38% of those who gave a negative answer did so [16].

Aside from expectation, motivation is also of utmost importance. In a study on return to work after a first myocardial infarction, motivation was, in fact, found to be he only significant factor. Of patients with good motivation, 92% returned to work compared to only 83% of those with poor motivation [17].

5. Social aspects of quality of life and their influence on return to work

Aside from such personal factors as cognitive function and psychological state, which refer primarily to the patient himself and indicate his subjective experience with his chronic disease and the operation, interpersonal relationships and factors having to do with the working place itself also influence the rate of returning to work. Return to work may be regarded in the framework of an improved quality of life after CABG of which marital happiness, sexual activity, and an enjoyable relationship between couples and the nuclear family are essential components.

A correlation of resumption of sexual activity and postoperative reemployment has been mentioned by several authors [18–20].

The Psychosocial Adjustment to Illness Scale (PAIS) has been performed in 96 patients pre- and six months postoperatively, in order to examine adjustment to illness in a variety of quality of life domains. A diminished interference of illness with job activity was found without any change in the attitude toward work. This improvement in vocational status went parallel with an increase in sexual function and frequency of sexual activity; however, the capacity for sexual pleasure, satisfaction, and the quality of marital relationship were not changed. The relationship with the nuclear family was strengthened though not with the extended family. While psychological distress was unaltered general concerns about health increased. These results were interpreted as indicating an improvement in the psychosocial adjustment to illness at six months after CABG [21].

Using the PAIS in 89 patients, Langeluddecke et al. found a high level of psychosocial impairment preoperatively, but, 1 year after coronary bypass, 84% of patients reported a significant improvement in their marital relationship, 85% an increased interest in sexual activities, and 2/3 greater involvement in leisure activities. Almost half of the initially unemployed resumed paid employment postoperatively [22].

Among patients working before surgery, 77% of those returning to work resumed sexual activity compared to only 60% not working after the operation. Non-medical, but rather psychosocial factors may play an important role in resuming both work and sexual activity, because there was no difference in symptomatic improvement between patients who resumed these activities and those who did not. Up to now physicians have played a rather limited role in the resumption of sexual activity. Although 2/3 of patients received sexual instructions before leaving the hospital, only 20% received these instructions at the instigation of a physician [20]. Thurer found that only 1/3 of patients were counseled at all regarding sexual activity [23]. The advisability of including sexual counseling into a comprehensive rehabilitation program is strongly suggested by the fact that the emotional relationship of sexually active couples became closer twice as frequently as in sexually inactive couples [20].

A coronary bypass operation may be felt by the patient and his partner to be such an earth-shattering experience that not returning to work becomes acceptable without having to lose face. This can yield a convenient excuse for avoiding any frustration that had existed at work [24]. Overprotection by the family which thinks that working might be bad for the patient could, of course, also lead to further unemployment after surgery. Thus the patient may get strong support in his desire not really to go back to work [25]. When there is subjective negative perception of working conditions, a patient be stimulated not to return to work because retirement will likely improve the quality of life. Examples of such negative situations are a poor personal relationship with colleagues, the subjective impression of not being able to make any useful contribution to the success of the company, and a noisy, smoky or otherwise uncomfortable working place. Even job modification may not be sufficient to improve pleasure at work because colleagues may be changed and income reduced [26].

The stigma attached to heart disease and to the heart operation may unfortunately influence employers not to re-employ the patient after his recovery. Informing them of their employees' capacity and ability to work may influence the employer to take them back. If working conditions are facilitated postoperatively (part-time work or less strenuous work), the possibility of going back to work at all may increase.

Physicians' attitudes towards postoperative employment and their advice to their patients may have a far reaching effect on return to work. In fact, in a study of 1602 patients having undergone coronary bypass surgery, the essential reason for failure to return to work was physician's advice, which was cited in 59%, followed by cardiac symptoms, blamed in 52% of the 542 patients not working postoperatively [27].

Liddle et al. have shown that psychological preparation of the patients by their physicians and employers could lead to an increase in postoperative employment. Their results were truly excellent: 95% of patients not working preoperatively returned to work, whereas 87% of those who were disabled preoperatively returned to work. This was accomplished by explaining to the patients before their operation that the primary goal of surgery was the possibility of returning to work. The authors assumed that the attitudes of physicians, families and employers was of utmost importance in attaining this goal. Stimulating the patients to return to work is justified by the fact that returning to work does not adversely influence survival or health. In fact, in the same study, 16% of patients were able to work up to 10 years beyond retirement age [28] (Figure 2).

Under certain circumstances voluntary retirement may be an acceptable alternative to returning to work. This is especially so if income is assured either through a well-developed national welfare system or through local company incentives [29–33]. When, however, retirement is forced upon the patient, morbidity increases. Zyzansky et al., for instance, found almost twice as much hospitalization after bypass surgery in those forced to retire than in those voluntarily retired. In those working, of course, hospitalization rate was even lower [34].

In a study of a 100 patients by Kornfeld et al., overall satisfaction and improvement in the quality of life at $3\frac{1}{2}$ years post-surgery was found, compared to pre-surgery. Family relations improved in 48%. In addition general pleasure ameliorated in 65% and mood in 42%. Corresponding to these benefits in quality of life after open heart surgery, the 9-month postoperative

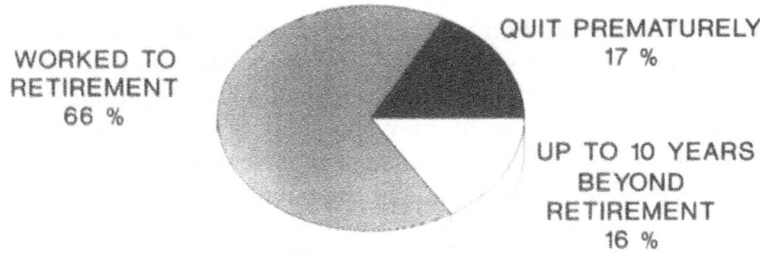

WORKED TO
RETIREMENT
66 %

QUIT PREMATURELY
17 %

UP TO 10 YEARS
BEYOND
RETIREMENT
16 %

Figure 2. Post-op rehabilitation. Working after myocardial revascularization in the elderly (USA) (from Liddle *et al.* [28]).

rate of return to work was 76%, quite similar to the 77% working at the time of surgery [35].

6. Strategies for improving postoperative employment as one facet of a patient's life quality

Boulay and colleagues, using psychosocial, economic, and social factors, as well as the functional capacity of patients measured pre- en postoperatively, were able to determine a prognosis of returning to work. They identified a group of patients unlikely to return to work. It may be assumed that by concentrating efforts and counseling on this group of patients, the rate of return to work might increase significantly [36]. Therefore early identification and treatment of those patients at risk for psychosocial disorders should be done in a preoperative phase. Unrealistic expectations and sexual problems should be discussed both with the patient and his or her partner. Studying quality of life parameters in 79 patients after coronary bypass surgery, Mayou and Bryant found that it was not medical factors, but mental state and a conscious passive approach to illness which were the main preoperative factors related to global social outcome. Although there was an improvement in mental state, leisure activity, and satisfaction in family life, dissatisfaction with sexual relations increased in about 20%, and the job situation deteriorated in 36% [37].

Patients' expectation of work resumption are greatly influenced by their knowledge of the benefits of returning to the job. The personal physician plays an important role in delivering sufficient knowledge about his patient's postoperative physical abilities supporting positive expectation and beliefs in his patient and therefore stimulating the patient's attitude towards return to work. Intensive communication between general practitioners, cardiologists, hospital physicians, cardiac surgeons and occupational physicians, e.g., to provide the patient and his family with consistent advice regarding resumption of postoperative employment, may ultimately result in increased confidence in the medical profession [26]. Stein et al. have shown that cooperation between the rehabilitation physician and the patient's personal physician is of the utmost importance in early return to work after acute myocardial infarction. In a prospective study of 124 patients, inability to work was shortened from an average from 4.3 months to an average of 7 weeks by optimal coordination of efforts by the doctors concerned and their emphasis on the real possibility of speedy reemployment [38].

Transient cognitive dysfunction appears frequently after bypass surgery and may lead to a period of mental depression or emotional instability. Pre- and postoperative teaching sessions with the patient and a family member on how to cope with cognitive dysfunction will help convince the patient that the feeling of being mentally slow is only a transient problem. These sessions may be performed by a cardiac surgical liaison nurse in cooperation with the cardiologist, a psychologist and the patient's private physician in order to increase motivation for postoperative employment [39].

Certain interventions may provide some improvement in life quality. Depression is the most common psychological aftermath of coronary bypass surgery, affecting approximately 30% of patients, and results in failure to achieve the quality of life consistent with good surgical outcome. Pimm and Jude, who have investigated intervention strategies for coronary bypass patients, have demonstrated that short-term counseling, i.e., crisis intervention, during the hospital stay and for eight weeks after discharge from the hospital results in significantly lower depression scores on the Beck Depression Inventory when these patients are compared to a non-intervention group. Depression occurred in 20% of control patients before surgery, increasing to 30% three years after surgery. In the group provided with psychological counseling in the form of crisis intervention, depression was found to occur in only 5% of patients three years after bypass surgery. Similar benefits were attained in patients receiving a handbook rather than personal counseling, lowering depression from 20% before the operation to about 10% 3 months after [40] (Figure 3).

Informed family participation in a comprehensive rehabilitation program gives patient and partner security concerning the level of physical activity possible and avoids frustration resulting from overprotection. It also inspires confidence in the patient's ability to earn his living. Preoperative instructions to patients' spouses on how to provide support in the postoperative period, for instance, resulted in fewer psychological problems [41]. Moreover, when positive expectation of the physical, psychological and social benefits of work

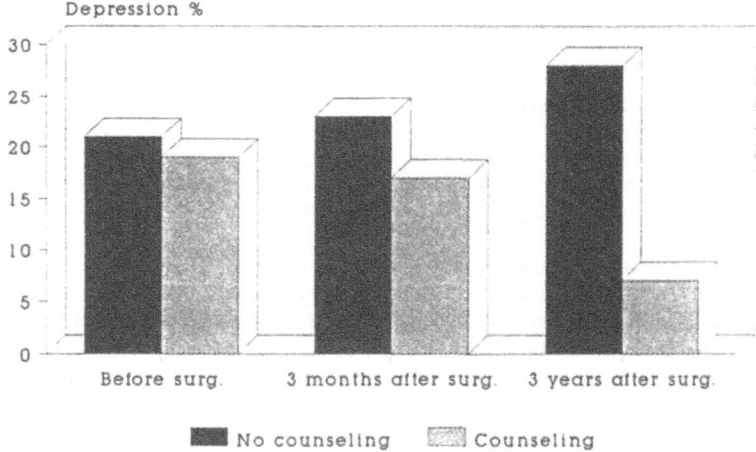

Figure 3. Effect of psychological intervention on depression after coronary bypass surgery (from Pimm and Jude [40]).

are shared by both partners and combined with realistic perception of the patient's illness, then postoperative employment can be expected [42].

7. Conclusion

There is a clear discrepancy between objectively measured functional improvement, personally felt ability to work, and definitive employment rate. Cognitive dysfunction and psychosocial abnormalities in the perioperative phase may discourage patients from returning to work after coronary artery bypass surgery. In order to attain increased postoperative employment, which may be seen as one factor of our patients' quality of life, strategies for comprehensive cardiac rehabilitation, including early identification of patients at risk and broad psychosocial counseling, must be developed.

References

1. Hacker RW, Riedl H, Guggenmoos-Holzmann I, Torka M: Employment status of patients after coronary artery bypass surgery. In: Walter PJ. (ed.) Return to work after coronary artery bypass surgery. Berlin, Heidelberg, New York, Tokyo: Springer-Verlag, 1985;38–45.
2. Hammermeister DE, De Rouen TA, English MT, Dodge HT: Effect of surgical versus medical therapy on return to work in patients with coronary artery disease. Am J Cardiol 1979;44:105–111.

3. Gundle MJ, Reeves BR, Tate S, Raft D, McLaurin LP: Psychosocial outcome after coronary artery surgery. Am J Psychiatry 1980;137-12:1591–1594.

4. La Mendola WF, Pellegrini RV: Quality of life and coronary artery bypass surgery patients. Soc Sci Med 1979;13A:457–461.

5. Newman S, Klinger L, Graham V, Smith P, Harrison M, Treasure T: Subjective reports of cognition in relation to assessed cognitive performance following coronary artery bypass surgery. J Psychosom Res 1989;33:227–233.

6. Cohen F, Lazarus RS: Coping with the stresses of illness. In: Stone GS, Cohen F, Adler NE (eds.) Health Psychology – A Handbook. San Francisco: Jossey-Bass Publishers, 1980;217–254.

7. Garrity TF: Behavioral adjustment after myocardial infarction: a selective review of recent descriptive, correlational, and intervention research. In: Weiss SM, Herd JA, Fox BM (eds.) Perspectives on behavioral medicine. New York; Academic Press 1981;67–68.

8. Krantz DS, Schulz R: A model of life crisis, control and health outcomes: cardiac rehabilitation and relocation of the elderly. In: Baum A, Singer I (ed.) Advances in environmental psychology. Hillsdale N J. Lawrence Erlbaum Ass. 1980;23–57.

9. Moos RH, Tsu VD: The crisis of physical illness: an overview. In: Moos RH (ed.) Coping with physical illness. New York: Plenum Medical Books, 1978;3–21.

10. Gutmann MC, Knapp DN, Pollock ML, Schmidt DH, Simon K, Walcott G: Coronary artery bypass patients and work status. Circulation 1982;66(suppl III):33–42.

11. Cay EL, Vetter N, Philip A, Dugard P: Return to work after a heart attack. J Psychosom Res 1973;17:231–243.

12. Garrity TF: Vocational adjustment after the first myocardial infarction: comparative assessment of several variables suggested in the literature. Soc Sci Med 1973;7:705–707.

13. Kushnir B, Fox KM, Tomlinson IW, Portal RW, Clive PA: The influence of psychological factors and an early hospital follow-up on return to work after first myocardial infarction. Scand J Rehabil Med 1975;7:158.

14. Brown JS, Rawlinson ME: Psychosocial status of patients randomly assigned to medical or surgical therapy for chronic stable angina. Am J Cardiology, 1979;44:543–554.

15. Maeland JG, Havik OE: Psychological predictors for return to work after a myocardial infarction. J Psychosom Res 1987;31–4:471–481.

16. Stanton BA, Jenkins CD, Denlinger P, Savageau JA, Weintraub RM, Goldstein RL: Predictors of employment status after cardiac surgery. JAMA 1983;249-7:907–911.

17. Guiry E, Conroy RM, Hickey N, Mulcahy R: Psychological response to an acute coronary event and its effect on subsequent rehabilitation and lifestyle change. Clin Cardiol 1987;10:256–260.

18. Jenkins CD, Stanton BA, Savageau JA, Delninger P, Klein MD: Coronary artery bypass surgery. Physical, psychological, social and economic outcomes six months later. JAMA 1983;250:782–788.

19. Kinchla J, Weiss T: Psychologic and social outcomes following coronary artery bypass surgery. J Cardiopulmonary Rehabil 1985;5:274–83.

20. Papadopoulos C, Shelley SI, Piccolo M, Beaumont C, Barnett L: Sexual activity after coronary bypass surgery. Chest 1986;90:681–685.

21. Folks DG, Blake DJ, Fleece L, Sokol RS, Freeman III AM: Quality of life six months after coronary artery bypass surgery: a preliminary report. South Med J 1986;79-4:397–399.

22. Langeluddecke P, Fulcher G, Baird D, Hughes C, Tennant C: A prospective evaluation of the psychosocial effects of coronary artery bypass surgery. J Psychosom Res 1989;33-1:37–45.

23. Thurer S: Sexual adjustment following coronary bypass surgery. Rehab Counseling Bull 1981;24:319–322.

24. Bunzel B, Eckersberger F: Arbeitswiederaufnahme nach koronarchirurgischen Eingriffen. Acta Chirurgica Austriaca 1988;20-2:36–40.

25. Ross JK, Diwell AE, Marsh J, Monro JL, Barker DJP: Wessex cardiac surgery follow-up survey: the quality of life after operation. Thorax 1978;33:3–9.
26. Cay EL, Walker DD: Psychological factors and return to work. Heart Journal 1988;9 supplement L:74–81.
27. Wenger NK, Almeida D, Bradford JM, King SB, Hurst JW: Return to work after coronary bypass surgery: Problems and prospects. In: Walter PJ (ed.) Return to work after coronary artery bypass surgery. Berlin, Heidelberg, New York, Tokyo: Springer-Verlag, 1985;323–331.
28. Liddle HV, Jones PD, Gould B, Clayton PD: The rehabilitation of patients following coronary revascularization surgery: social and economic aspects. In: Walter PJ.(ed.) Return to work after coronary artery bypass surgery. Berlin, Heidelberg, New York, Tokyo: Springer-Verlag, 1985;341–353.
29. Gregori AN, Hetzer R, Schwarz B *et al*: Change in quality of life after coronary revascularization. Z. Kardiol. 1983;72:12–17.
30. Hymowitz Z, Freiman I, Borman J, Applebaum A, Gotsman MS: Work status before and after coronary artery bypass surgery. Public Health 1985;99:367–374.
31. Bass C: Psychosocial outcome after coronary artery bypass surgery. Br J Psychiatry 1984; 145: 526–532.
32. Wallwork J, Potter B, Caves PK: Return to work after coronary artery surgery for angina. BMJ 1978;2:1680–1681.
33. Sergeant P, Lesaffre E, Flameng W, Suy R: How predictable is the postoperative work resumption after aortocoronary bypass surgery? Acta Cardiologica 1986;XLI-1:41–52.
34. Zyzanski SJ, Rouse BA, Stanton BA, Jenkins CD: Employment changes among patients following coronary bypass surgery: social, medical, and psychological correlates. Public Health Rep 1982;97-6:558–565.
35. Kornfeld DS, Heller SS, Kenneth AF, Scott NW, Malm JR: Psychological and behavioral responses after coronary artery bypass surgery. Circulation 1982;66(suppl III):24–28.
36. Boulay F, David P, Danchin N, Bourassa MG: Can we improve work status after surgery? In: Walter PJ (ed.) Return to work after coronary artery bypass surgery. Berlin, Heidelberg, New York, Tokyo: Springer-Verlag, 1985; 332–340.
37. Mayou R, Bryant B: Quality of life after coronary artery surgery. Q J Med 1987;62:239–248.
38. Stein G, Jungmann H, Krasemann EO, Zothner M: Inability to work after myocardial infarction: A 5-year follow-up study. In: Walter PJ (ed.) Return to work after coronary artery bypass surgery. Berlin, Heidelberg, New York, Tokyo: Springer-Verlag, 1985;375–379.
39. Raymond M, Conklin C, Schaeffer J, Newstadt G, Matloff JM, Gray RJ: Coping with transient intellectual dysfunction after coronary bypass surgery. Heart Lung 1984;13-5:531–539.
40. Pimm JB, Jude JR: Beck depression inventory scores of coronary bypass patients with and without psychological intervention. In: Willner AE, Rodewald G. (eds.) Impact of cardiac surgery on the quality of life. Neurological and psychological aspects aspects. New York and London: Plenum Press, 1990;447–454.
41. Chatham MA: The effect on family involvement on patient's manifestations of post cardiotomy psychosis. Heart Lung 1978;7:995–9.
42. Russel RO, Abi-Mansour P, Wenger NK: Return to work after coronary artery bypass surgery and percutaneous transluminal angioplasty: issues and potential solutions. Cardiology 1986;73:306–22.

20. The relationship between medical and occupational rehabilitation in two cohorts of coronary artery bypass patients ten years apart

UTA GERHARDT

1. Introduction

The imperfect fit between medical and occupational rehabilitation after coronary artery bypass surgery has long been noticed [1,3,12,14,17]. It has even been suggested that whether or not a patient receives surgical or medical treatment for his/her angina pectoris does not influence whether or not full-time employment is continued [5,9].

Recently, the unsatisfactory situation regarding documentation of beneficial outcome of CABS has led to research focussing on patients' perception of changes of severity of symptoms and ease of everyday living before and after surgery to emphasize CABS's clinical value [4,6]. While remarkable improvements of perceived state of health and reported scope of activities of daily living are thus shown, the question remains under what conditions quality of life due to CABS means a patient's full occupational rehabilitation.

A frequent tacit assumption in the literature is that occupational rehabilitation were more frequent if the welfare state would not provide disability pensions even for medically improved patients who prefer early retirement to continuation of employment in an uncertain labour market [11,13]. On the other hand, Anderson et al. argue that probability of postoperative retirement of CABS patients is elevated by only 10 percent over that of the general population for men aged under 55 years as measured by the U.S. Bureau of Labor Statistics [2, p. 11].

In order to settle the controversy, the following three issues may be addressed: *first*, while different rates of return to work of white-collar and blue-collar workforce have been documented worldwide, their changes since the 1960s have not been investigated on a longitudinal basis. *Second*, while surgery has improved remarkably over the last two and a half decades, patients' return to work has not been conceptualized in its relationship to medical rehabilitation on a case basis. *Third*, while the impact of the family, especially spouse, has been recognized, it is mainly deemed psychological,

Paul J. Walter (ed.): *Quality of Life after Open Heart Surgery*, 215–226.
© 1992 Kluwer Academic Publishers.

not economic; however, the latter is relevant for a patient's occupational rehabilitation [8].

2. Patients and methods

Our study looks at the problem from three angles different from epidemiology. *First*, emulating the case orientation of clinical practice, we focus on case analysis, thus establishing whether discrepancy or adequacy between medical and occupational rehabilitation prevail in each individual case. *Second*, we consider rehabilitation an ongoing process over time which is partly related to the prognosis of symptom reduction due to the operation, and partly liable to reflect changes and developments of the labour market. The ongoing-process nature of rehabilitation has been recognized for mortality, and, to a certain extent, for medical and occupational rehabilitation separately in such well-known longitudinal research as CASS, and the European Multicenter Study [5,15,16]. *Third*, we incorporate the spouse and also the physician into the study. In the study 'Coronary artery bypass surgery and return to work' conducted at Justus Liebig University Giessen Medical School, the general research question is: Can discrepancy between medical and occupational rehabilitation after CABS be accounted for by general biographical or marital aspects of patients' life-situation?

Two study populations are contrasted with each other, namely 30 cases each of a retrospective and a prospective sample some ten years apart in date of operation but carefully selected to match four common criteria indicating maximum likelihood of postoperative return to work: Age at operation not exceeding 55 (57) years, preoperative employment status, LVEF > 50 percent preoperatively, and angiographically confirmed coronary artery disease. Both study populations were drawn from an interview population of 40 (39) cases of patients presently or previously married, or living with a partner. While the prospective interview population was recruited as consecutive cases fulfilling at least three of the four criteria and receiving coronary artery bypass surgery at University Hospital after April 1st, 1987 (until September, 1988), the retrospective interview population was constituted in a two-step procedure. First, all names of patients fulfilling at least two of the four criteria were drawn from the register of patients angiographed at the Max-Planck Cardiovascular Unit after January 1st, 1976, and questionnaires mere mailed to the physicians of the 147 suitable cases who had been angiographed up to 1980. Of these, 115 were returned of which 107 were analysable documenting that 92 patients were alive and could be contacted. Second, 40 patients (patient couples, spouses) as well as their physicians were interviewed using a conversation-like format mostly during a visit to the home or surgery.

While patient couples and their doctors were interviewed once in the

Table 1. Some medical and social characteristics of the retrospective and prospective patient populations.

	Retrospective pilot study	Retrospective study pop.	Prospective study pop.
Age at operation	$N = 107$	$N = 30$	$N = 30$
Up to 50 years	52 (49%)	17 (57%)	15 (50%)
Over 50 years	55 (51%)	13 (43%)	15 (50%)
Disease status	$N = 147$	$N = 30$	$N = 30$
One-vessel disease	20 (14%)	3 (10%)	3 (10%)
Two-vessel disease	33 (22%)	5 (17%)	6 (20%)
Three-vessel disease	71 (48%)	20 (67%)	21 (70%)
Main-stem stenosis	17 (12%)	1 (3%)	–
Multiple/unknown	6 (4%)	1 (3%)	–
Sex	$N = 147$	$N = 30$	$N = 30$
Male	138 (94%)	29 (97%)	28 (93%)
Female	9 (6%)	1 (3%)	2 (7%)
Socio-economic status	$N = 85$	$N = 30$	$N = 30$
Professional, manager	9 (11%)	3 (10%)	–
Higher employee	12 (14%)	5 (17%)	2 (7%)
Middle employee, self-empl.	22 (26%)	7 (23%)	3 (10%)
Upper-class status	43 (51%)	15 (50%)	5 (17%)
Supervisor, low-level empl.	14 (16%)	4 (13%)	10 (33%)
Skilled worker	14 (16%)	5 (17%)	3 (30%)
semi-sk., unskilled worker	14 (16%)	6 (20%)	3 (20%)
Lower-class status	42 (49%)	15 (50%)	25 (83%)
Employment status postop	$N = 85$	$N = 30$	$N = 30$
Return to work	43 (51%)	22 (73%)	14 (47%)
Retirement	42 (49%)	8 (27%)	16 (53%)

retrospective study, covering 7–11 years of postsurgery biography, those in the prospective study were interviewed up to three times, that is, preoperatively, postoperatively after 3 months, and after 18 months; the postoperative physician interview at 3 months was conducted with a member of the surgical team. Furthermore, data on preoperative and postoperative clinical status were elicited from clinical records. In all, 303 tape-recorded interviews were conducted; those with patient couples were on average 60 minutes long, and those with physicians were some 20 minutes long; 76 documentations of clinical records were also established.

The retrospective as well as prospective study populations represent cohorts of 30 surviving married (partnership) cases homogeneous on four criteria, each cohort being investigated through 30 clinical documentations, and 60 tape-recorded interviews for the retrospective cohorts and 180 for the prospective cohorts. Table 1 describes the sample of the retrospective pilot

Table 2. Biographical interview schedule (medical-occupational-family).

Past history occupation and family

Occupation
Explanation of illness ("cause")
Myocardial infarction, diagnosis
Family structure and situation
Marital division of labour re health management
Decision pro surgery

Operation
Perioperative events and in-hospital stay
Rehabilitation hospital stay
Marital health management postoperatively
Marital decisions regarding spouses' occupation(s)
Decision to return to work

Return to work
Marital occupational division of labour
Decision to retire from work

Retirement
Consequences of retirement
Marital health (illness) management today
Marital occupational and domestic division of labour today
Explanation of illness today
Family structure today
Clinical state and health situation today
Family's (patient's) economic situation today

---

study and the two study populations in terms of their medical and social characteristics.

The interview schedule for patients and spouses consisted of a 24-step guideline of topics covering medical history plus occupational and family biography over the entire period after onset of symptoms in chronological order. The interviews followed the schedule as closely as the conversation format permitted but the main topics had to be covered extensively. The interview schedule for physicians covered the same issues in less depth and concentrated on medical history, medication, prognosis, and physician's explanation of patient's coronary artery disease as well as physician's involvement in and evaluation of patient's postoperative history regarding employment. The guideline used to interview patient couples is shown in Table 2.

The tape-recorded interviews with patients and their spouses were either transcribed verbatim or paraphrased in detail with respect to contents and sequence of topics. All interviews with physicians were transcribed. The transcripts were submitted to two steps of data analysis. On the one hand, profiles of patients' medical and occupational rehabilitation were constructed from patient couple narratives, physician interviews, and data elicited from clinical records. These yielded case-based documentation of changes of severity of symptoms preoperatively and postoperatively as well as over time, and related to work before and after CABS. The medical and occupational rehabilitation profiles were combined into case profiles of composite rehabilitation. On the other hand, profiles of family rehabilitation were established, focusing on the relationship between spouses in terms of their contribution to family income through involvement in the labour force. Family rehabilitation is a dynamic concept focusing on whether spouses are employed full-time or part-time, enter or leave the labour force, or remain outside it during various phases of a patient's case biography [7,8].

3. Results

The course of *medical rehabilitation* for the retrospective cohort was determined using a five-point index measurement covering absence or presence of preoperative myocardial infarction, degree of preoperative coronary impairment, quality of operation, clinical state at 18 months postoperatively and at interview, that is, 7–11 years after surgery; for the prospective cohort, the last measurement point was omitted. Indicators of preoperative coronary impairment were number of diseased vessels, left ventricular ejection fraction, and extent of medication directly impinging upon myocardial function; quality of operation was determined through absence or occurrence of perioperative complications as well as revascularization effect; indicators for postoperative clinical state at 18 months were symptomatology as measured through NYHA categorization, extent of medication of direct cardiac impact, and level of ergometric performance; indicators regarding postoperative clinical state 7–11 years after surgery were duration of symptom-free interval, severity of symptoms, and extent of medication with direct cardiac significance.

Figures 1 and 2 show the course of medical rehabilitation for the retrospective and prospective cohorts covering the time period up to 18 months after surgery.

It emerges that the two cohorts operated on ten years apart were remarkably similar with regard to the number of cases with satisfactory and unsatisfactory clinical status 18 months after surgery. As regards the retrospective cohort, no drastic changes as compared with 18 months postoperatively happened to most patients until today; 7–11 years postoperatively the clinical condition of 16 patients was satisfactory while that of 14 patients was unsatisfactory, with 21 of them having remained in the same category while 3 had improved and 6 had deteriorated.

Occupational rehabilitation was measured at 18 months postoperatively for both cohorts (and at 7–11 years after surgery for the retrospective cohort). Since all patients in the two cohorts were employed preoperatively, differences between their postoperative occupational status invoke contexts

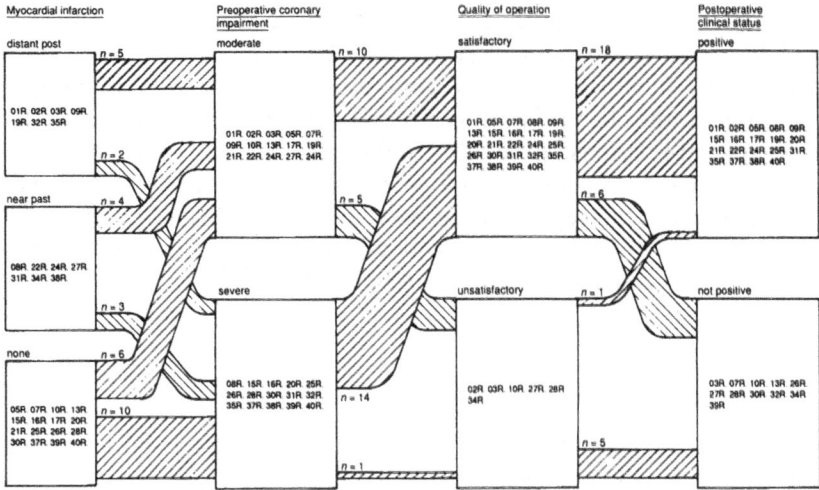

Figure 1. Medical rehabilitation, retrospective cohort (*N* = 30).

favourable or unfavourable to postoperative resumption of occupational work. Since manual work is known to decrease the likelihood of postoperative return to work and blue-collar occupations are mostly lower class, while non-manual work is known to improve the chances of postoperative return to work in white-collar occupations usually of upper-class standing, return to work as opposed to early retirement at 18 months after surgery was analysed by social class. The 34-level scale measuring socio-economic status developed by Handl [10] for the generation born 1920–1940 was divided into six groups of status strata; I–III indicate upper-class status, and IV–VI indi-

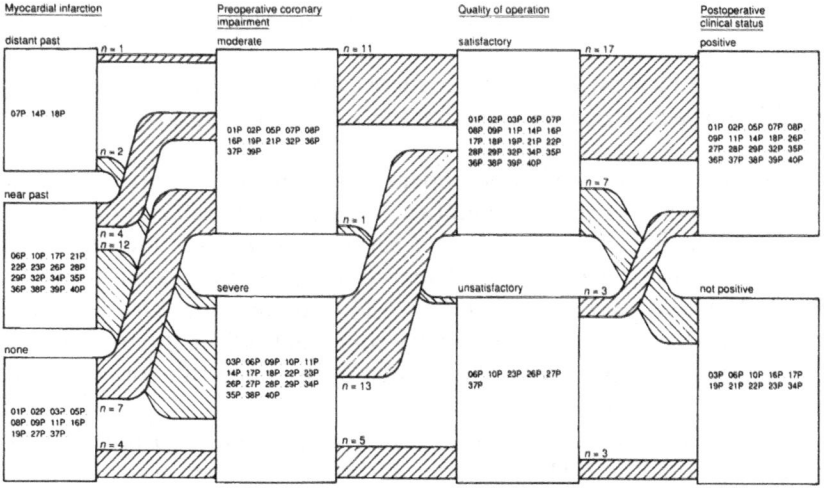

Figure 2. Medical rehabilitation, prospective cohort (*N* = 30).

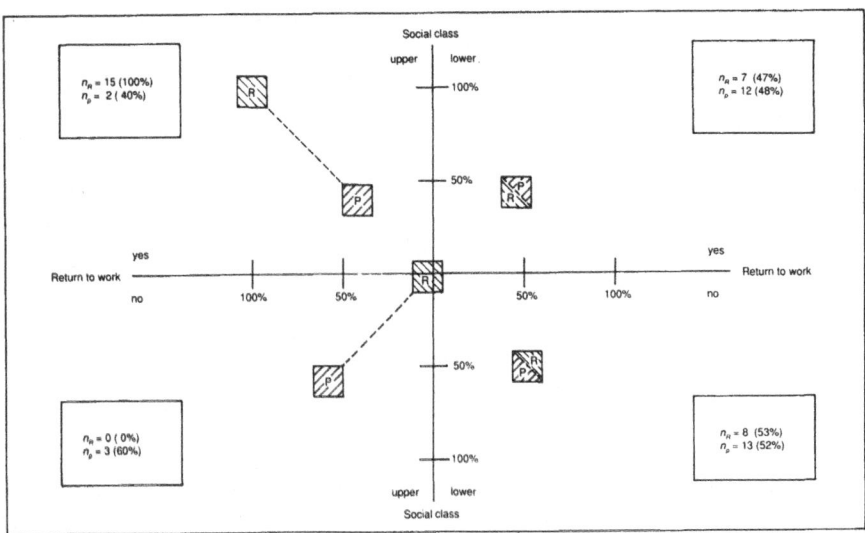

Figure 3. Occupational rehabilitation by social class in the retrospective and prospective cohorts.

cate lower-class status. Figure 3 shows that likelihood of return to work or early retirement remains nearly the same for the lower classes while it undergoes considerable change in the upper classes between the operative period of the retrospective and the prospective cohorts. Although the number of cases in the upper classes is small in the prospective cohort, a tendency of decreasing likelihood of occupational rehabilitation in white-collar occupations is visible.

If *medical and occupational rehabilitation* are considered *together* for each case, four types of composite rehabilitation emerge. First, medical as well as occupational status may be positive, which characterizes *positive adequacy*. Second, both may be negative, which signifies *negative adequacy*. Third, discrepancy may prevail combining unsatisfactory clinical status with positive occupational rehabilitation, which is called *positive discrepancy*. Fourth, satisfactory clinical rehabilitation may go together with early retirement, which is termed *negative discrepancy*. The frequency of the four types of rehabilitation varies if the retrospective cohort is compared with the prospective cohort. This is shown in Figure 4.

It emerges that the number and proportion of cases with negative discrepancy increased dramatically between the retrospective and the prospective cohorts. Furthermore, negative adequacy increased slightly while positive discrepancy decreased at about the same rate as positive adequacy. The distribution of the four types of overall rehabilitation status by social class (upper-class and lower-class status) in the cohorts operated 1976(1977)–1980 and 1987–1988 are shown in Figure 5.

Family rehabilitation was ascertained preoperatively and postoperatively

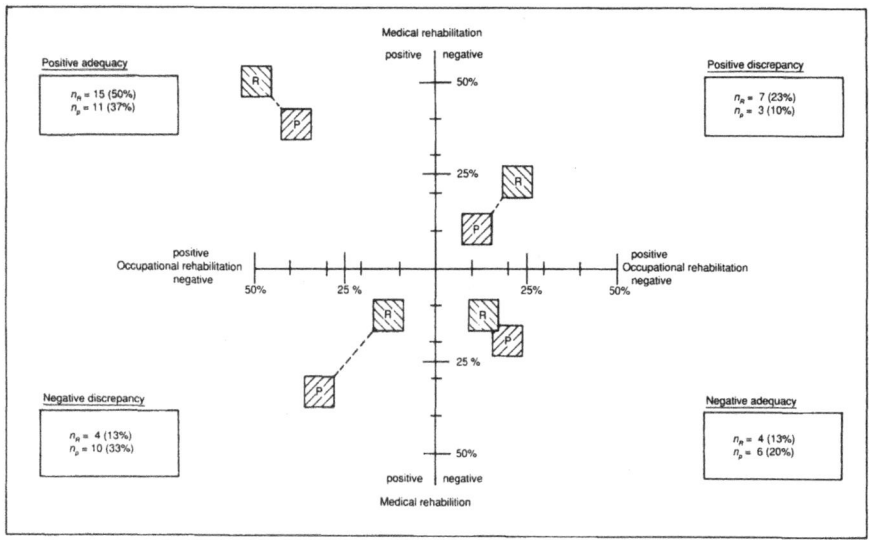

Figure 4. Four types of rehabilitation in the retrospective and prospective cohorts.

for both cohorts. Three basic types may be distinguished: first, traditional marriage means husband's role as sole or main breadwinner, with spouse as housewife, employed part-time, or working in husband's business. Second, dual-career marriage means that both spouses are employed full-time or receive an early-retirement pension from previous full-time employment. Third, wife-related marriage means that the wife is the sole breadwinner, working full-time or part-time, while the husband has either retired early from his employment, is on unemployment or supplementary benefit, or has no income of his own. These are condensed into two types according to

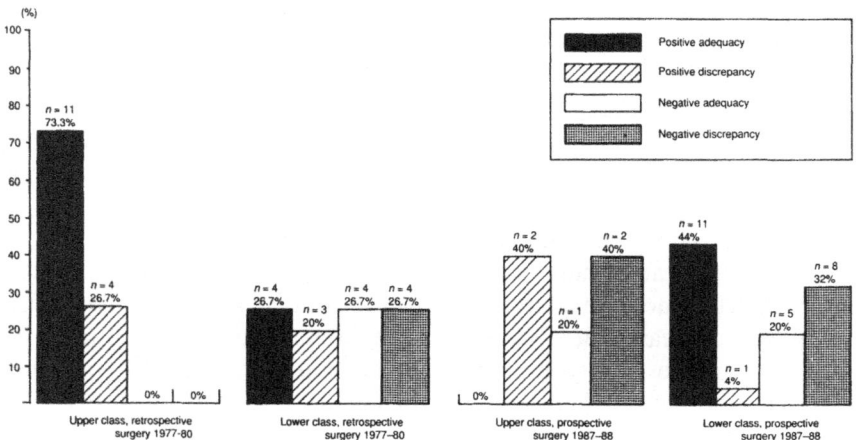

Figure 5. Rehabilitation types by social class in the retrospective and prospective cohorts.

Table 3a,3b. Family rehabilitation in the 1970s and 1980s, by case numbers.

RETROSPECTIVE COHORT

		post-operative		
		traditional	companionship	n
pre-operative	traditional	01R, 02R. 03R. 05R. 07R. 08R. 09R. 13R. 16R. 17R. 18R. 20R. 21R. 24R. 26R. 27R. 28R. 30R. 31R. 34R. 22R. 35R. 37R. 39R. 40R.	15R. 32R. 38R.	28
	companionship		10R. 25R.	2
	n	25	5	30

PROSPECTIVE COHORT

		post-operative		
		traditional	companionship	n
pre-operative	traditional	08P. 16P. 18P. 21P. 23P. 26P. 28P. 29P. 35P. 37P. 38P. 39P. 40P.	03P. 06P. 09P. 10P. 11P. 11P. 22P. 27P.	21
	companionship		01P. 02P. 05P. 07P. 14P. 19P. 32P. 34P. 36P.	9
	n	13	17	30

▨▨▨ upper class
☐ lower class

the wife's contribution to the economic livelihood of the marriage/family: *Traditional* or *companionship* marriage, the latter comprising dual-career and wife-related marital structure. Tables 3a and b show dramatic changes between the second half of the 1970s and of the 1980s, documented through preoperative and postoperative family rehabilitation in the retrospective and prospective cohorts.

It emerges that between the preoperative and postoperative life-situation the frequency of traditional family rehabilitation changed in the retrospective cohort from 28 to 25 cases, and that of companionship marriages from 2 to 5 cases; but in the prospective cohort the number of traditional marriages decreased from 21 to 13 cases, and companionship marriages increased from 9–17 cases. While in both cohorts the number of cases with companionship structure doubled between the preoperative and the postoperative measurement points, the likelihood of the prospective cohort to live in a companionship marriage prior to surgery was four times that of the retrospective cohort.

4. Discussion

Our study populations are homogenous on one socio-medical, two medical, and two social criteria, namely, relatively young age at operation, high preoperative LVEF, angiographically confirmed coronary-artery disease, preoperative full-time employment, and married status (living with a partner). Our research is particularly interested in discrepancies between medical and occupational rehabilitation in this patient population of high likelihood of postoperative return to work.

Our data show that while the proportion of cases with satisfactory postoperative clinical status (positive medical rehabilitation) was nearly the same in the retrospective and prospective cohorts (see Figures 1 and 2), the proportion of cases postoperatively returning to employment decreased by a quarter from 73 percent in the retrospective study to 47 percent in the prospective study (Table 2). This means that despite the quality of revascularization remaining unchanged over the decade, the outcome of successful occupational rehabilitation occurred in considerably fewer cases in the late 1980s than 1970s.

The research question was whether biographical and marital life-situation can account for discrepancies between the two sides of rehabilitation.

Positive and negative discrepancy vary over time. If the data for 18 months after surgery are considered for the cohorts operated on in the 1970s and 1980s, return to work despite negative clinical condition (positive discrepancy) and early retirement despite positive clinical condition (negative discrepancy) reverse their positions among the four types of rehabilitation (see Figure 4). In the retrospective cohort, positive discrepancy occurred in 7 cases, but in the prospective cohort, only in 3 cases. At the same time, negative discrepancy occurred 4 times in the retrospective cohort but 10 times in the prospective cohort. Thus, while the likelihood of discrepancy in general increased slightly over the decade, that of negative discrepancy increased two-and-a-half-fold while that of positive discrepancy decreased to about one half between the two cohorts.

Can it be argued that the increased frequency of companionship marital structure in the prospective study population means that a facilitation context is discovered for negative discrepancy? Among the 9 preoperative companionship marriages in the prospective cohort are 4 cases of postoperative negative discrepancy, and among the 8 cases changing to companionship structure after surgery are a further 2 with negative discrepancy. Taken together, 17 cases of companionship marriage include 6 cases of negative discrepancy while 13 cases of traditional marriage include 4 cases. Among the latter, as the tape-recorded interview data reveal, 3 of the wives are also working although not in regular employment but on an hourly basis as part of what is often called shadow economy. In comparison, only 2 of the 8 wives do this who live in traditional marriages where the relationship between the patient's medical and occupational rehabilitation is either positive or negative adequacy.

To conclude, the known increase of frequency of wives' employment over the last decade in the general population may throw some light on the increase of companionship and the decrease of traditional marital patterns as observed in our retrospective and prospective study populations operated on in the late 1970s and the late 1980s. The tendency away from husband's sole responsibility for family livelihood forms a background to the prospective cohort husbands' increased preference for early retirement, often when successfully revascularized, frequently in cases where wives continue or take up employment. At the same time, likelihood of positive discrepancy regarding postoperative rehabilitation status is decreasing while traditional marriages become less frequent in the general population.

Acknowledgement

The research project is funded by the German Research Council (Deutsche Forschungsgemeinschaft) under grant No. Ge 313/1-4. Co-researcher is Dr. phil. Beate Rachstein. For advice and support we wish to thank Prof. Dr. Friedrich Wilhelm Hehrlein, Director of the Department of Cardiovascular Surgery at Justus Liebig University Medical School Hospital Giessen, and Prof. Dr. Martin Schlepper, Director of the Kerckhoff-Klinik and the Max-Planck Institute of Cardiovascular Disease Research, Bad Nauheim (Germany).

References

1. Almeida D, Bradford M, Wenger NK, King SB, Hurst W: Return to work after coronary artery bypass surgery. Circulation 1983;68:(Suppl. II):295313.
2. Anderson AJ, Barboriak JJ, Hoffman RG, Mullen DC, Walter JA: Age- and sex-specific incidence and main factors. In: Walter PJ ed. Return to work after coronary artery bypass surgery. Heidelberg: Springer, 1985.
3. Blachy PH, Blachy BJ: Vocational and emotional status of 263 patients after heart surgery. Circulation 1968;38:524–532.
4. Caine N, Harrison SCW, Sharples LD, Wallwork J: Prospective study of quality of life before and after coronary artery bypass grafting. Brit Med J 1983;302:511–516.
5. CASS Principal Investigators and Their Associates. Coronary Artery Surgery Study (CASS): A randomized trial of coronary artery bypass surgery. Quality of life in patients randomly assigned to treatment groups. Circulation 1983;68:951–960.
6. Gerhardt U: The discrepancy between social and medical rehabilitation of patients with coronary heart disease. In: Walter PJ ed. Return to work after coronary artery bypass surgery. Heidelberg: Springer 1985a.
7. Gerhardt U:,Family rehabilitation in end-stage renal failure. In: Stevens E, Monkhouse P eds. Proceedings of the European Dialysis and Transplant Nurses Association. Vol. 13. London: Pitman Medical, 1985b.
8. Gerhardt U: Family rehabilitation and longterm survival of chronic renal failure patients. In: Albrecht GL, Levy JA eds. Advances in medical sociology II: Chronic illness. Greenwich, CT: JAI Press, 1991.
9. Hammermeister KE, DeRouen TA, English MT, Dodge HT: Effect of surgical versus medical therapy on return to work in patients with coronary artery disease. Am J Cardiol 1979;44:105–111.
10. Handl J: Sozioökonomischer Status und der Prozess der Statuszuweisung – Entwicklung

und Anwendung einer Skala. In: Handl J, Mayer KU, Müller W eds. Klassenlagen und Sozialstruktur. Frankfurt/New York: Campus, 1977.

11. Killip T: Twenty years of coronary bypass surgery. N Engl J Med 1988;319:366–368.

12. Klonoff H, Campbell C, Kavanagh-Gray D, Mizgala H, Munro I: Two-year follow up of coronary artery bypass surgery. J Thorac Cardiovasc Surg 1989;97:78–85.

13. Niles NW, Vander Salm TJ, Cutler BS: Return to work after coronary artery bypass operation. J Thorac Cardiovasc Surg 1980;79:916–921.

14. Russell RO, Abi-Mansour P, Wenger NK: Return to work after coronary artery bypass surgery and percutaneus transluminal angioplasty: Issues and potential solutions. Cardiology 1986;73:306–322.

15. Varnauskas E and the European Coronary Surgery Study Group. Survival, myocardial infarction and employment status in a prospective randomized study of coronary bypass surgery. Circulation 1985;72:(Suppl. V):90–101.

16. Varnauskas E and the European Surgery Study Group. Twelve-year follow-up of survival in the Randomized European Coronary Surgery Study. N Engl J Med 1988;319:332–337.

17. Wallwork J, Potter B, Caves PK: Return to work after coronary artery surgery for angina. Brit Med J 1978;i:1680–1681.

21. Factors influencing quality of life after CABG: a prospective study

VADIM P. ZAITSEV, TATYANA A. AIVAZYAN,
NATALIYA I. GRACHEVA and DMITRY S. DEKIN

1. Introduction

The concept of a patient's quality of life (QL) naturally covers first of all those dimensions which are affected by a disease and its treatment. Usually researchers focus on such big areas of QL as functional capacity and symptoms [3,5,6]. However, another important component of QL – perception of changes of life due to disease, level of well-being and satisfaction with life – has not yet been paid proper attention. A decrease of QL does not necessarily mean negative changes of life style as a result of the disease, however. First such changes may be perceived by a patient not as something unpleasant, threatening, disabling and so forth, but sometimes even as something positive for him. Second, a patient may suffer not only from actual changes to his mode of life: he may also suffer from the possibility of negative changes, even though they may not occur. In this connection, some years ago, our team developed a QL Scale measuring *level of a patient's dissatisfaction with regard to real and/or expected negative changes in his life* related with a cardiovascular disease [4]. This scale was validated and shown to discriminate patients with a variety of conditions [1].

QL of patients after coronary artery bypass graft surgery (CABG) is an area of special interest for investigators, since operative risk, physical and psychological suffering during the first days after the operation, and financial expenses, may not be covered by any positive influence on mortality and morbidity and, therefore, changes in different aspects of QL after the operation should be taken into account among the other important outcomes. The least studied aspect of QL after CABG is the perception of changes in life, the level of well-being, and satisfaction with life, after the operation. The factors influencing QL in this dimension after CABG have been even less well studied. The aim of our study was to investigate some of them.

Paul J. Walter (ed.): Quality of Life after Open Heart Surgery, 227–234.
© 1992 Kluwer Academic Publishers.

2. Subjects and methods

A group of 154 inpatients (males) with CHD were examined 2–3 days before CABG. Forty-eight of the patients were invited for a one-year follow-up examination; five of them did not participate for a variety of reasons (heart failure – 2, cerebral tumor – 1, relocation to another city – 1, refused to collaborate – 1). Thus 43 patients were followed-up (age 27–65, mean 49.1 ± 1.3 years).

The clinical examination performed at the Department for Cardiovascular Surgery (Professor R.S. Akchurin, head) of the National Cardiology Research Centre included: (a) coronary angiography; (b) standardised progressive exercise stress test performed on an electrically braked bicycle ergometer; and (c) registration of frequency of angina pectoris episodes.

Psychological examination included the Quality of Life Scale [4], Mini-Mult [7] and Interpersonal Relation Test [2]. The data obtained were analyzed using the SPSS statistical package.

3. Results

Analysis of *QL changes during the one-year follow-up* revealed an increase (improvement) of total QL index in 60% of the patients and a decrease in 35% of the patients. The total QL index before CABG was −8.6 ± 0.6, and one year later it was −6.5 ± 0.7 ($p < 0.05$). The improvement of QL was mainly due to a perceived decrease of restrictions ($p < 0.05$): in everyday life (the subscale index increased in 44%, decreased in 16% of the patients), in physical activity (40% and 9%), in leisure activity (33% and 2%) and in sexual life (37% and 12% of the patients, respectively).

Analysis of correlations of QL changes and clinical and psychological indicies changes duirng follow-up revealed interrelations between the QL total index and Mini-Mult scale 4 ($r = − 0.62$, $p < 0.01$) and between QL subscales and Mini-Mult scales (Table 1). One can see that the different QL subscales correlate with different sets of Mini-Mult scales. All the correlations are negative, except one. Viewed as a whole, this means that the improvement of QL was based on an improvement of the patient's psychological condition (decrease of Mini-Mult profile on clinical scales).

Correlations between QL subscales changes and physical tolerance changes during follow-up were also found (Table 2). The correlations between QL changes due to all the restrictions, changes of friends' attitudes and smoking limitation shows that QL improvement parallels a decrease of the number of angina pectoris episodes and vice versa. But QL improvement due to social status and/or income parallels a *decrease* of physical capacity.

An analysis of causes of paradoxical relation of QL social status/income subscale with physical capacity and with Mini-Mult scale 1 (Figure 1) revealed

Table 1. Correlations between QL and Mini-Mult index changes during 1 year follow-up.

QL subscales	Mini-Mult scales	r	p <
* All the restrictions	4	−0.61	0.01
* Restrictions of	1	−0.51	0.05
physical activity	3	−0.51	0.05
	4	−0.67	0.01
	7	−0.56	0.01
* Social status/income lowering	1	+0.73	0.001
* Necessity to be under	4	−0.66	0.01
treatment	6	−0.57	0.01
	7	−0.56	0.01
	8	−0.57	0.01

two different subgroups of patients. *In one subroup* the increase of QL social status/income subscale paralleled a decrease of Mini-Mult scale 1 and an increase of physical capacity during the one-year follow-up. *In the other subroup* increase of QL social status/income subscale was connected with an increase of Mini-Mult scale 1 and a decrease of physical capacity.

Changes in a QL subscale do not necessarily parallel changes in the QL scale as a whole. Thus (Figure 2), in patients whose QL social status/income subscale paralleled an increase of Mini-Mult scale 1 and a decrease of physical capacity, the total QL index decreased during the one-year follow-up (-2.0 ± 1.5). In patients whose increase of QL social status/income subscale was connected with a decrease of Mini-Mult scale 1 and an increase of physical capacity, total QL index increased ($+6.6 \pm 0.8$, $p < 0.01$).

The QL total index improved after CABG in both: *pre-CABG employed* (initially -7.6 ± 0.6, 1 year later -4.8 ± 0.5) and *pre-CABG unemployed* patients (-8.5 ± 0.5 and -7.1 ± 0.7 scores, respectively).

In pre-CABG unemployed patients an improvement of QL total index did not depend on whether a patient returned to work after the operation (in-

Table 2. Correlations of dynamics of QL and physical tolerance indices during follow-up.

QL changes due to:	Factors	r	p <
* All the restrictions	AP at rest & on effort	−0.39	0.10
* Changes of attitude of friends or colleagues	AP on effort	−0.39	0.10
* Smoking reduction or cessation	AP on effort	−0.36	0.10
* Lowering of income and/or social status	physical capacity	−0.41	0.05

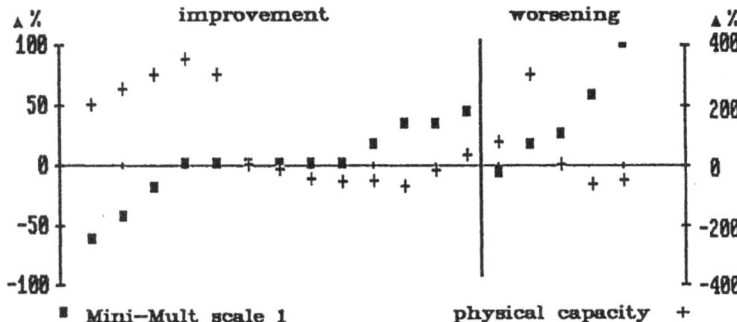

Figure 1. Interrelations of QL social status/income subscale, physical capacity and Mini-Mult scale 1 changes at one-year follow-up.

itially -6.3 ± 1.7, 1 year later -5.1 ± 0.6) or not (-9.9 ± 0.9 and -7.5 ± 0.8, respectively).

Among the pre-CABG employed patients, QL improved dramatically for those who returned to work after CABG (initially -9.8 ± 1.3, 1 year later -4.5 ± 0.7), whereas the picture was the reverse for those who did not return (-5.8 ± 0.7 and -8.4 ± 0.4, respectively). The differences between those subgroups of patients in QL changes were highly significant ($p < 0.001$).

In order to discover *predictors of QL changes* we compared pre-CABG data of 26 patients with *QL total index improvement* and 15 patients with *QL total index worsening at one-year follow-up*. Initially the groups were comparable in respect of age, physical capacity and coronary angiography data, but differed in pre-CABG QL and psychological characteristics. Thus, in patients with QL total index improvement after CABG, this index was initially much lower (-10.0 ± 0.8) than in patients with QL total index

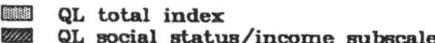

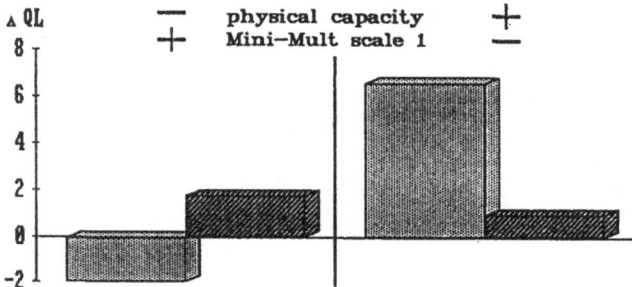

Figure 2. Interrelations of QL total index and QL social status/income subscale changes at one-year follow-up.

Table 3. Correlations between pre-CABG Mini-Mult scores and 1 year follow-up QL indices changes (total QL index improved).

QL subscales	Mini-Mult scales	r	$p <$
Restrictions			
* of leisure activity	F	+0.52	0.01
	K	−0.42	0.05
* of physical activity	F	−0.50	0.01
	4	+0.44	0.05
* on work	6	+0.44	0.05
* Smoking reduction	7	+0.61	0.01
or cessation	7	+0.40	0.05
* Lowering of income	7	+0.45	0.05

worsening at one-year follow-up (-5.6 ± 0.6). This difference was highly significant ($p = 0.0003$). Significant differences were also revealed in QL subscales as follows: necessity for treatment (-1.2 ± 0.2 and -0.4 ± 0.2, $p = 0.002$), all the restrictions (-1.4 ± 0.2 and -0.9 ± 0.1, $p = 0.03$), in particular: at work (-0.8 ± 0.2 and -0.3 ± 0.1, $p = 0.03$), in physical activity (-1.0 ± 0.2 and -0.5 ± 0.1, $p = 0.03$) and in daily activity (-1.4 ± 0.2 and -0.8 ± 0.1 scores, $p = 0.009$, respectively).

According to Interpersonal Relation Test data patients with QL total index improvement during follow-up had an initial conflict level lower ($p < 0.1$) than patients with QL total index worsening after CABG: at work (25.1 ± 3.2 and 26.7 ± 6.0) and with wife (10.3 ± 1.0 and 14.5 ± 2.8).

Analysis of correlations of *pre-CABG clinical and psychological status data* with *QL changes after the operation* was performed separately for patients with QL total index improvement and QL total index worsening during foliow-up. In patients with improvement of QL total index, the index changes correlated with pre-CABG Mini-Mult scale 9 ($r = +0.52$, $p < 0.001$). Correlations of pre-CABG Mini-Mult scales and different QL subscale changes during follow-up were also revealed (Table 3). In patients with worsening of QL total index, besides correlations of pre-CABG Mini-Mult scales with QL subscales changes (Table 4), pre-CABG exercise tolerance correlated with changes in the QL social status/income subscale during follow-up ($r = +0.87$, $p < 0.01$).

4. Discussion

As expected, in the majority of the patients QL improved 1 year after CABG. The improvement of QL was mainly due to a decrease of restrictions in everyday life. Analysis of correlations between changes of QL and Mini-Mult indices during follow-up revealed that improvement of QL was con-

Table 4. Correlations between pre-CABG Mini-Mult scores and 1 year follow-up QL indices changes (total QL index worsened).

QL subscales	Mini-Mult scales	r	p <
* All the restrictions	L	+0.64	0.01
	K	+0.59	0.05
Restrictions			
* of daily activity	L	−0.58	0.05
* on work	4	+0.54	0.05
* Smoking reduction or cessation	K	−0.65	0.01
* Necessity to be under treatment	6	+0.55	0.05
	7	+0.56	0.05

nected with reduction of conflict level, aggressiveness, impatience, impulsiveness (reduction in Mini-Mult scale 4). In other words, the patients became more socially adapted and felt more integrated into the community.

It is also important to note that the different QL subscales correlated with different sets of Mini-Mult scales. For example, improvement of QL due to perceived decrease of restrictions in physical activity paralleled a decrease of anxiety, fears about health condition, complaints and neuroticism (Mini-Mult scales 1, 3, 4 and 7). Improvement of QL due to a decrease of the dependency on treatment was associated with a reduction of sensitivity, tension, impatience, hostility, aggressiveness, and improving interpersonal relations (Mini-Mult scales 4, 6, 7 and 8).

One most interesting finding was the paradoxical correlations: a QL improvement in social status/income subscale paralleled a decrease of physical capacity and increase of hypochondriasis. We could think of only one explanation: bodily preoccupation (which *per se* may worsen performance during the bicycle test or may be conditioned by lowered physical capacity) leads to an increase position of *health* in the patients' value system and – as a result – to a decrease of negative experiences concerning social status and income, perceived as being less important in this situation. As a result of this, QL in this particular subscale may improve just because problems concerning social status and income do not bother the patient, much, any more.

Further analysis revealed, in regard to improvement of QL in social status/income subscale, two different subgroups hide behind the same phenomenon: either with improvement of both physical and psychological conditions, or with their worsening.

It appeared that improvement of QL in the social status/income subscale did not necessarily mean an improvement of QL as a whole. According to the data obtained, a decrease of physical capacity together with an increase of hypochondriasis leading to an improvement of the index in that QL subscale was accompanied by a worsening of the QL total index. Improvement of physical and psychological condition naturally led to an improvement of both QL indicies: total and in the subscale.

After CABG, QL improved in patients who were both employed and unemployed before the operation. However, in those who worked before and returned to work after CABG, QL was surprisingly lower at the baseline but much better at the one-year follow-up than in patients who had worked before but not returned to work after the operation. It is likely that the patients who had worked before the operation and returned to work after CABG initially had had a higher level of demands, which had governed their more intensive disatisfaction with existing restrictions related with the disease. This could govern their higher motivation for returning to work after the operation. Return to work, as well as a quite favourable perception of even the slightest improvement of their condition after the operation by those patients, may explain the dramatic improvement of their QL.

As to those patients who worked before CABG but did not return to work after the operation, they were likely to have lower motivation for work even before the operation and – as a result – their pre-CABG QL was not too low, despite the restrictions related with the disease. After the operation the patients were able to justify their unwillingness to work in their own eyes as well as in the eyes of significant third parties. In turn, being on a disability pension did not allow any increase of QL proportionally to clinical improvement after the operation.

Analysis of predictors of QL changes revealed that the strongest one was the pre-CABG QL total index: a lower QL predicts its improvement, whereas considerably higher QL predicts a worsening one year after the operation. A higher level of interpersonal conflict at work and with the spouse before the operation is likely to predict a worsening of QL after CABG.

In patients with QL improvement, pre-CABG Mini-Mult scales correlate with changes during follow-up – in particular QL subscales in different ways – which may reflect different patterns of value hierarchies (QL subscales) which relate with personality traits (Mini-Mult scales). The correlation patterns in patients with a worsening of total QL index differed from those in patients with a improvement of the total QL index at follow-up.

5. Conclusion

1. After CABG, quality of life improves due to the perceived reduction of everyday life restrictions.
2. Quality of life after the operation is influenced by: pre-CABG quality of life, employment, psychological factors and initial physical tolerance.

References

1. Aivazyan TA, Zaitsev VP: Life quality in patients with essential hypertension. Kardiologiia 1989;9:43–46.
2. Dzhaginov EA, Vorobiov GV, Sheremeta VM: Method of studing interpersonal relations in patients with myocardial infarction,. Psykhologicheski Zhurnal 1982;3:93–99.
3. Fletcher AE, Hunt BM, Bulpitt CJ: Evaluation of quality of life in clinical trials of cardiovascular disease. J Chron Dis 1987;40:557–566.
4. Gladkov AG, Zaitsev VP, Aronov DM, Sharfnadel MG: Quality of life assessment in patients with cardiovascular disease. Kardiologiia 1982;2:100–103.
5. Walter PJ, ed. Return to Work after Coronary Artery Bypass Surgery: Psychosocial and Economic Aspects. Springer-Verlag. Berlin, Heidelberg, 1985;395 pp.
6. Wenger NK, Mattson ME, Furberg CD, Elinson J: Assessment of quality of life in clinical trials of cardiovascular therapies. Am J Cardiol 1984;54:908–913.
7. Zaitsev VP: A version of psychological test Mlni-Mult. Psykhologicheski Zhurnal 1981;3:118–123.

22. Changes of coronary risk factors in women after elective coronary bypass surgery

FRANK LOSKOT, BERND HARTMANN, PETRUS NOVOTNY and
NIKOLAS MOUSELIMIS

1. Introduction

Abnormal serum lipid concentration and elevated blood pressure are the two established risk factors which have a major influence on the development of atherosclerosis. Two other important determinants of atherosclerosis are male sex and increasing age. Coronary artery disease (CAD) in younger women is less frequent than in males and shows some peculiarities when compared with CAD in males. Most risk factors are of similar importance in men and women, but some have a stronger influence in women.

Cigarette smoking has a similar implication in males and females and corresponds to an increased risk of sudden coronary death and myocardial infarction. Smoking further aggravates the effect of other risk factors such as hypercholesterolaemia. Increased awareness that serum lipids and smoking are the major coronary artery disease risk factors has led to their prospective screening in the women referred for coronary bypass surgery (CABG).

2. Methods

Analysis of atherogenic risk factors was taken in relation to following two parameters: hypercholesterolaemia and cigarette smoking. The lipid profile and smoking habits were determined before CABG, within 6–7 weeks, 6–7 months and 30–32 months after operation in 48 premenopausal women (group A) between the ages of 39 and 53 years (mean 46.7 ± 5.5) and 54 postmenopausal women (group B) aged 52 to 66 years (mean 56.8 ± 7.2). In each of the examinations the women were asked about their menstrual status. Postmenopausal women were defined as having had no menstruation during the last 6 months before CABG. There was no woman who developed secondary amenorrhrea or who had bilateral oöphorectomy or oestrogen treatment.

All women were asked on admission to determine their awareness of prior

Paul J. Walter (ed.): Quality of Life after Open Heart Surgery, 235–241.
© 1992 Kluwer Academic Publishers.

risk factor evaluation and of any therapy. On the basis of this interview, patients were placed into one of three subgroups. In subgroup 1 blood lipids were normal; women in subgroup 2 had been referred to the physician to help correct the lipids by dietary low cholesterol intervention; and women in subgroup 3 had been started on pharmacological therapy.

Information about smoking habits was obtained by interview.

All patients were examined by quantitative coronary angiography 3–5 months before and 30–32 months (31.5 ± 0.6) after CABG.

Coronary stenosis was determined quantitatively after administration of 0.8 mg nitroglycerin in order to prevent coronary spasm. The percentage diameter stenosis of coronary lumen obstructions was quantified using a Vernier.

Total cholesterol and the serum triglyceride level were determined enzymatically by an automated analyzer. The level of low density lipoprotein cholesterol (LDL) was calculated as the difference between the level of total cholesterol and the sum of HDL cholesterol and one-fifth of the triglyceride level.

3. Statistical analysis

The results have been reported as the arithmetic mean $\pm$ the standard error of the mean. The significance of differences between mean values was estimated with the Student's t-test. The hypothesis of no difference in frequencies between groups was tested with the χ^2-test. Differences were considered statistically significant for values of $p < 0.05$.

4. Results

The results of lipid analysis are illustrated in Tables 1, 2 and 3. Thirty-five (64.8%) and 39 (72.2%) women, respectively, referred for coronary artery bypass grafts (CABG) in the postmenopausal group B had high serum cholesterol, compared with 16 (33.3%) and 21 of 48 (43.8%) patients in the premenopausal group A, respectively. The difference was statistically significant ($p < 0.001$–0.003). Total serum cholesterol, high density lipoprotein (HDL), low density lipoprotein (LDL) and serum triglycerides (TG) in both groups (A,B) were significantly lower within four to seven weeks after CABG. The differences between groups A and B were not significant. By contrast there was a significantly lowering of total serum cholesterol and HDL cholesterol within seven weeks and 32 months, respectively, in group A after CABG compared with the preoperative period.

The number of atherogenic risk factors is listed in Tables 3a and 3b.

If one looks at the lipid profile with respect to smoking habits in all groups,

Table 1. Prevalence of coronary risk factors – *high serum cholesterol.*

		Group A ($n = 48$)	Group B ($n = 54$)	*p*-value
Before CABG	chol.	33.3% (16)	64.8% (35)	0.001
	chol./HDL	43.8% (21)	72.2% (39)	0.003
After CABG	chol.	16.7% (8)	24.1% (13)	n.s.
7 weeks	chol./HDL	22.9% (11)	31.5 (17)	0.04
7 months	chol.	29.2% (14)	55.6 (30)	0.003
	chol./HDL	33.3% (16)	66.7% (36)	0.001
32 months	chol.	25.0% (12)	61.1%	0.001
	chol./HDL	20.8% (10)**	74.1% (40)	0.001

High blood cholesterol $\geqslant 240$ mg/dl respectively cholesterol/HDL $\geqslant 4.5$.
** Significantly lowering period in relation to preoperative period.

it can be seen that, after CABG (Table 3b), there was a significant reduction of blood lipids and cigarette smokers in premenopausal women (group A/1,2,3) compared with group B. In group A there were 34 (71%) cigarette smokers before CABG (23 ± 11 cigarettes/day) compared with 20 women (37%; 19 ± 9 cigarettes/day) in group B (Table 4). The differences between both group were significant ($p < 0.001$). In relation to smoking status, after CABG (7 and 32 months), there was a significant lowering of serum lipids ($p < 0.002$) by comparing those women who smoked before CABG (Table 4; group A and B) and later stopped (group A 85.3%; group B 25.0%) with those who contined to smoke after CABG (group A 14.7%; group B 75.0%). The greatest reduction of serum lipids was seen in women who stopped smoking and started on drug therapy (group A3,B3).

Angiographic findings are summarised in Tables 3 and 5.

A total of 102 women (group A and B) have completed quantitative coronary angiography before and 30–32 months after CABG. There were no significant differences in the number of coronary arteries involved (V/pt) in premenopausal (group A) and postmenopausal women (group B) before and after CABG (Table 5). All patients underwent repeated angiography in 31.5 ± 0.6 months after CABG and 35.3 ± 1.1 months after the first

Table 2. Prevalence of coronary risk factors – *high serum triglycerides.*

	Group A ($n = 48$)	Group B ($n = 54$)	*p*-value
Before CABG	56.3% (27)	29.6% (16)	< 0.01
After CABG 7 weeks	18.8% (9)	20.4% (11)	n.s.
7 months	29.2% (14)	31.5% (17)	n.s.
32 months	35.4% (17)**	37.0% (20)	n.s.

High serum triglycerides $\geqslant 200$ mg/dl.
** Significantly lowering in relation to preoperative period.

Table 3. Extent of coronary disease and blood lipids in patient groups before (Table 3a) and after (Table 3b) coronary surgery (32 months).

Table 3a

Group/ subgroup	n	chol (mg%)	chol/ HDL	LDL/ HDL	TG (mg%)	Cigarette smokers	V/pt
A/1	32	229.5 ± 10.7	5.88 ± 0.71	4.38 ± 0.32	194.3 ± 17.9	24	2.8 ± 0.3
A/2	13	228.4 ± 7.0	5.00 ± 0.30	4.47 ± 0.48	181.8 ± 31.4	8	2.8 ± 0.6
A/3	3	227.5 ± 9.4	5.02 ± 0.25	3.88 ± 0.31	173.5/14.4	2	2.4 ± 0.4
B/1	18	239.2 ± 8.7	5.89 ± 0.84	4.23 ± 0.45	219.5 ± 16.9	4	2.9 ± 0.4
B/2	24	233.2 ± 11.8	5.79 ± 0.27	4.57 ± 0.66	196.7 ± 27.6	8	3.3 ± 0.5
B/3	12	231.3 ± 6.7	5.74 ± 0.71	3.87 ± 0.53	201.3 ± 34.1	8	2.8 ± 0.4

Table 3b

Group/ subgroup	n	chol (mg%)	chol/ HDL	LDL/ HDL	TG (mg%)	Cigarette smokers	V/pt
A/1	13	222.7 ± 7.7	4.18 ± 0.39	3.99 ± 0.42	169.4 ± 19.2	–	2.9 ± 0.5
A/2	21	221.5 ± 11.8	3.88 ± 0.42	3.87 ± 0.38	167.3 ± 18.2	2	3.1 ± 0.4
A/3	15	216.3 ± 11.2	3.79 ± 0.30	3.63 ± 0.18	162.6/11.8	3	2.1 ± 0.2
B/1	15	242.7 ± 15.6	5.03 ± 0.69	4.17 ± 0.52	218.7 ± 11.1	–	3.3 ± 0.5
B/2	22	231.3 ± 14.5	5.11 ± 0.33	4.22 ± 0.50	190.2 ± 20.2	8	3.6 ± 0.4
B/3	17	229.8 ± 18.3	4.82 ± 0.31	3.81 ± 0.68	178.7 ± 0.19	7	2.7 ± 0.5

Chol. (total cholesterol); HDL (high density lipoprotein); LDL (low density lipoprotein); TG (triglycerides); V/pt. (number of involved coronary vessels per patient); cigarette smoking (>10 cigarettes/day).

Table 4. Prevalence of coronary risk factors – *cigarette smoking.*

	Group A (n = 48)	Group B (n = 54)	p-value
Before CABG	71% (34)	37% (20)	< 0.01
After CABG** 7 weeks	4.2% (2)	7.4% (4)	n.s.
7 months	6.2% (3)	18.5% (10)	<0.03
32 months	10.4% (5)	27.8% (15)	< 0.02

** Currently smokes more than 10 cigarettes per day.

Table 5. Involved vessels per patient (V/pt.) and changes in the percentage diameter stenosis of new coronary lesions (%NL/pt) and the average percentage diameter showing increased stenosis per subject (%D) after CABG.

		Group A (n = 48)	Group B (n = 54)	p-value
Before CABG	V/pt.	2.7	3.5	n.s.
Repeat Angiography	V/pt.	2.8	3.8	n.s.
	%D	37.1	44.8	p = 0.03
	%NL/pt	27	42	p = <0.02

(preoperative) angiogram. The progression was defined as lumen obstruction of ⩾25%. Changes in the average percentage diameter stenosis (% D) also as percentage diameter stenosis of new coronary lesions (% N/pt) per patient progressed significantly in postmenopausal women (group B, Table 5). As opposed to this, among 15 subjects (group A3) who started the pharmacological therapy treatment produced a significant reduction in the progression of atherosclerosis in native coronay arteries.

The average number of arteries involved regressed from 2.4 to 2.1/patient ($p < 0.02$, Table 3). In groups A2–B2 and A3–B3 diet and treatment significantly reduced the percentage of women with any adverse changes in bypass grafts ($p < 0.02$) compared with changes in bypass grafts in group A1 and B1.

5. Discussion

The results from different studies about whether or not there is a relationship between menopausal women and CAD are still contradictory. An increase in CAD has been described, following either natural or surgical menopause in women [1]. The reason for the resistance of women in their reproductive years to coronary atherosclerosis remain poorly understood, as are the reasons for loss of this advantage after the age of menopause. There is no doubt that there are associations between menopause and different risk factors for CAD such as serum cholesterol, serum triglycerides, smoking habits and blood pressure [2]. In most trials treatment of hypercholesterolaemia by diet or by drugs reduced the incidence of CAD. Statistical analyses have shown that reducing total or LDL cholesterol levels consistently reduces the incidence of myocardial infarction or coronary death [3]. The effect is graded: the greater the cholesterol reduction, the larger the benefit. The effect of blood pressure on cardiovascular morbidity and mortality has been well described [4], as has the interaction between blood pressure and serum cholesterol levels. The interrelation of blood lipids and hypertension has been suggested as a partial explanation for the lack of a continued decline in CAD mortality [5]. There is an additional dimension to the lipid–hypertension interaction – antihypertensive drug-induced changes in lipid profile [6–8]. Antihypertensive drugs may be divided into three categories, depending on their effect on either total lipids or a given lipid subfraction: lipid neutral, atherogenic or antiatherogenic. Antihypertensive agents that decrease HDL cholesterol may reduce or even negate the benefits of therapy that successfully reduce blood pressure. With this in mind, proatherogenic antihypertensive agents should be avoided, lipid neutral agents are acceptable, and antiatherogenic agents are preferable.

Serum lipids were significantly lower following CABG. The reduction in serum cholesterol, of HDL, LDL and serum triglycerides after CABG, and the gradual increase in serum lipids within 6–8 weeks may be analogous to the reduction of lipoproteins that occurs after plasma exchange [9,10]. The reduction in serum cholesterol affected by plasma exchange can mimic the decrease in serum lipids observed in patients following CABG.

Angiographic studies [11] have also revealed a relationship between hyperlipidemia and the extent of CAD. In patients after CABG the majority of venous bypass grafts with atheromatous involvement also are correlated with increased LDL and decreased HDL levels. Strict dietary and drug control of hyperlipidemia also retarded progression and induced regression of native vessel and venous bypass graft vessel atherosclerotic lesions after CABG [12,13].

Cigarette smoking provides perhaps the strongest and most consistent correlation with the increased incidence of atherosclerotic disease and appears to be a major contributor to increased risk of disease, generally in combination with other risk factors. Cigarette smoking may induce atherosclerosis by a number of mechanisms [14].

Apparently, cessation of cigarette smoking decreases the risk for development of the clinical sequelae of atherosclerosis and possibly may augment regression of lesions. Cigarette smoking also unequivocally alters lipid levels. Men and women who smoked more than 15 cigarettes daily had lower HDL levels and higher LDL cholesterol and triglyceride levels than the exsmokers and nonsmokers [15]. Cessation of cigarette smoking increases the HDL/LDL ratio [16] and lowers the plasma fibrinogen level [17].

6. Conclusions

Serum cholesterol and triglycerides were significantly lower following CABG. The decrease in serum lipids after CABG appears to be due to the dilutional effect of the pump prime on serum lipids analogous to the reduction of lipids after plasma exchange. Regardless of the precise etiology of lipid reduction after CABG, the authors suggest that lipid screening should not be performed within the first postoperative weeks after open heart surgery.

The clinical implications of these results are that drug therapy of hypercholesterolaemia and stopping of cigarette smoking in premenopausal women are able significantly reduce serum lipids and induce regression of atherosclerotic lesions of native vessels or any adverse changes in bypass grafts. In view of the decisive role of HDL-cholesterol percentage as a coronary risk indicator that significantly surpasses the predictive value of total cholesterol it would seem advisable to consider elevation of the HDL cholesterol as a major goal of any coronary artery disease prevention program.

References

1. Gordon T, Kannel WB, Hjortland MC: Menopause and coronary heart disease. The Framingham Study. Ann Intern Med 1978;89:157–167.
2. Lindquist O, Bengtsson C: Menopausal age in relation to smoking. Acta Med Scand 1978;205:73–77.
3. Peto R, Yusuf S, Collins R: Cholesterol-lowering trial results in their epidemiological context. Circulation 1985;72:(suppl. 2):451–458.
4. Castelli WP: Epidemiology of coronary heart disease: the Framingham Study. Am J. Med 1984;76:4–12.
5. Chobanian AV: Overview: hypertension and atherosclerosis. Am Heart J 1989;116:1:319–322.
6. Ames RP: The effects of antihypertensive drugs on serum lipids and lipoproteins. I. Diuretics. Drugs 1986;32:260–278.
7 Ames RP: The effects of antihypertensive drugs on serum lipids and lipoproteins. II. Non-diuretic drugs. Drugs 1986;32:335–357.
8. Chobanian AV: Hypertension, antihypertensive drugs, and atherogenesis: mechanisms and clinical implications. J Clin Hypertens 1986;3:suppl:148S–157S.
9. Thompson G, Myant N, Kilpatrick D, Oakley C, Raphael M, Steiner R: Assessment of long-term plasma exchange for familial hypercholesterolemia. Br Heart J 1980; 43:680–688.
10. Stein E, Glueck C, Wesselmann A, Owens E, Nichols S, Vink P: Repetive intermittent flow plasma exchange in patients with severe hypercholesterolemia. Atheroclerosis 1981;28:149–164.
11. Thompson ER: Evidence that lowering serum lipids favourably influences coronary heart disease. Q J Med 1987;62:87–95.
12. Blankenhorn D, Nessim SA Johnson RL, Sanmarco ME, Azen SP, Cashin-Hemphill L: Beneficial effects of combined colestipol-niacin therapy on coronary atherosclerosis and coronary venous bypass grafts. JAMA 1987;257:3233–3240.
13. Barndt R Jr, Blankenhorn DH, Crawford DW: Regression and progression of early femoral atherosclerosis in treated hyperlipoproteinemic patients. Ann Intern Med 1977;86:139–144.
14. Klein LW: Cigarette smoking, atherosclerosis and the coronary hemodynamic response: A unifying hypothesis. J Am Coll Cardiol 1984;4:972–6.
15. Brischetto CS, Connor WE, Connor SL, Matarazzo JD: Plasma lipid and lipoprotein profiles of cigarette smokers from randomly selected families: Enhancement of hyperlipidemia nad depresion of high-density lipoprotein. Am J Cardiol 1983;52:675–680.
16. Tyroler HA (ed.): Epidemiology of plasma high-density lipoprotein cholesterol levels. The Lipid Research Clinics Program Prevalence Study. Circulation 1980;(suppl. IV, part II):1–9.
17. Meade TW, Imeson J, Stirling Y: Effects of changes in smoking and other characteristics on clotting factors and the risk of ischaemic heart disease. Lancet 1987;2:986–992.

E: Summary

Quality of life after coronary bypass surgery

BERNARD J. GERSH

1. Late results of CABG – survival and 'quality of life'

This session provided a comprehensive review of coronary bypass surgery upon survival, the relief of symptoms, and upon other less tangible manifestations of the quality of life. Coronary bypass surgery (CABG) is now in its third decade, and the mass of information emanating from the large multicenter, randomized trials, numerous registry studies, and individual series have taught us a great deal about the indications for the procedure and its impact upon late outcome and, in particular, late survival. Much has been made of the differences between the three large randomized trials which compared coronary bypass surgery with medical therapy [the Veterans Administration Trial, the European Coronary Artery Surgery Study (ECSS), and the National Heart, Lung, and Blood Institute Coronary Artery Surgery Study (CASS)] and the patient populations which were entered into these trials *do* differ in regard to the severity of symptoms, the distribution of the coronary anatomy (particularly in relationship to the frequency of left anterior descending coronary artery disease), and left ventricular function. Less emphasized but of equal, if not greater, importance, however, is the consistent message delivered in *each* of the three trials; namely, that the greatest benefit of coronary revascularization upon survival is achieved among subsets of patients at *higher risk*. The latter can be categorized on the basis of the severity of ischemia, the presence of left ventricular dysfunction, and the number of vessels diseased and their location.

Over time, the differences in survival between medically and surgically treated patients in the Veterans Administration [1] and the European Coronary Surgery Study diminished [2]. Although this may be due in part to the impact of graft attrition (in a patient population receiving saphenous vein grafts in the main) and progression of disease in ungrafted native vessels, the impact of 'crossovers' on the *differences* in survival cannot be discounted when the results are analyzed on an 'intention to treat' basis. In the CASS study at ten years, 37 percent of patients initially assigned to medical therapy

Paul J. Walter (ed.): *Quality of Life after Open Heart Surgery*, 245–249.
© 1992 Kluwer Academic Publishers.

had undergone CABG, and 8 percent of surgically assigned patients never underwent operation. Moreover, among subsets with triple-vessel disease, crossovers occurred in approximately 50 percent of the patients [3]. Nonetheless, among this subset with mild, stable angina and triple-vessel disease in whom left ventricular dysfunction was present, the CASS ten-year data show that the benefits of surgery over medical therapy upon survival, which were initially present at five to seven years, were maintained after ten years. Despite this, however, it must be appreciated that the 'intention-to-treat principle', which reflects a clinical *strategy* in the short-term, must be affected in the long-term by a substantial crossover rate, which would reduce the *difference* in outcome between strategies. This cannot be ignored in the interpretation of data dealing with late outcome.

Indices of the quality of life, such as angina relief, increased physical activity, and a reduction in the use of antianginal medications, are initially superior in surgically assigned patients. Nonetheless, after ten years, differences between surgical and medical groups are less apparent – due in part to a recurrence of symptoms in surgically treated patients and, of more importance, the performance of late surgery in a substantial portion of patients initially treated medically [4].

2. Role of risk factor modification

There is increasing evidence to suggest that risk factor modification, e.g., control of hyperlipidemia, hypertension, and the cessation of cigarette smoking, are important, if not essential, steps which will improve the outcome of both surgical and medical therapy. Several presentations emphasized the role of the comprehensive rehabilitation of patients after CABG, and risk factor modification is an integral part of the process.

3. Results in women

Surgical mortality is increased in women, and the long-term effects upon the quality of life and recurrence of symptoms appear less impressive than in men [5]. Technical factors, including the smaller diameter of the coronary vessels in the majority of women, may account for some, but not all, of the differences in results according to gender [6]. There is, however, accumulating and disturbing evidence from several studies in the United States of America which imply that a referral bias is operative in women, leading to underutilization of CABG and referral later in the course of their disease [7,8].

4. Return to work

As society becomes aware of the burgeoning cost of medical care in relationship to limited resources, the potential for a procedure to return individuals to the work force is a secondary, but increasingly important, issue. There is a wide variation in the rate of return to work after CABG, and this reflects the cultural, social, and economic heterogeneity of patients undergoing coronary bypass surgery around the world. Nonetheless, in general, the rate of return to work after CABG has been disappointing when taken in conjunction with the degree of symptomatic relief. Psychological and social problems and the overall emotional state of the patient are significant determinants of the low incidence of return to work. Other major factors include increasing age, the employment status of the patient and of the patient's spouse preoperatively, and socioeconomic status.

5. Cognitive function

Documentation of abnormalities in cognitive function during the early postoperative period after CABG are disturbing. It is clear that the impairment of neuropsychological performance based upon objective testing is greater than what would be expected based upon the patient's own perception of cognitive changes. It is encouraging that the deterioration appears to improve over time, and serious disability six months after surgery is very unusual. Moreover, the association with advanced age, techniques of cardiopulmonary bypass, and peripheral vascular disease raises the issue of intraoperative microemboli, including atheroemboli, as a significant and potentially preventable cause.

6. Psychological reaction

Several presentations drew attention to derangements in psychological and emotional function after coronary bypass surgery. This is an area that has tended to be neglected by cardiologists and surgeons, whose natural tendency is to focus upon the impact of coronary obstructive disease upon survival and cardiac symptoms. Nonetheless, the psychosocial adaptation to CABG may exert a profound influence upon the effect of the procedure on the 'quality of life' and warrants attention to this aspect of management, both preoperatively and during the period of rehabilitation. Realization and acceptance of the problem could enhance the potential for CABG to influence the quality of life, in addition to survival.

7. Age

The aging of the population in many countries and the expanding use of invasive cardiovascular procedures in the elderly are issues with enormous socioeconomic and ethical implications for society. The benefits of CABG upon survival and symptom relief in the 'young old' is accepted. Among the 'old old' (e.g., octogenarians), the *feasibility* of such an approach is well documented, and in selected patients in expert hands, mortalities are surprisingly low [9]. Nonetheless, as the elderly comprise an expanding proportion of the population, it must also be realized that the maximum age of survival has changed little, if at all, and among patients of advanced age, particularly in the face of other features of extensive cardiovascular disease, the potential for CABG to alter survival to a substantial and meaningful extent is limited. This is a difficult area in which to provide strict guidelines, and there is a dire need to establish a database of invasive cardiovascular procedures among elderly patients in their 80s and 90s. The issues are complex, but the implications of the expansion of complex medical technologies among patients of advanced age need to be addressed now. If rational decisions are to be formulated, it is imperative that the relevant data be *prospectively* obtained and that such studies focus upon the quality of life, in addition to survival.

References

1. Varnauskas E and the European Coronary Surgery Study Group: 12–year follow-up of survival in the randomized European Coronary Surgery Study. N Engl J Med 1988;319:332–337.
2. The Veterans Administration Coronary Artery Bypass Surgery Cooperative Study Group: Eleven-year survival in the Veterans Administration randomized trial of coronary bypass surgery for stable angina. N Engl J Med 1984;311:1333–1339.
3. Alderman EL, Bourassa MG, Cohen LS, Davis KB, Kaiser GG, Killip T, Mock MB, Pettinger, and Robertson TL for the CASS Investigators: Ten-year follow-up of survival in myocardial infarction in the randomized Coronary Artery Surgery Study. Circulation 1990;82:1629–1646.
4. Rogers WJ, Coggin J, Gersh BJ, Fisher LD, Myers WO, Oberman A, and Sheffield LT for the CASS Investigators: Ten-year follow-up of quality of life in patients randomized to receive medical therapy or coronary artery bypass graft surgery in the Coronary Artery Surgery Study (CASS). Circulation 1990;82:1647–1658.
5. Gersh BJ, Kronmal RA, Schaff HV, Frye RL, Ryan TJ, Myers WO, Athearn MW, Gosselin AJ, Kaiser GC, Killip T: Long-term (5–year) results of coronary bypass surgery in patients 65 years old or older: A report from the Coronary Artery Surgery Study. Circulation 1983;68:(Suppl. II):190–199.
6. Fisher LD, Kennedy JW, Davis KB, Maynard C, Fritz JK, Kaiser G, Myers WO, and the participating CASS clinics: Association of sex, physical size, and operative mortality after coronary artery bypass in the Coronary Artery Surgery Study (CASS). J Thorac Cardiovasc Surg 1982;84:334341.
7. Tobin JN, Wassertheil-Smoller S, Wexler JP, Steingart RM, Budner N, Lense L, Wachspress J: Sex bias in considering coronary bypass surgery. Ann Int Med 1987;107:1925.

8. Kahn SS, Neesim S, Gray R, Czer LS, Chaux A, Matloff J: Increased mortality of women in coronary artery bypass surgery: Evidence for referral bias. Ann Int Med 1990;112:561567.
9. Mullany CJ, Darling GE, Pluth JR, Orszulak TA, Schaff HV, Ilstrup DM, Gersh BJ: Early and late results after isolated coronary artery bypass surgery in 159 patients aged 80 years and older. Circulation (Suppl) 1990;82:IV-229–IV-236.

PART THREE

QUALITY OF LIFE AFTER SURGICAL CORRECTION OF CONGENITAL HEART DISEASE

A: Physiological State

23. Quality of life 30 to 36 years after closure of isolated ventricular septal defects in 341 patients

C. WALTON LILLEHEI, CEEYA PATTON and JAMES H. MOLLER

1. Introduction

In 1954 at the University of Minnesota Hospital intracardiac correction began for ventricular septal defects (VSD) on March 26 utilizing extracorporal circulation (ECC). Cross circulation [1–3] was utilized for the first 27 patients, and then beginning in 1955 the DeWall-Lillehei bubble oxygenator [4–6] was utilized routinely through December 31, 1960. During that time period 341 patients had VSD closure with 45 hospital deaths (13%) leaving 296 who were discharged from the hospital.

Many of these patients are alive 30 to 36 years later. Sets of these patients have been the subject of previous reports [7–12], but this study represents an attempt to determine the status of each of the survivors operated upon during the period 1954 through 1960. While there have been a number of reports of patients following repair of VSD, often concerned with specific post-operative aspects, such as pulmonary vascular resistance [12–21] or conduction disturbances [22–28], none of these studies has extended for 30–36 years or covered as large a sample of patients from this early era of cardiac surgery.

The specific purposes of this long term follow-up study are indicated in Table 1.

2. Materials and methods

The hospital records of 341 patients who underwent repair of VSD in the years 1954 through December 31, 1960 were reviewed and tabulated. The clinical status of patients following hospital discharge was determined through individual patient evaluation, correspondence with the patient, his/her relatives, personal physicians, or records from other hospitals. A cardiac catheterization was recommended to each patient post-operatively [11]. Current information was sought from all patients operated upon during this period.

Paul J. Walter (ed.): Quality of Life after Open Heart Surgery, 253–265.

Table 1. Ventricular septal defect, 30–36 year follow-up.

Purposes:
· Late deaths: Frequency/cause
· Morbidity: Frequency/cause
· Assess Life Styles, Offspring, Education, Employment

Table 2. Ventricular septal defect, 30–36 year follow-up.

Age at operation	No. patients	Long term survivors	
Under 2 years	26	23	(88%)
2–5 years	94	76	(81%)
6–10 years	111	84	(76%)
Over 10 years	59	48	(81%)
Totals	290	231	

If a patient had died, information was obtained from the family, personal physician or medical records regarding the circumstances of death, health status prior to death, and details of the post-mortem examination, if performed.

3. Results

Between March 26, 1954 and December 31, 1960, 341 patients with VSD underwent repair at the University of Minnesota hospital. Their age at operation is shown in Table 2. An overview of the results is presented in Table 3. The current status of 290 of the 296 survivors is known, with only 6 (2%) being lost to follow-up. A total of 7912 postoperative years of follow-up is reported (Table 3).

4. Late mortality

Of the 296 survivors, 59 (20%) have died from 1 month to 33 years after their operation. Thirty-one deaths occurred in the first postoperative decade, 13 in the second, 14 in the third, and I in the fourth. These numbers equate

Table 3. Ventricular septal defect, 30–36 year follow-up.

Patients operated 1954 through 1960			341
Hospital Mortality: 45 Pts. (13%)			
Survivors/Discharged:			296
Follow-up complete	290	(98%)	
Alive (actuarial surv. at 35 yrs. = 83%)	231		
Late deaths	59		
Total follow-up			7912 pt. yrs.

Table 4. Cause and decade of death in 59 patients, ventricular septal defect 30–36 year follow-up.

Cause	0–9	10–19	20–29	>30	Total
Heart block	7	2	1	–	10
Reoperation	8	–	1	–	9
PVOD	5	6	5	–	16
Accident	2	1	3	–	6
Infection (3 Cardiac)	3	–	1	–	4
Cardiac failure	1	–	–	–	1
Sudden (unexplained)	2	0	2	1	5
Unknown	3	4	1	–	8*
Totals	31	13	14	1	59

The table has a spanning header "Interval from operation (yrs.)" over columns 0–9, 10–19, 20–29, >30.

PVOD = pulmonary vascular obstructive disease.
* All 8 had closed defects.

to 11 deaths per 1000 patient years during the first decade, and 5 deaths per 1000 patient years for the second, and third decades following operation.

Late deaths occurred from a variety of causes (Table 4). In 10 patients, death presumably was form heart block, 7 of the 10 having complete heart block, and the other 3 transient heart block postoperatively. Only 1 of the latter 3 had a history of syncope. Eight of the 10 did not receive a cardiac pacemaker, for these patients were treated in an era before pacemakers were developed [33,34,39]. In the other 2, a pacemaker was placed and death occurred presumably from pacemaker failure. Nine other patients died during an operation for residual cardiac abnormality. They were among 19 patients in whom a cardiac reoperation was performed. In 8 of the 9, death occurred 6 months to 9 years following the initial operation. The ninth patient died 21 years after the closure of the VSD, following aortic and mitral valve replacement for valvar disease associated with coexistent Marfan's syndrome.

Another 16 patients, each with a pre or postoperative pulmonary resistance >8 mmHg/L/min/M^2 died from 2 to 24 years postoperatively. Eight of the 16 showed a major rise in pulmonary vascular resistance postoperatively.

Six of the 59 patients died accidentally – two each from drowning and automobiles, another from boating, and the last patient from a cervical cord injury in a trampoline accident. None of these 6 patients showed transient heart block postoperatively, and only 1 had an elevated pulmonary vascular resistance (10 mmHg/L/min/M^2.

Four patients died of complications of infections. Three were related to complications of infective endocarditis – 2 of these from rupture of an intracranial mycotic aneurysm, and the other from aortic insufficiency. The fourth patient, a 5 year old, died 3 months postoperatively of staphylococcal sepsis.

One patient with a residual VSD and a perforation in the septal leaflet of the tricuspid valve died in congestive cardiac failure 3 months postoperatively.

Table 5. Sudden and unexpected deaths. Details in 5 patients, ventricular septal defect, 30–36 year follow-up.

Patient	Age of death (Yrs.)	Postoperative duration (Yrs.)	Postoperative electrocardiogram	Block at initial operation
1	24	3	QRS = 0.18 Sec.	0
2	11	8	CRBBB	0
3	24	22	CRBBB	0
4	39	29	Normal	Transient
5	38	33	LAD + CRBBB	0

CRBBB = Complete right bundle-branch block; LAD = left axis deviation; 0 = absent.

Five patients died suddenly and unexpectedly, having had no cardiac symptoms (Table 5); one of the deaths occurred following exercise (patient l) and another in the postpartum period (patient 2).

Eight other patients (Table 4), each with a closed defect, died form an unknown cause or the circumstances regarding their deaths could not be fully ascertained. Only one of the eight had transient heart block post-operatively. The pulmonary vascular resistance was 6 mmHg/L/min/M^2 in 1 patient, and normal in the remaining.

5. Late non-fatal major complications (Table 6)

5.1. *Arrhythmias*

Twenty patients have had an arrhythmia post-operatively. Among the 20, there were eight with episodes of supraventricular tachycardia, two others with atrial flutter, and an additional three with atrial fibrillation. One patient had a single episode of ventricular tachycardia 23 years post-operatively. Another four experienced premature ventricular contractions, three of whom were treated. In the remaining two of the 20 patients, an arrhythmia was

Table 6. Ventricular septal defect, 30–36 year follow-up.

Non-fatal major medical problems:		
· Cardiac Arrhythmias		20
Supravent tachyarrhymia	13	
P.V.C.	4	
Vent. tach.	1	
· Bacterial endocarditis		6 (in 5 Pts.)
· Diabetes mellitus		5
· Malignancy		4
· Cardiomyopathy		3 (K arrest)
· Late pacemaker		2
· Miscellaneous		4

Table 7. Bacterial endocarditis details of 9 episodes in 8 patients, ventricular septal defect, 30–36 year follow-up.

Years postoperative	Anatomic details
4	No defect
4	No defect
7 (died)	Mycotic aneurysm
7 (died)	Mycotic aneurysm
8	Residual VSD
8 (died)	Aortic valve abnormality
19 (died)	Aortic valve abnormality
12 & 21	No defects

VSD = ventricular septal defect.

reported but not described. Of 13 patients with supraventricular tachyrhythmia, five had a major cardiac residual problem (cardiomyopathy in two, replacement of either the mitral or tricuspid valve in one each, and obstructive pulmonary vascular disease in the fifth).

5.2. *Bacterial endocarditis*

Nine episodes of infective endocarditis occurred in 8 patients from 4 to 22 years following the operation (Table 7). This occurrence was 11/10 000 patients years. Three of the eight patients died of complications of endocarditis and were described above (Table 4). In 3 of the 8, post-operative cardiac catheterization showed neither a residual defect nor a shunt. These episodes of endocarditis occurred before echo cardiography was available to identify the site of infection.

There were few other serious illnesses among the survivors. Five have developed diabetes mellitus (current ages 34, 40, 40, 55, and 65 years). There were single instances of the following conditions: Hodgkin's disease, breast cancer, multiple sclerosis, and rheumatic fever. Two patients have mildly restrictive pulmonary disease.

In three patients, dilated cardiomyopathy has been diagnosed. Each patient developed congestive cardiac failure 20 to 30 years post-operatively and echocardiograms show ventricular dilatation. Cardiac transplantation has been performed in one, and is being considered in two. A probable cause for the cardiomyopathy has been identified as the (Melrose) potassium cardioplegia [29] that was used briefly on our service.

Table 8. Ventricular septal defect, 30–36 year follow-up.

Cardiac reoperations:	19 patients
· Residual Septal Defect	13
· Tricuspid Regurgitation	2
· Aortic Valve Replacement	2
Repair	1
· Infundib. Obstruction	1

6. Cardiac reoperation (Table 8)

In 19 patients (6% of the survivors), a second cardiac operation was performed; 17 of the reoperations were performed within the first 10 years, 10
primarily for a residual shunt, two for tricuspid regurgitation and one for an
aortic abnormality. In the remaining two of the 19, the aortic valve was
replaced at 20 and 21 years, respectively, after the initial operation to close
the VSD. As indicated in Table 4, death occurred following 9 of these 19
reoperations.

7. Postoperative hemodynamic studies

Cardiac catheterization was performed on 161(55%) of the 290 patients
followed. These studies were done as part of the routine follow-up in order
to determine: (1) efficacy of closure; (2) physiologic responses. Catheterization was not limited to patients with symptomatology or suspected shunts.

The defect was found to be completely closed in 134 patients (83.2%)
(Table 9). Included among these closed defects, were five patients who had
a second operation to achieve closure Another patient who had a small
residual defect, had a spontaneous closure by the second recatheterization.

A residual left to right was found in 27 patients (Table 9). Among the 27
patients with residual defects, there were 11 with small left to right shunts

Table 9. Ventricular septal defect, 30–36 year follow-up, success measured by postoperative
recatheterization.

Pulmonary Artery Pressure (mmHg at Recath.)	Number of patients		
	Closed defect	Residual shunt	Totals
less 30	80 (87%)	12	92
30–70	45 (76%)	14	59
over 70	9 (90%)	1	10
TOTALS	134 (83%)	27	161

(L–R) of under 30%, and no further surgical treatment was considered necessary. The residual shunt was between 30% to 49% in 7 patients, and between 50 and 75% in 9. In the former group observation has been carried out; and reoperation has been recommended or carried out in the latter group.

8. Exercise status

Survivors were asked to rate their exercise ability according to the New York Heart Association criteria. Among the 232, 208 were class 1 (89.6%) and 18 were class 2 (7.7%). Only four (1.7%) described themselves as class 3 – one is a patient in a group home, another has gross obesity, a third has severe scoliosis, and the fourth, despite this self-classification, performs manual labor. Two were in class 4: one with multiple sclerosis, and the other with severe developmental delay.

9. Offspring

Amongst the 296 survivors of operations performed from 1954–1960 to repair VSD, there have been 222 patients choosing to reproduce. Of the 348 pregnancies, 311 have resulted in live births (including two sets of twins). There were 36 spontaneous abortions (10.3%) and two elective abortions. Four pregnancies have not yet reached term. Ten of the 311 live births (3.2%) have a documented cardiac malformation. Seven of these have required surgical intervention, with one death occurring in an infant with pulmonary atresia, (PA) and VSD.

Malformations include VSD (4), VSD, PA (1), pulmonary stenosis (1), partial anomalous pulmonary venous return (1), coarctation (1), atrioventricular canal (1), unknown cardiac malformation (1). Of the affected offspring, 3 had fathers with VSD and 7 had mothers with VSD. These findings are summarized as follows:

Sex	# of pregnancies	# of live births	Abortions
Females	206	175	30
Males	142	136	6

In this group of adults with VSD, there have been more spontaneous abortions and offspring with cardiac malformations in affected mothers compared to fathers.

Table 10. Ventricular septal defect, 30–36 year follow-up.

Education status*	Beyond high school
	No. of Patients
Technical school	25
Attended college	52
College graduate	44
Masters degree	24
Doctoral degree	12
(Ph.D. = 6, M.D. = 5, D.D.S. = 1	157

* From 232 of 290 Survivors.

10. Educational status

The educational status of 232 survivors was ascertained; 23, including 7 in special education classes, did not complete high school. Another 52 had no formal education following receipt of a high school diploma. In Table 10 the achievements of those 157 patients that sought, education beyond high school is portrayed. Twenty-five attended a technical school following high school. Finally 132 (57%) attended college, with 44 (19%) receiving a bachelor degree, another 24 (10%) a master's degree, and 12 (5%) a doctoral degree (including 5 physicians).

11. Discussion

On March 26, 1954, the first VSD was closed by surgeons at the University of Minnesota Hospital [1–12]. Over the next 6 years, a total of 341 patients underwent this operation at our hospital. In this paper, we describe at 30 to 36 years the current status of 290 of the 296 postoperative survivors (98% follow-up). Fifty-nine deaths have occurred among the 290 operative survivors. Deaths have occurred in each decade since the operation, with more occurring within the first 10 years. In analyzing the groups of patients who had better survival rates, there were those who were operated upon under the age of 2 years, and those with a pulmonary vascular resistance less than $7 \, mmHg/L/min/M^2$. While intracardiac repair of VSD during infancy is considered a new development, 26 of our patients were under 2 years of age at the time of operation, the youngest being 4 months of age. Of these 26, only 3 subsequently died, none from obstructive pulmonary vascular disease. Among the patients operated upon after the age of 2 years, 79% survived and all the deaths from obstructive pulmonary vascular disease occurred in this age group of patients.

The effects of elevated pulmonary vascular resistance on survival following VSD closure has been studied [11–13,17–19] and mortality found greater in patients with a resistance $>7 \, mmHg/L/min/M^2$ (18) or $>8 \, mmHg/L/min/M^2$

[13,17,19]. Among our patients, we found a late mortality of 51% for a preoperative level $>7\,\mathrm{mmHg/L/min/M^2}$, and 11% for those below this level. The higher mortality occurred not only from pulmonary vascular disease but from all causes. Pulmonary vascular disease may have been an important factor in death of patients from other causes. We could attribute only one death to obstructive pulmonary vascular disease among patients with a low preoperative level of pulmonary vascular resistance. Because of its unique nature, that case was previously described [12]. Sixteen deaths were attributed directly to obstructive pulmonary vascular disease and its complications. Each of these 16 patients was at least 5 years of age when operated upon. The deaths occurred from 2 to 24 years following VSD closure.

Conduction abnormalities have been a major concern in postoperative patients [22–28,30]. Patients with coexistent complete right bundle-branch block and left axis deviation are not considered to develop complete heart block unless transient heart block is present in the perioperative period [23,26,31,32]. Our data support this thought and provides a longer duration of follow-up. Among our 9 patients with coexistent right bundle-branch block and left axis deviation, two have died, both suddenly. One of the two had transient heart block in the operating room.

Postoperative heart block has important implications. Of our 37 patients with transient block postoperatively, two subsequently developed complete heart block at 6 and 25 years, respectively. Eight of these 37 patients have died – 3 from obstructive pulmonary vascular disease, two suddenly and unexpectedly, two from unknown causes, and the remaining patient from complete heart block for which a pacemaker had not been placed. Ten other patients with complete heart block have died. In 8 of these 10 patients, a pacemaker had not been placed because either pacemakers had not been developed or were newly available [33,34], and the indications for their placement were still being explored. In two of the 10, a pacemaker was placed, and death occurred because of pacemaker failure. Our study confirms the serious and life-threatening nature of operatively-induced complete heart block, which fortunately is an uncommon complication in the current era of cardiac surgery. Nineteen patients underwent a second cardiac operation, 14 for a residual shunt and 2 others for significant tricuspid regurgitation. With improvements in operative techniques, a significant residual shunt or tricuspid regurgitation are now uncommon. Nine of our 59 deaths occurred in patients following a cardiac reoperation, a situation which would rarely occur today. Another patient who died with congestive heart failure can be considered in the same category, for his death was related to a large residual defect.

Thus, these 36 deaths – 10 from heart block, 9 from cardiac reoperation, 1 from heart failure, and 16 from obstructive pulmonary vascular disease – would largely be avoided using current management principles. The tendency to operate before the age of 2 years avoids the development of pulmonary vascular disease, and the current techniques usually result in complete closure without damage to the conduction system.

The health status of our survivors is excellent, with few patients indicating the presence of major medical problems. One concern is the apparent cardio-myopathy in three survivors. The origin of this cardiac problem is believed to be related at least in part to the method of cardioplegia [29].

Infective endocarditis occurred in 9 of our patients (11.4/10 000 patient years), a rate similar to the 11.7/10 000 in unoperated children ages 2–17 years [35], and 12/10 000 patient years for children ages 2–14 years, some of whom had undergone cardiac surgery [36]. Three of our patients who developed endocarditis had no residual shunt. A previous report described infective endocarditis in patients with successfully closed VSD [28]. This occurrence again emphasizes the recommendation for antibiotic prophylaxis for dental, oral surgical, and other procedures in patients with structural cardiac disease. Seven of the episodes of endocarditis which occurred among our patients were in the era before there were uniform recommendations for antibiotic prophylaxis concerning postoperative patients.

Another postoperative problem has been the occurrence of arrhythmias in 20 patients, most of whom received treatment, and in each instance, with a single medication. In patients with sustained rhythm disturbance, particularly if unusual, for example atrial flutter, atrial fibrillation, or ventricular tachycardia, further investigation is indicated.

The 83% incidence of complete closure by recatheterization in this very early series, when so much had to be learned about the pathologic anatomy and surgical techniques, has been gratifying, and compares favorable with the experiences of others.

Kirklin, McGoon, and Dushane [37] reported a hospital mortality of 17.8% in 320 patients having closure of VSD's between 1955–1960. Amongst the survivors, 84.7% of patients were judged to have complete closure based upon catheterization or clinical study. in a subsequent study from the Mayo Clinic upon patients operated upon from 1960–1965 [38], the complete closure rate was reported at 73% (again, a total of recatheterization cases plus clinical judgement).

In a series of 36 VSD patients repaired at Hammersmith Hospital between 1958 and 1967, all with pulmonary hypertension and pulmonary resistance of not less than 8 units, closure was found complete by recatheterization in 56% [15].

Finally, in a collected series from 6 major institutions [21] repaired in the '60s, complete VSD closure was reported in 47% to 60% of patients (again, some were deemed completely closed on a clinical basis without recatheterization).

The incidence and severity of pulmonary vascular disease in these patients and their responses to the closure of their VSD's reported herein have also been subjects of previous reports by us [7–12].

The educational achievements of this early group was far above average. There were obviously other factors responsible for this surprising finding (heredity, environment, the motivation provided by recovery from a serious illness), but it is further confirmation that even the very early perfusion techniques did not adversely affect intellectual capacity. Their employment records were also reviewed, but were not detailed herein because, as expected, there was a close correlation with their education levels. Nonetheless, good educations and rewarding occupations both added significantly to their quality of life.

There were many major obstacles, to open heart surgery in the 1950s such as: new and untested perfusion methods, frequent errors in preoperative diagnoses, unfamiliar intracardiac pathology, lack of external defibrillators, pacemakers, and no respiratory assist equipment for infants/children. Even pH and blood gas measurements were not available clinically during most of this period. Despite all of these deficiencies, the hospital mortality was only 13%, and the closure rate was high.

Today virtually all of these great deficiencies in our knowledge, as enumerated above, have been eliminated by the spectacular progress that has occurred during these 36 years. Thus, the outlook for an infant born today, with even a large ventricular septal defect, is very close to normal.

12. Conclusions

(1) 290 of 296 survivors (98%) were followed 30–36 years.
(2) 231 patients are alive. Actuarial survival at 35 years is 83.3%.
(3) 59 late deaths occurred, many now avoidable.
(4) 83% of 161 patients recatheterized have *closed* defects.

Amongst the survivors there are: few medical problems with excellent records for quality of life, offspring, education, and employment.

References

1. Warden HE, Cohen M, Read RC, Lillehei CW: Controlled cross circulation for open intracardiac surgery. Physiologic studies and Results for creation and closure of ventricular septal defects. J Thoracic Surg 1954; 28:331–343.
2. Warden HE, Read RC, DeWall RA, Aust JB, Cohen M, Ziegler NR, Varco RL, Lillehei CW: Direct vision intracardiac surgery by means of a reservoir of 'arterialized venous' blood. Description of a simple method and report of the first clinical case. J Thoracic Surg 1955;30:649–657.
3. Lillehei CW, Varco RL, Cohen M, Warden HE, Patton C, Moller JH: The first open-heart corrections of ventricular septal defect, atrio-ventricular communis, and tetralogy of Fallot utilizing extracorporeal circulation by cross-circulation; A 30-year follow-up. Ann Thor Surg 1986; 41:4–21.

4. Lillehei CW, DeWall RA, Read RC, Warden HE, Varco RL: Direct vision intracardiac surgery in man using a simple disposahle artificial oxygenator. Diseases of the Chest 1956; 29:1–8.

5. DeWall RA, Warden HE, Read RC, Gott VL, Ziegler NR, Varco RL, Lillehel CW: A simple, expendable, artificial oxygenator for open heart surgery. Surgery Clinics of North America 1956; 36:1025–1034.

6. Gott VL, Sellers RD, DeWall RA, Varco RL, Lillehei CW: A disposable unitized plastic sheet oxygenator for open heart surgery. Diseases of the Chest 1957; 32:615–625.

7. Adams P Jr, Anderson RC, Meyne N, Lillehei CW: Physiologic changes after closure of ventricular septal defects. Lancet 1961;81:497–501.

8. Lillehei CW, Anderson RC, Wang Y: Clinical and hemodynamic changes after closure of ventricular septal defects. JAMA 1968;205:822–827.

9. Lillehei CW, Anderson RC, Eliot RS, Wang Y, Ferlic RM: Pre and postoperative cardiac catheterization in 20() patients undergoing closure of ventricular septal defects. Surgery 1968;63:69–76.

10. Lillehei CW, Levy MJ, Adams P, Anderson RC: High-pressure ventricular septal defects. JAMA 1969;188:246–260.

11. Allen HD, Anderson RC, Noren GR, Moller JH: Post-operative follow-up of patients with ventricular septal defect. Circulation 1974;50:465–471.

12. Braunlin EA, Moller JH, Patton C, Lucas RV Jr, Lillehei CW: Predictive value of lung biopsy in ventricular septal defects: Long-term follow-up. J Am Coll Cardiol 1986;8:1113–1118.

13. Clarkson PM, Frye RL, DuShane JW, Burchell HB, Wood EH, Weidman WH: Prognosis for patients with ventricular septal defect and severe pulmonary vascular obstructive disease. Circulation 1968;38:129–135.

14. Gotsman MS, Beck W, Barnard CN, Schrire V: Hemodynamic studies after repair of ventricular septal defect. Br Heart J 1969;31:63–71.

15. Hallidie-Smith KA, Hollman A, Cleland WP, Bentall HH, Goodwin JF: Effects of surgical closure of ventricular septal defects upon pulmonary vascular disease. Br Heart J 1969;31:246–260.

16. Keith JD, Rose V, Collins G, Kidd BSL: Ventricular septal defect. Incidence, morbidity, and mortality in various age groups. Br Heart J 1971;33:81–87.

17. Weidman WH, DuShane JW: Closure of pulmonary hypertension following surgical closure of ventricular septal defect. Adv Cardiol 1974;11:131–134.

18. Friedl B, Kidd BSL, Mustard WT, Keith JD: Ventricular septal defect with increased pulmonary vascular resistance. Late results of surgical closure. Am J Cardiol 1974:33:403–409.

19. DuShane JW, Krongard E, Ritter DG, McGood DC: The fate of raised pulmonary vascular resistance after surgery in ventricular septal defect. In: Rowe RD, Kidd GSC (eds.) The child with congenital heart disease after surgery. Mt. Kisco, New York: Futura Publishing Company, 1976:299–312.

20. Hallidie-Smith KA, Wilson RS, Hart A, Zeidifard E: Functional status of patients with large ventricular septal defect and pulmonary vascular disease 6 to 16 years after surgical closure of their defect in childhood. Br Heart J 1977;39:1093–1101.

21. Weidman WH, Blount SG Jr, DuShane JW, Gersony WM, Hayes CJ, Nadas AS: Clinical course in ventricular septal defect. Circulation 1977;56(Suppl I):I56–I69.

22. Kulbertus HE, Coyne JJ, Hallidie-Smith KA: Conduction disturhances before and after surgical closure of ventricular septal defect. Am Heart J 1969;77:123–131.

23. Downing JW Jr, Kaplan S Bove KE: Post-surgical left anterior hemiblock and right bundle-branch block. Br Heart J 1972;34:263–270.

24. Goodman MJ, Roberts NK, Izukawa T: Late postoperative conduction disturbances after repair of ventricular septal defect and tetralogy of Fallot. Circulation 1974;39:214–221.

25. Ziady GM, Hallidie-Smith KA, Goodwin JF: Conduction disturbances after surgical closure of ventricular septal defect. Br Heart J 1972;34:1199–1204.

26. Pahlajani DB, Serrato M, Mehta A, Miller RA, Hastreiter A, Rosen KM: Surgical bifasicular block. Circulation 1975;52:82–87.
27. Okoroma EO, Guller B, Maloney JD, Wideman WM: Etiology of right bundle-branch block pattern after surgical closure of ventricular septal defects. Am Heart J 1975;90:14–18.
28. Blake RS, Chung EE, Wesley H, Hallidie-Smith KA: Conduction defects, ventricular arrhythmias, and late death after surgical closure of ventricular septal defect. Br Heart J 1982;47:305–315.
29. Melrose, DG, Dreger B et al: Elective Cardiac Arrest. Lancet 1955;2:21.
30. Kirklin JW, Harshbarger HG, Donald DE, Edwards JE.: Surgical correction of ventricular septal defect: Anatomic and technical consideration. J Thorac Cardiovasc Surg 1957;33:45–59.
31. Wolff GS, Rowland TW, Ellison RC: Surgically induced right bundle-branch block with left anterior hemiblock: An ominous sign in postoperative tetralogy of Fallot. Circulation 1970;46:587–594.
32. Steeg CN, Krongard E, Davachi F. Bowman FO Jr, Mann JR. Gersony WM: Postoperative left anterior hemiblock and right bundle branch block following repair of tetralogy of Fallot. Clinical and etiologic considerations. Circulation 1975;51:1026–1029.
33. Weirich WL, Paneth M, Gott VL, Lillehei CW: Control of complete heart block by the use of an artificial pacemaker and a myocardial electrode. Circ Res 1958;6:410–415.
34. Lillehei CW, Gott VL, Hodges PC, Long DM, Bakken EE: Transistor pacemaker for treatment of complete atrioventricular dissociation. JAMA 1960;172:2006–2010.
35. Shah P, Singh WS, Rose V, Collins G, Keith JD: Incidence of bacterial endocarditis in ventricular septal defect. Circulation 1966;34:127–131.
36. Corone P, Doyon F, Gaudeau S, Guerin F, Vernant P, Ducam H, Rumeau-Rouquette C, Gaudeul P: Natural history of ventricular septal defect. A study involving 790 cases. Circulation 1977;55:908–915.
37. Kirklin VW, McGoon DC, DuShane VW: Surgical treatment of ventricular defect J Thorac Cardiovasc Surg 1960;40:763–775.
38. Cartmill TB, DuShane VW, McGoon DC, Kirklin VW: Results of repair of ventricular septal defect. J Thorac Cardiovasc Surg 1965;52:486–501.
39. Thevenet A, Hodges PC, Lillehei CW: The use of a myocardial electrode inserted percutaneously for control of complete atrioventricular block by an artificial pacemaker. Diseases of the Chest 1958;34:621–631.

24. Long-term results after atrial correction of transposition of the great vessels

MARKO TURINA, MIRALEM PASIC, MONIKA FRY and LUDWIG VON SEGESSER

1. Introduction

Surgical correction of transposition of the great vessels (TGA) is today possible both on the atrial and arterial level. The first successful operation for TGA was performed by Senning in 1958 [1], utilizing an atrial rerouting of the blood flow by an operation which nowadays carries his name. Arterial correction, considered by many to be a more physiological procedure, was first described by Jatene in 1976 [2]. Both methods can be considered as physiological, but not true anatomical corrections: in the atrial procedure the right ventricle must function as systemic ventricle and the tricuspid valve functions as systemic atrio-ventricular valve; in the arterial switch procedure the pulmonic valve becomes the aortic valve. Current low operative mortalities do not allow a true comparison between these two methods of correction of TGA by looking only at the immediate surgical risk. The only acceptable analysis of surgical results must involve an extended follow-up, which might disclose late problems not visible when examining only short- or mid-term results. This report analyzes the extended survival after atrial correction of TGA and focuses on the significant problems emerging long after surgery.

2. Patients and methods

A retrospective analysis of late survival and complications after atrial correction of TGA performed at the University Hospital of Zurich was undertaken in 254 consecutive 30-day survivors of Senning's procedure and its numerous modifications utilized during this period. Surgery was performed between 1965 and 1988. All survivors were contacted either by letter or by telephone; physicians' reports were obtained whenever possible. For patients residing in Switzerland, the follow-up was performed in most cases by the Childrens' Hospital in Zurich. This follow-up was complete in 231 patients (91.7%).

Paul J. Walter (ed.): Quality of Life after Open Heart Surgery, 267–275.

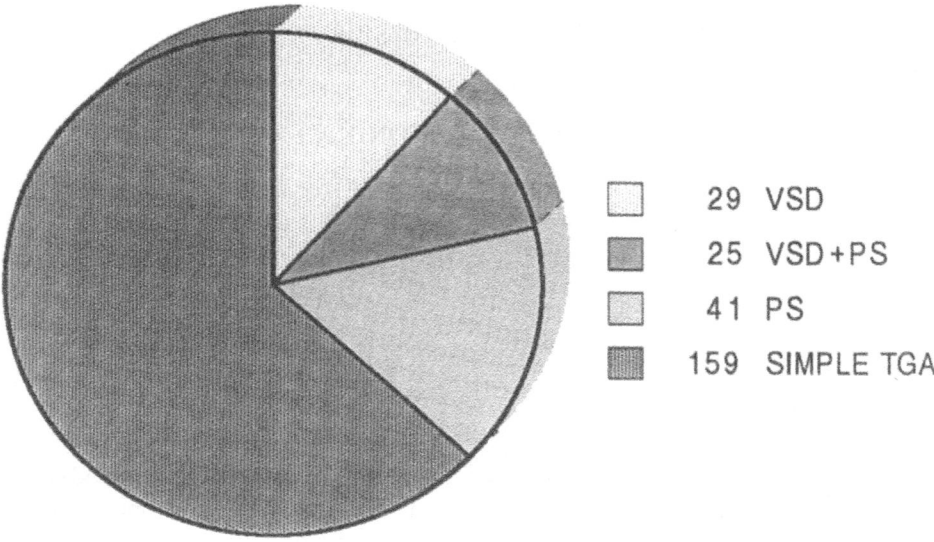

Figure 1. Clinical classification of the total patient group. VSD: ventricular septal defect; PS: pulmonary stenosis. Only relevant malformations (requiring surgical correction) were tabulated.

The total spectrum of malformations is shown in Figure 1. The greatest majority of survivors (63%) had a simple TGA; 16% had an additional pulmonary stenosis (PS), 11% had a ventricular septal defect (VSD), and in 10% TGA was combined with PS and VSD.

Survival was analyzed by the actuarial method; $2 x k$ contingency tables and chi-square statistics were utilized when testing for differences between the groups. BMDP statistical software was employed for univariate and multivariate analysis.

3. Results

3.1. *Survival*

Survival was similar for simple and complex TGA; 95% of patients surviving 5 years after operation, 91% at 10 years and 88% at 15 years; there was a late fall of survival at 20 years, with only 81% surviving. The data are not reliable at this very late point, due to the small number of patients followed for such a long interval (Figure 2). Actuarial analysis showed no significant difference in late survival for simple vs. complex TGA, for TGA with intact septum vs. those with VSD; nor was survival different for those patients operated on after 1978 as opposed to those operated on prior to that year.

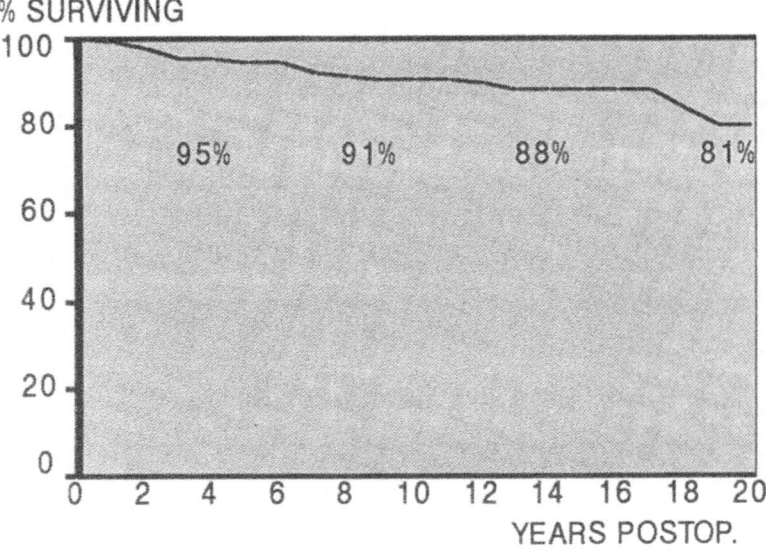

% SURVIVING

USZ, 1965 - 88, 254 Pts.

Figure 2. Late survival of all 30-day survivors of atrial correction of TGA (simple and complex), calculated by actuarial method.

The only demonstrated difference was better survival of patients when the total correction was performed before the age of 1 year (Figure 3).

Univariate analysis demonstrated an age (at total correction) of younger than 1 year as the only significant predictor for late survival. The other variables examined (simple and complex TGA, presence of VSD, surgery after 1978) did not reach statistical significance.

3.2. *Reoperations*

Thirty-nine reoperations were performed in the total patient group. Residual ASD or VSD were the most common indication, followed by stenosis of superior or (rarely) inferior vena cava (Figure 4). Tricuspid valve repair became necessary in 7 patients, and in 3 patients heart transplantation had to be performed due to failure of the systemic ventricle.

Reoperation-free suvival was calculated according to the atuarial method: 88% survived free of reoperation at 15 and 87% at 20 years (Figure 5).

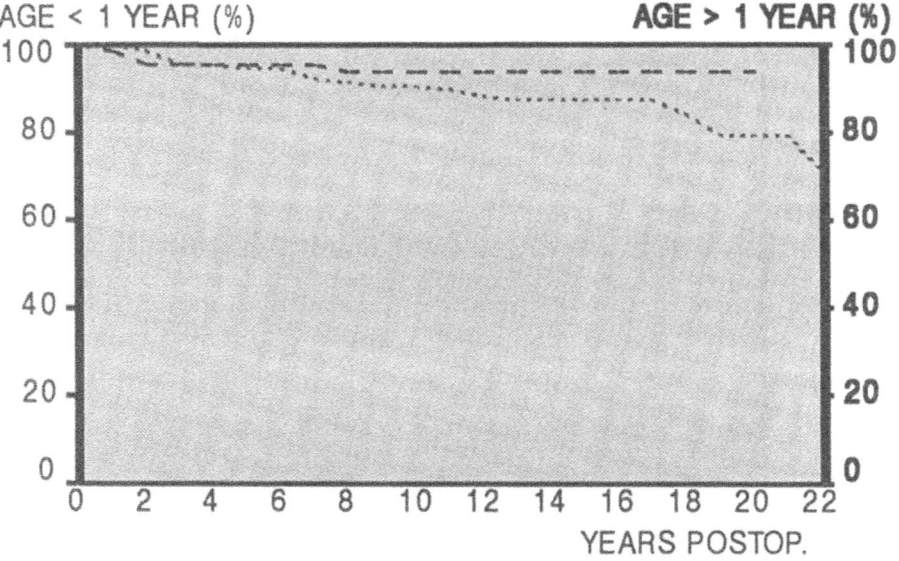

AGE < 1 YEAR (%) AGE > 1 YEAR (%)

YEARS POSTOP.

USZ, 1965-88; 94 TGA < 1 YEAR, 160 TGA > 1 YEAR

Figure 3. Difference in survival when the operation was performed below age of 1 year, as opposed to the survival of children who were older than 1 year at time of atrial correction. Note the virtual absence of very late mortality (beyond 7 years) for the age group of less than 1 year. (– – – age below 1 year; · · · · · · age more than 1 year)

3.3. *Social integration*

A very large proportion of our patients attended normal schools (86%); only 1% were mentally retarded and 13% attended special schools (Figure 6). At the last census among 82 adults, all long-term survivors of total correction of TGA, 13.4% were university graduates, 43.9% were employed as white-

Residual VSD or ASD	12
Stenosis SVC and IVC	8
Tricuspid valve repair	7
Pulmonary stenosis	5
Stenosis of pulmonary atrium	4
Heart transplantation	3

USZ, 1964-90 (271 PTS)

Figure 4. List of reoperations performed after total correction. ASD: atrial septal defect; SVC: superior vena cava; IVC: inferior vena cava.

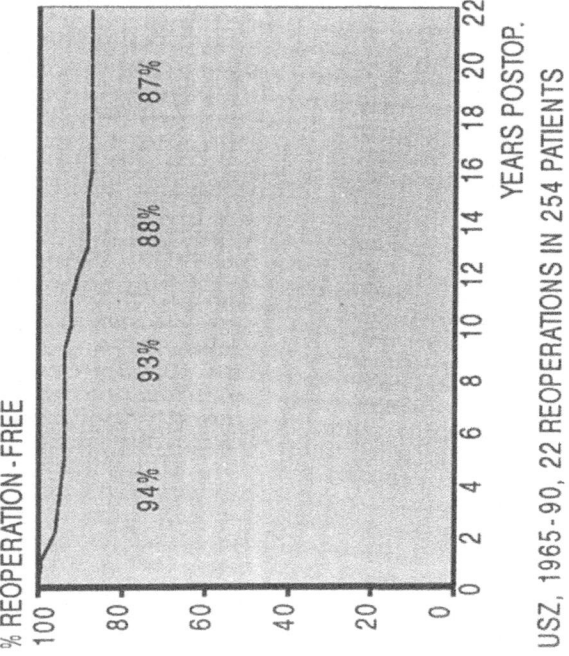

Figure 5. Reoperation-free rate for the total group.

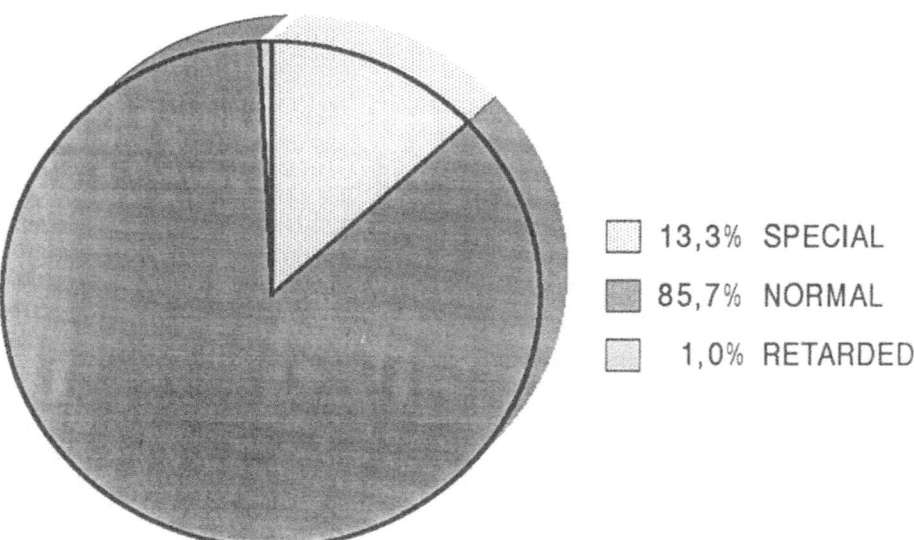

Figure 6. School attendance for 205/254 survivors of total correction. Only 1% had to attend the school for retarded children, but 13.3% went to special schools, indicating some intellectual impairment.

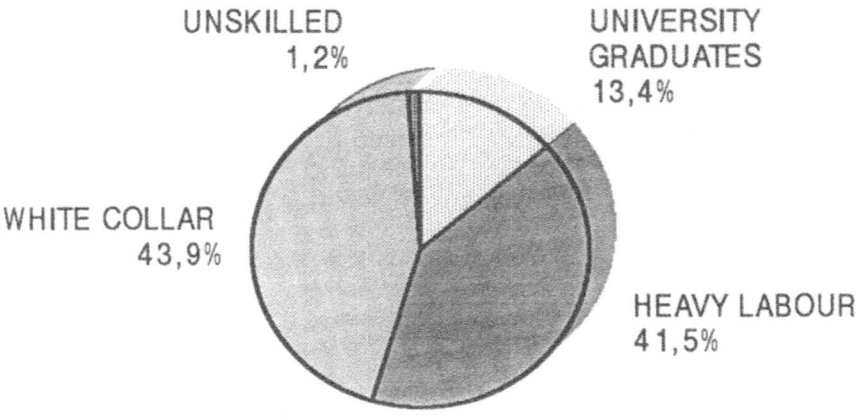

UHZ, 1964 - 88 (82 ADULT SURVIVORS)

Figure 7. Analysis of the type of work presently being performed for 82 adult survivors: 13.4% of university graduates were all involved in white collar work or belonged to professions; only 1.2% were considered as unskilled labor due to lack of formal education. Fully 41.5% were involved in heavy manual labor, denoting excellent functional capacity.

collar workers, and 41.5% performed heavy manual labour; only 1.2% were listed as unskilled labourers (Figure 7).

4. Discussion

This study represents one of the longest follow-ups of the atrial total correction of TGA. Since its description by Senning [1], this method has remained an attractive surgical option due to its potential for growth and the relative paucity of long-term problems. In the seventies and early eighties in particular, when the benefits of early total correction of TGA became obvious, Senning's operation became the method of choice, as opposed to the method of Mustard [3], which had a considerable potential for complications when foreign material was used for intra-atrial rerouting of the blood flow. Today, the results of atrial correction have to be compared to the results gained with arterial correction described by Jatene [2]. It is not really possible to perform a true comparison between these two methods: the results obtained with arterial switch represent the level of cardiac surgery in the nineties, and when several centers compare their results in the recent era, no difference between arterial and atrial correction can be found in the early and intermediate follow-up [4].

The results of surgery in complex congenital corrections can be evaluated only after the patients have reached adulthood; furthermore, many significant problems tend to become apparent much later (dysrhythmias, failure of systemic ventricle, caval stenosis etc.). A thorough evaluation of late results in long-term survivors of TGA correction has become very important in recent years, with the awareness of systemic ventricle failure as a significant late complication in patients where the morphologically right ventricle has to perform systemic work [5]. Nevertheless, very long observations of surgical results – 25 years or more, as in our study – must be viewed with caution: there were major changes in the surgical technique and postoperative treatment (use of cardioplegia, correction of TGA at a very early stage of life, improved pharmacotherapy, intensive care management etc). With respect to the logistic of follow-up, it becomes difficult to keep track of patients when they reach adulthood; the physicians who took care of them are already retired or died; and just the study of clinical records going back for a quarter of a century or more makes one aware of the general improvements in medicine in recent years.

The operative mortality for the total correction of TGA, especially of its complex forms, was very high in the pioneering years. It is very well possible that some of the problems encountered by these patients today are not due to their malformation as such, but to the insufficient myocardial protection and poor perioperative management in that era.

Potential disadvantages of atrial correction of TGA are numerous, and they have been spelled out frequently by the proponents of arterial switch: late arrhythmias, systemic atrio-ventricular valve incompetence, late failure of systemic ventricle, persistent late mortality, complex operation in newborns (growth problems), stenosis of superior and inferior vena cava, stenosis of pulmonary veins or of pulmonary atrium, and the general fact that atrial correction is not an anatomic correction in narrow sense. Without going into the relative merits of atrial vs. arterial correction for TGA – and a similar list of disadvantages can be made for arterial switch as well – there are definite advantages to atrial correction. This procedure is nowadays carried out with an extremely low operative risk, even in the first weeks of life; cummulative mortality of balloon septostomy followed by atrial correction at the age of 2–3 months lies around 5% [6]; this procedure has been demostrated to enable satisfactory growth of the heart after correction – which still has to be proven for coronary anastomoses and pulmonary valve in arterial switch procedure; preparative operations like banding or aorto-pulmonary shunt are not necessary; and – probably most important of them all – atrial correction has been proved to be successful in a great majority of patients 10–20 years after surgery.

The functional results of atrial correction, although not perfect, can still be considered as very good. When evaluating late life achievements and their present position in the society, patients must be evaluated not only with respect to their actual work capacity, usually determined by the ability of the heart to increase cardiac output during exercise, but also by the level of their intellectual development. Our data show no clear-cut trend: most of the patients attended normal schools and some even continued to the universities, but 13% were sent to special schools, denoting some degree of intellectual impairment. The reason for this deficiency is not quite clear, and probably multifactorial; it is well known in other cyanotic malformations as well [7]. All these patients had a longer period of low arterial oxygen saturation with its deficient brain development; in some of the children – before the era of balloon septostomy – the hypoxia was extreme, sometimes coupled with longer periods of acidosis. The reactive hyperglobulia in cyanotic patients leads to the formation of venous thrombi, which can become dislodged and cause cerebral infarctions, well known in all cyanotic malformations with right–left shunting [8]. And finally, difficult postoperative course in the sixties might have also caused some cerebral damage. Early total correction of TGA might improve the cognitive function of these children [9].

In conclusion, atrial correction provides very good results in a great majority of patients with simple and complex TGA; the results seem to be better in the present era. Failure of systemic ventricle and sudden death remain the principal problems in the extended follow-up; it is difficult to decide how many of those problems are related to either the procedure or to malformations.

Our present management of TGA is as follows: arterial switch in newborns with or without VSD; balloon septostomy in children with major associated anomalies, sepsis or neurological problems. This is followed by atrial correction at the age of 3–6 months in simple TGA. PA banding is practiced only in multiple VSDs or in the problem cases mentioned above. In patients with TGA and organic PS, atrial correction with PS repair is again done after Rashkind procedure, preferably beyond neonatal age.

References

1. Senning A: Surgical correction of transposition of the great vessels. Surgery 1959;45:966–980.
2. Jatene AD et al.: Anatomic correction of transposition of the great vessels. J Thorac Cardiovasc Surg 1976;72:364–370.
3. Mustard WT: Successful two-stage correction of transposition of the great vessels. Surgery 1964;55:469–472.
4. Norwood WI et al.: Intermediate results of arterial switch repair. J Thorac Cardiovasc Surg 1988;96:854–863.
5. Turina M et al.: Late functional deterioration after atrial correction for transposition of the great arteries. Circulation 1989;80(suppl I):I-162–I-167.
6. Bender HW et al.: Ten year's experience with the Senning operation for transposition of great arteries: physiological results and late follow-up. Ann Thorac Surg 1989;47:218–223.

7. Tyler HR, Clark DB: Incidence of neurological complications in congenital heart disease. Arch Neurol Psychiatry 1957;77:17–22.
8. Cottrill CN, Kaplan S: Cerebral vascular incidents in cyanotic congenital heart disease. Am J Dis Child 1973;125:484–487.
9. Newburger JW, Silbert AR, Buckley LP, Fyler DC: Cognitive function and age at repair of transposition of the great arteries in children. N Engl J Med 1984;310:1495–1499.

25. Congenital heart disease: an analytic approach to functional outcome after open heart surgery

CATHERINE A. NEILL and EDWARD B. CLARK

1. Introduction

Quality of life is ephemeral, mysterious, and ultimately a secret known only to the individual heart. Yet we seek, in following our patients, to go beyond survival curves, to ask, as we do of our friends: 'What really happened to them, how well are they, what is their quality of life?'

Every adult who has undergone open heart surgery for a congenital heart defect has passed through a series of thickets which may affect later quality of life [1]. These thickets are often thought of as involving only the timing and technical success of anatomic cardiac repair. We who have been fortunate enough to know a number of these adults are very aware of their own remarkable achievements; many of those who underwent repair of tetralogy of Fallot in the 1960s had already had one or more prior operations, and at least one other hospitalisation for cardiac catheterisation. They have had more exposure to hospitals and to hazards than many persons experience in a lifetime. That so many have gone on to successful careers and productive lives is a continuing source of happiness, a tribute to surgical skill and to the strength and resilience of these pioneering patients and their families. As we think of and remember the mathematicians, the lawyers, the teachers and the nurses who have grown from these formerly cyanotic small children, as we study the photographs of their own healthy children (and even grandchildren), we are moved and inspired by their quality of life. Yet there continue to be gaps in our understanding of the spectrum of how children born with cardiac defects perform in adult life.

Miettinen [2], at a symposium on the postoperative cardiac child, stated that problem conceptualisation in research into post-surgical course 'involves considerable complexity and subtlety'. In this chapter we discuss some of these complexities, summarising some of the few published studies; our major focus is on the need in the future for more sophisticated analyses of the new cohorts of patients who will reach adulthood in the 21st century.

The group of patients already followed presents several special problems

Paul J. Walter (ed.): Quality of Life after Open Heart Surgery, 277–291.

in analysis: first, having been born with a heart defect, and undergone surgery in childhood, they cannot compare adult life before and after intervention; they thus differ from transplant patients or those with hypertension, who have been more extensively studied [3,4]. Second, some feel themselves to be entirely well even if objective signs of impaired ventricular function or exercise capacity are present; their perceived quality of life is normal, yet their cardiopulmonary function is not. Third, many published series concern outcome in pioneer patients whose parents travelled to distant centres to obtain help, journeys involving possibly exceptional motivation and devotion; the very high achievement levels reported may not be entirely representative. Despite these caveats, quality of life studies are valuable and need to be continued and amplified. The use of standardised instruments, such as the Quality of Well Being Index [5,6], will assist future interstudy comparisons.

1.1. *Prior studies*

These have often dealt with patients and their cardiac defects in isolation, without mention of other influences on their lives: most have described specific cardiac defects, followed by one centre over one or more decades after surgery. In the early years following open heart repair, most follow-up studies emphasised, very reasonably, clinical status and hemodynamic results. It is perhaps not surprising that the words 'vocation' 'career' and 'family' are lacking from the index of some text books dealing with congenital heart disease in the adult.

Combining published reports on the 'classic' defects of tetralogy [6–15], and atrial [16] and ventricular septal defects [17,18], studies to date confirm the clinical impression that such children do well in adult life. The Natural History Study II, involving patients with ventricular septal defect, aortic stenosis and pulmonic stenosis followed over a 25-year period, shortly to be published [19], shows that patients' self-assessment of health, employment status, and ability to lead an independent life closely parallels the members of an age-matched population. Questions remain regarding the pioneering group of patients operated before the 1980s, as to completeness of psychosocial adaptation [20,21], the true incidence of defect recurrence in the next generation [22–25], the role of early postoperative exercise programs, and the best methods of improving the patient's understanding of his own defect. Furthermore, a consensus has not been reached on the optimal frequency and type of cardiac follow up. There is as yet no systematic information on reaction and adjustment to mid-life crises, nor on response to aging.

1.2. *The changing cohort*

As the success rate of surgery continues to improve, and as repair is undertaken at progressively younger ages [26,27], the cohort of patients reaching adult life is steadily increasing. For example, by the year 2000, some infants who have had an arterial switch procedure for transposition [28,29] will be reaching their early 20s; their survival, ventricular function, freedom from reoperation and quality of life can then be compared with those surviving atrial switch operations [30,31].

Children born with tetralogy of Fallot can be the paradigm for those with severe defects. Prior to the surgical era, less than 20% of such children survived to twenty years of age [32]; now [26], approximately 95% of infants who undergo tetralogy repair survive, and late deaths are rare, characteristically 3% or less over a ten to fifteen year period of follow up. (Survival rates in tetralogy with pulmonary atresia remain significantly lower [33,34]). Roberts [35] has calculated that by the year 1995 there will be over 15 000 children with tetralogy between one and twenty years of age alive in the USA. Hoffman [36] has estimated an overall benefit:cost ratio of successful surgical treatment of heart defects to be at least 2.5:1, since the overwhelming majority of survivors will become productive members of society. Figure 1 shows schematically some of the historic landmarks that have led to this extraordinary change in outcome. The full impact of the management changes in the 1980s, allowing successful repair in infancy without prior shunt procedures, has yet to be felt, since of necessity such children are still in their first or second decade of life. This cohort will differ from those in the

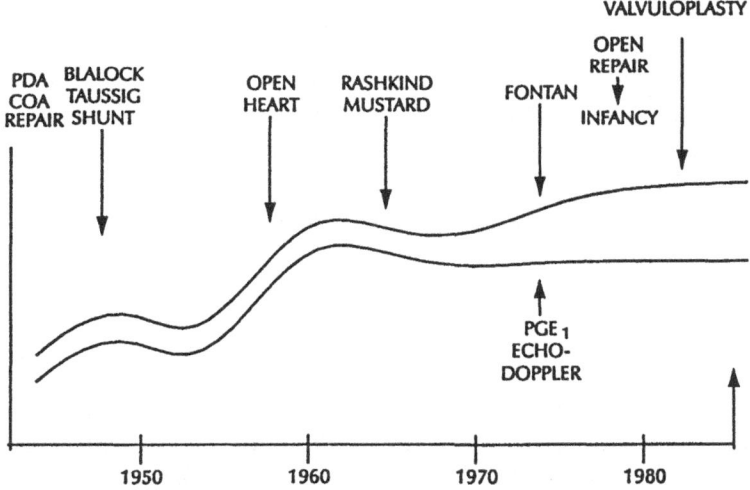

Figure 1. Schematic rendering of milestones contributing to expanding numbers of patients born with heart defects reaching adult life.

CARDIAC

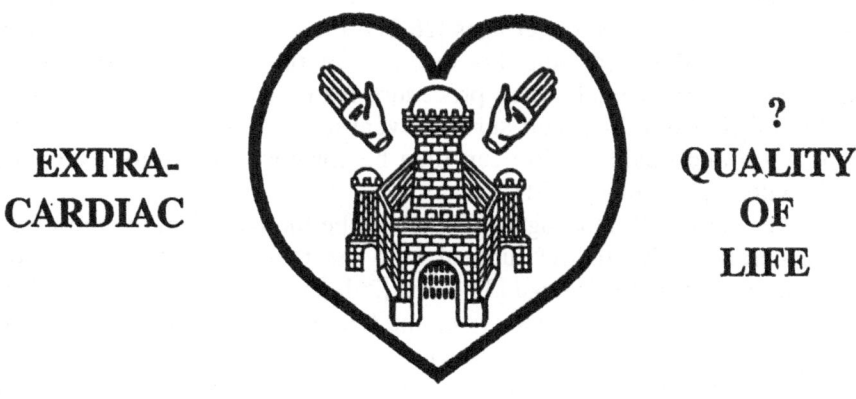

EXTRA-
CARDIAC

**?
QUALITY
OF
LIFE**

ENVIRONMENT

Figure 2. Input variables contributing to quality of life in adults after repair of congenital heart defects.

past; they will have had less prolonged hypoxia and will benefit from continuing surgical advances. However, they will more closely resemble regional cohorts of live born infants, and may include more with extracardiac and environmental problems. There are thus a number of 'input variables' which might affect quality of life in the adult.

2. Input variables

Using the coat of arms of Antwerp as an illustration (Figure 2), every child who has had heart surgery and reached adulthood will, like his peers with normal hearts, attempt to spend the next six decades building his own castle and a new independent life. Attempts to do this are influenced by cardiac, extracardiac and environmental factors.

2.1. *Cardiac factors*

The cardiac factors, including the timing and type of prior surgical shunt procedures, were a major focus in past studies; most have excluded complex tetralogy variants, including those with atrioventricular canal and absent pulmonary valve, and have assessed outcome separately for tetralogy with pulmonary stenosis or atresia. Although no study has shown adult quality of life to be affected by age at open repair or the performance of prior shunt procedures, there is accumulating evidence that late ventricular arrhythmias are more common in patients who have had prolonged myocardial hypoxia [37].

2.2. *Extracardiac factors*

These may include defined syndromes or extracardiac anomalies, complications of the defect or of therapy, and other illness. Recent studies [38,39] of infants with tetralogy have shown that 25% have *extracardiac* anomalies, including 9% with chromosomal syndromes, mainly trisomy 21; many of these in future can be expected to reach adult life. Tetralogy is associated with abnormalities of mesenchymal cell migration [40], specifically cells derived from the neural crest; such abnormalities may be of clinical and genetic significance [41].

Extracardiac Factors

- Syndromes
    Chromosomal: Down, other
    Neural crest: di George, other
- Congenital defects, mental retardation
- Complications of defect or therapy
- Other illness (e.g., malignancy, endocrine)
- Aging

In this age of microbiology it may not be too fanciful to think of cardiac factors as comparable to DNA, analysable by 'Northern blot' techniques: extracardiac factors as RNA Western blot), environment as 'Southern blot', and the quality of life as the unknown Eastern blot, yet to be discovered. These speculative analogies are only mentioned to suggest that though we, as cardiologic teams, have little or no influence on problems outside the heart, they may nevertheless profoundly affect the child's later life and future.

Fyler [42], in a report on 126 children five years following cardiac surgery, found lower IQ scores correlated with the presence of extracardiac anomalies and with a lower family social index, but not with previous cyanosis. This was the first study to evaluate the possible impact of extracardiac and environmental factors on potential quality of life. Excellent analyses of subsequent psychosocial [20], and neurologic [43] studies are available.

Presbitero [44], reporting on 40 patients undergoing tetralogy repair in adult life, found preoperative *complications* including endocarditis and scoliosis in over one third of subjects: many, if not all, of these complications should be absent in future cohorts repaired in infancy.

The effect of *aging* on the heart with a cardiac defect is not yet known: but it is sobering to realise that some patients with repaired congenital defects may shortly feature in one of the numerous studies of geriatric quality of life!

Environmental variations may profoundly affect the quality of life.

Environmental factors

- Family
- Socioeconomic
- Health care: Access and quality
- 'Land mines'

A child's *family* provides both genetic and environmental input into his development. A few studies have compared intellectual achievement in cardiac children [45] with their siblings, and in adults [13] with that of other family members. Donovan [20] has discussed the complex relationship between family anxiety and cardiac severity. Though the over-protective family, and particularly the anxious mother, may sometimes play a negative role, the positive aspects of having a parent who notes subtle changes in the child's well being and brings him back for needed treatment is seldom discussed. Behind every functional twenty-year-old born with a severe heart defect, now successfully repaired, there lies not only a good cardiac team, but a caring family; the long term outcome in the increasing numbers of children born into dysfunctional families or to single mothers is still unknown. Further studies of outcome in the context of family education and achievement levels [13] are needed.

In the Western world, access to good pediatric cardiac *health care* is almost universal; the network of such facilities is one of the triumphs of modern medicine; adults may encounter problems related to lack of such a special network [46,47], or to inadequacy of health insurance [48].

As we have recently been reminded by the desperate plight of the Kurdish refugees, sudden catastrophe, or 'land mines' may overwhelm even those with normal or successfully repaired hearts. The interaction of cardiac with other *input variables* is complex; incorporation of their effects into future studies of the spectrum of quality of life of birth cohorts of infants undergoing cardiac repair presents a significant challenge.

3. Outcome measures

Early long term studies [49] described clinical status, including heart size, murmurs and electrocardiographic changes; some included post operative cardiac catheterisations. The absence of cyanosis and heart failure was commented on, and the overall health assessment by parents, children and cardiologist was usually described as 'good to excellent'. Taussig [50] reported that 53 of 180 patients who had had a shunt procedure between November 1944 and January 1951 were active in professions, and 'one young man received his appointment as a full professor of law before his thirtieth birthday.' This appears to be the first mention of vocational outcome.

Later outcome studies have included self assessment of activity, objective measures of cardiopulmonary status, analysis of vocational and educational achievement, and in some cases, assessment of the new independent family unit. Until recently hemodynamic status was assessed at cardiac catheterisation, but Doppler-echocardiography is now the major method used. There has been steadily increasing use of exercise studies.

Cardiopulmonary status

- Somerville Ability Index
- Echo-Doppler Studies
- Exercise testing
- Holter monitoring
**Progressive problem*

Although in the early years after open repair of tetralogy was available, a number of patients had significant residual outflow obstruction or ventricular septal defects, the major hemodynamic problem now is pulmonary valvar insufficiency; mild degrees are well tolerated over many years: in only about 1% of patients does such insufficiency cause cardiac disability, and then usually only in those with extensive outflow patches, severe pulmonary arterial stenosis, or associated pulmonary vascular disease.

Reoperation for residual defects is needed in only between three and five percent of patients in most long term follow-up studies [7,9,11,12,14]. Although early and late mortality and reoperation rates are higher for tetralogy with pulmonary atresia, nevertheless 86 of 90 surviving patients were classified as NYHA I at ten year follow-up [51]. Since the recognition that a few patients (less than 1% per year), followed for ten or more years died suddenly from probable ventricular arryhthmias [52], there have been many efforts to document risk factors for significant ventricular ectopy [53,54]. In a recent study from The Johns Hopkins Medical Institutions, Zahka [55] examined 59 patients who underwent open repair of tetralogy in the first decade of life, and were studied a mean of eighteen years postoperatively. No patient had sudden death or symptomatic arrhythmias; however, ventricular couplets and episodes of ventricular tachycardia were more frequent in those with moderate pulmonary regurgitation and right ventricular dilatation (Figure 3). Rowe [56] performed exercise testing on the same group of patients and found moderate pulmonary regurgitation and increased right ventricular diastolic area were both inversely related to exercise duration and capacity. Nearly one half of patients had a vital capacity less than 80%

VENTRICULAR COUPLETS / TACHYCARDIA

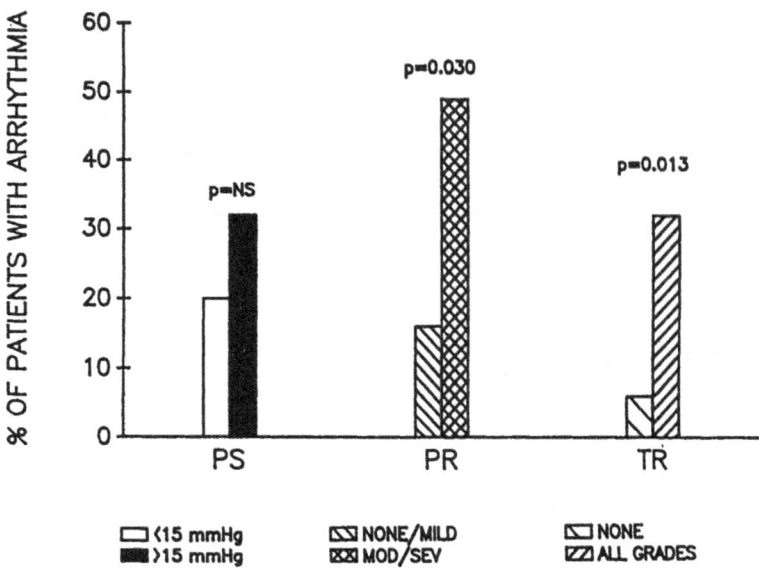

Figure 3. Percentage of post operative tetralogy patients with ventricular couplets or tachycardia: PS pulmonary stenosis: PR pulmonary regurgitation: TR tricuspid regurgitation. Adapted, with permission, from Zahka et al. Circulation 1989 [55].

of predicted; nevertheless, over 90% had exercise duration within the normal range. Perrault [57] reported subnormal cardiac index and chronotropic limitation in response to submaximal exercise ten years postoperatively in 13 patients repaired before 5 years of age, despite asymptomatic clinical status.

Pulmonary regurgitation, studied by many different techniques [58,59], has not been a useful index of quality of life, since it is present in many asymptomatic patients. Calza [12], in a clinical and hemodynamic study of 150 operated patients, found 96% to be socially active, 92% to have good exercise tolerance, and 79.3 % to be participating in sports; and found minor degrees of pulmonary insufficiency to be well tolerated. Redington [59], using pressure volume loops to analyse the relationship between right ventricular dysfunction and pulmonary regurgitation, has stressed the need for further long term studies. Right ventricular dilatation and dysfunction is not solely a function of pulmonary insufficiency. New strategies are needed for recognising the rare progressive myocardial dysfunction and for treating the damaged myocardium by cellular implants or by stimulating myocardial cell growth.

It seems probable that there is a specific degree of pulmonary insufficiency and right ventricular outflow dyskinesis severe enough to progress over time and result in right ventricular dilatation, possibly ventricular arrhythmias and gradual decrease in exercise capacity and quality of life; there is as yet no consensus on such a definable end point separating the overwhelming majority with trivial pulmonary insufficiency from the much rarer form resulting in complications.

3.1. *Somerville's ability index*

This is useful, and can include input variables already outlined. Recent long term studies of tetralogy show 85–90% of patients to be in her Groups I or II, leading normal lives, some with mild restriction in exercise capacity or mild pulmonary insufficiency. In following patients we prefer to include in Group III all those patients who may be asymptomatic and have an excellent quality of life when seen at a cross section in time, but whose problem, cardiac or extracardiac is known to be *progressive*. Although a consensus on the group may not yet be available, we include all individuals with homografts or prosthetic valves [10,56], all with aortic valve disease or major aortic dilatation, and all with severe pulmonic insufficiency or right ventricular dysfunction. Because long term outcome is not well established, we also include all adults with transposition following atrial baffle procedures and postoperative Fontan patients though many are asymptomatic and leading normal lives.

3.2. *Vocational studies*

Such studies [7,8,10,11,13,15,55] have shown between 75 and 85% of repaired tetralogy patients to be fully employed: in Zahka's study [55] 84% were either fully employed or still receiving graduate or postgraduate education. Hallali [15] detailed socio-professional integration of 104 patients and reported 79 (76%) were employed or students, 19 were unemployed or chose not to work, and six had 'poor integration into society'. He also tabulated survival and reoperation rates in six previous long term studies, and discusses some of the problems of inter-study comparisons. Shampaine [13] found IQ to be stable in 21 subjects over a 20-year period; there was good correlation between intelligence, academic achievement and type of employment. Only two subjects (9.5%) did not work. The level of same-sex parental and sibling education was comparable to the patients'. Since 'Time's wingéd chariot' is as audible to cardiac teams as to patients, a prolonged multidisciplinary study such as this represents great stability and quality of life in patients and academic investigators alike. Lillehei [7] has commented on the higher than average educational achievement levels of patients who underwent tetralogy repair in the early years. Future studies [60] may help resolve some of the continuing discrepancy between the excellent outcome in published series and the frequent graphic yet rarely published reports of the thickets an individual patient with a complex defect may encounter in obtaining and keeping employment [61].

Several authors have analysed the interaction of physical handicap and psychosocial well being. Kramer [62] found cardiac children with physical handicap had more basic anxiety and a greater sense of inferiority than those with no handicap. Garson [21] reported that neurotic symptoms in adults following tetralogy repair were increased in those with more frequent prior hospitalisations, but did not correlate with objectively measured severity of cardiac defect. The discrepancy between anxiety and severity has been noted by others.

New *family* units and an independent life are established at a slightly older age than usual, but the difference does not appear significant. Mothers with prior corrective surgery tolerate pregnancy well: the only caveats concern those with severe myocardial dysfunction or pulmonary vascular disease; those on anticoagulants present special management problems. The *genetic risk* of recurrence of a cardiac defect in the next generation is not usually included under quality of life, but deserves mention as a topic of intense interest and concern to patients, even those who have had a benign clinical course. The low overall recurrence risk of around 3–5% in offspring needs modification for parents with left heart flow defects including aortic stenosis and coarctation; their risk is probably closer to 15% [63], and counselling on obtaining fetal echocardiography before 20 weeks' gestation is indicated. Such studies help in the management of affected infants, and can be greatly reassuring in the normal majority. The risk of recurrence of tetralogy of Fallot in offspring has varied, and particular effort should be made to exclude genetic syndromes before counselling [64,65].

3.3. *Freedom from reoperation*

This is at a high level, and should continue to improve, as should freedom from risk of sudden arrhythmic death. Our patients, like ourselves, need the freedom from want and fear and the other freedoms defined by President Franklin D. Roosevelt; in addition, this special group needs freedom from iatrogenic anxieties, repetitive invasive cardiac procedures, and conflicting medical advice, referred to here as the 'Tower of Babel' syndrome. Affected patients may respond with anxiety and symptomatology, or by avoiding further cardiac visits for many years. Either outcome is undesirable, particularly as a normal life span may well lie ahead for many, and preventive cardiology and a heart healthy life style thus become of crucial long term importance.

**CARDIO-
PULMONARY
STATUS**

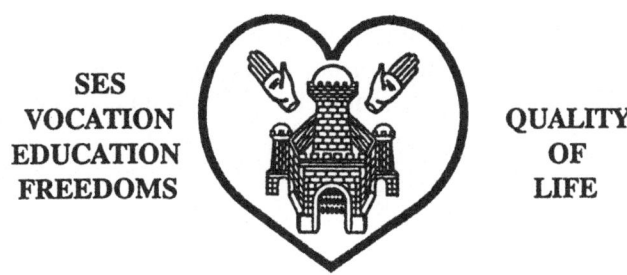

**SES
VOCATION
EDUCATION
FREEDOMS**

**QUALITY
OF
LIFE**

**FAMILY UNIT
PSYCHO-SOCIAL**

Figure 4. Outcomes assessed in studies of quality of life in adults after repair of congenital heart defects.

3.4. *Overall quality of life assessments*

To date, in operated patients, such studies are thus highly reassuring. In a pioneering analysis correlating cardiac status with the quality of well-being index in patients ten years following tetralogy repair, Torii [6] found an average well being score of 0.773 (range 0.58–1.0). Twelve of 47 patients with a normal well being score of 1.0 were free of any objective sign of cardiac disability. Lower well being scores correlated with cardiomegaly or high right ventricular/left ventricular pressure ratios, but not with arrhythmia status using the Lown grading system.

4. Future studies of adult quality of life (Figure 4)

Stimulated by this volume, such studies should be planned on a *regional* basis. This would permit analysis of the entire spectrum of outcome in defects such as tetralogy, rather than being limited to those who reached major super-regional surgical referral centers. Studies from such centers have already documented conclusively that the majority of patients with isolated cardiac defects can now become adults leading essentially normal lives. The new cohort of infants with transposition undergoing arterial switch procedures should show similar excellent outcome, since their freedom from extracardiac anomalies is well established; further studies of education and achievement compared to other family members are needed, in addition to other input variables and *extracardiac* problems not included in prior studies. New techniques for correlating the many input variables with outcome will have to be developed. Although the terminology of some quality of life literature is daunting, use of relatively simple and accepted instruments, such as the Quality of Well-Being Index [4–6] may help in making outcome findings comparable in different studies. Arranging outcome analysis in *age cohorts* by decades will make inter study group comparisons easier. The fourth decade of life, including patients from thirty to forty, will be particularly informative, since by that age schooling is usually completed and an independent life established.

Future studies

- Regional basis
- Input variables: Outcome correlations
- Groupings by age cohort (decades)
- Quality of Life standard instruments

The past 50 years have been a period of remarkable achievement by pioneering surgeons, cardiologists, patients and families. The focus of research is moving towards etiology and prevention of major congenital defects [25,38,39,40,65]. At the same time, analytic studies on quality of life, incorporating and building on prior work, could document the triumphs and occasional problems of operated cardiac patients as they enter the 21st century, and be an enduring monument to the foundations laid by the present volume.

References

1. Neill CA: Quality of life issues in the adult with congenital heart disease. Quality of Life and Cardiovasc Care 1987;3:5–14:Part II. The new generation ibid 57–61.
2. Miettinen O: Post-surgical course in congenital heart disease: Problem-conceptualisation for research. In: Kidd L, Rowe RD (eds.) The Child with Congenital Heart Disease After Surgery. New York: Futura Publishing 1976;439–445.
3. Kaplan RM: Health related quality of life in cardiovascular disease. J Consult Clin Psychol 1988;56:382–392.
4. Spilker B, Molinek FR, Johnston KA, Simpson RL, Tilson HH: Quality of life bibliography and indexes. Medical Care 1990;(suppl)28:DS1–DS77.
5. Kaplan RM, Anderson JP, Wu AW, Mathews WC, Kozin F, Orenstein D: The quality of well-being scale. Applications in AIDS, cystic fibrosis, and arthritis. Medical Care 1989;27:S27–S43.
6. Torii S, Suma K, Miyawaki F, Shiroma K, Inoue K: Postoperative long term quality of life at present after total correction of tetralogy of Fallot. Kyobu Geka 1990;43:620–624.
7. Lillehei CW, Varco RL, Cohen M et al.: The first open-heart corrections of tetralogy of Fallot: a 26–31 year follow-up of 106 patients. Ann Surg 1986; 204:490–501.
8. Garson A Jr, McNamara DG, Cooley DA: Tetralogy of Fallot. In: WC Roberts (ed.) Adult Congenital Heart Disease Philadelphia: FA Davis, 1987;493–518.
9. Fuster V, McGoon DC, Kennedy MA Ritter DG, Kirklin JW: Long term evaluation (12–22 years) of open heart surgery for tetralogy of Fallot. Am J Cardiol 1980;46:635–642.

10. Viart P, Deuvaert F, Gallez A, Primo G, Dramaix M: Résultats tardifs des cures de tetralogie de Fallot. Arch Mal Coeur 1990;83:653–657.

11. Shimada M, Tsunemoto M: Long term (10–23 years) clinical evaluation of quality of life in patients following open heart repair of tetralogy of Fallot. Kyobu Geka 1990;43:634–639.

12. Calza G, Pannizon G, Rovida S, Aigueperse J: Incidence of residual defects determining the clinical outcome after correction of tetralogy of Fallot: Postoperative late follow up. Ann Thorac Surg 1989;47:428–435.

13. Shampaine EL, Nadelman L, Rosenthal A, Behrendt D, Sloan H: Longitudinal psychological assessment in tetralogy of Fallot. Pediatr Cardiol 1990;10:135–140.

14. Lange PE: Long term results after surgical treatment of tetralogy of Fallot. Z Kardiol 1989;78(suppl 7):47–51.

15. Hallali P, Davido A, Corone P: Tetralogy of Fallot: 20 years experience concerning 144 cases. Arch Mal Coeur 1989;82:683–688.

16. Murphy JG, Gersh BJ, McGoon MD, Mair DD, et al.: Long term outcome after surgical repair of isolated atrial septal defect. Follow-up at 27 to 32 years. N Engl J Med 1990;323:1645–1650.

17. Otterstad JE, Tjore I, Sundby P: Social function of adults with isolated ventricular septal defects. Scand J Soc Med 1986;14:15–23.

18. Kagawa Y, Horiuchi T, Ito T, et al.: Long term results of open heart repair of ventricular septal defect. Tohoku J Exp Med 1987;151:1–14.

19. Gersony WM, Hayes CJ, Dricoll DJ et al.: The Second Natural History Study of congenital heart defects: Quality of life of patients with aortic stenosis, pulmonary stenosis or ventricular septal defect. Awaiting publication as supplement to Circulation 1992.

20. Donovan EF: Psychosocial considerations in congenital heart disease. In: Adams FH, Emmanouilides GC, Riemenschneider T (eds.) Moss' Heart Disease in Infants Children and Adolescents. 4th Ed. Baltimore: Williams and Wilkins 1989: 984–991.

21. Garson A Jr, Williams RB Jr, Reckless J: Long term follow-up of patients with tetralogy of Fallot: Physical health and psychopathology. J Pediatr 1974;85:429–433.

22. Whittemore R, Hobbins JC, Engle MA: Pregnancy and its outcome in women with and without surgical treatment of congenital heart disease. Am J Cardiol 1982;50:361–370.

23. Emanuel R, Somerville J, Inas A, Withers R: Evidence of congenital heart disease in the offspring of parents with atrioventricular septal defects. Brit Heart J 1983;49:144–147.

24. Ferencz C, Boughman JA, Neill CA, Brenner JB, Perry LW and the BWIS study group: Congenital cardiovascular malformations: Questions on inheritance. J Am Coll Cardiol 1989;14:756–63.

25. Pyeritz RE Murphy EA: Genetics and congenital heart disease: Perspectives and prospects J Am Coll Cardiol 1989;13:1458–68.

26. Kirklin JW: The movement of cardiac surgery to the very young. In: Crupi G, Parenzan L, Anderson RH (eds) Perspectives in Pediatric Cardiology vol 2 Pediatric Cardiac Surgery 1989;2:3–27.

27. Walsh EP, Rockenmacher S, Keane JF, Hougen TJ, Lock JE, Casteneda A: Late results in patients with tetralogy of Fallot repaired during infancy. Circulation 1988;77:1062–1067.

28. Norwood WL, Dobell AR, Freed MD, Kirklin JW, Blackstone EH and the Congenital Heart Surgeons Society: Intermediate results of the arterial switch repair: a 20 institution study. J Thorac Cardiovasc Surg 1988;96:854–63.

29. Planche C, Serraf A, Lacour-Gayet F, Bruniaux J, Bouchart F: Anatomic correction of complete transposition with ventricular septal defect in neonates: experience with 42 consecutive cases. Cardiol Young 1991;1:101–103.

30. Kirklin JW: The surgical repair for complete transposition. Cardiol Young 1991;1:13–25.

31. Redington AN: Functional assessment of the heart after corrective surgery for complete transposition. Cardiol Young 1991;1:84–9022.

32. Bertranou EG, Blackstone EH, Hazelrig JB, Turner ME, Kirklin JW: Life expectancy without surgery in the tetralogy of Fallot. Am J Cardiol 1978;42:458–466.

33. Shimazaki Y, Tokuan Y, Lio M, et al.: Pulmonary artery pressure and resistance late after repair of tetralogy of Fallot with pulmonary atresia. J Thorac Cardiovasc Surg 1990;100:425–440.

34. Hofbeck M, Trusler GA, Freedom RM et al.: Analysis of survival in patients with pulmonic valve atresia and ventricular septal defect. Am J Cardiol 1991: 67:737–743.

35. Roberts NK, Cretin S: The changing face of congenital heart disease. A method for predicting the influence of cardiac surgery upon the prevalence and spectrum of congenital heart disease. Medical Care 1980;18:930–939.

36. Hoffman JIE: Incidence, mortality and natural history. In: Anderson RH, Shineburne EA, Macartney FJ, Tynan M (eds.) Pediatric Cardiology. Edinburgh: Churchill Livingstone, 1987;1: 3–14.

37. Sullivan ID, Presbitero P, Gooch VM, Aruta E, Deanfield JE: Is ventricular arrhythmia in repaired tetralogy of Fallot an effect of operation or a consequence of the course of the disease? Br Heart J 1987; 58:40–44.

38. Ferencz C, Rubin JD, McCarter RJ, et al.: Cardiac and non-cardiac malformations: Observations in a population-based study. Teratology 1987;35:367–378

39. Voisin M, Doan B, Elboury S, Messner P, et al.: Extracardiac malformations in tetralogy of Fallot. Arch Mal Coeur 1989;82:689–692.

40. Clark EB, Takao A: Overview: a focus for research in cardiovascular development. In: Clark EB, Takao A (eds). Developmental Cardiology: Morphogenesis and Function. New York: Futura Publishing 1990;3–12.

41. Radford DJ Thong YH: Facial and immunological abnormalities associated with Tetralogy of Fallot. International J Cardiol 1989;22:229–236.

42. Fyler DC, Silbert AR, Rothman K: Five year follow up of infant cardiacs: Intelligence quotient. In: Kidd L, Rowe RD (eds.) The Child With Congenital Heart Disease After Surgery. New York: Futura Publishing, 1976;409–419.

43. Fishman MA Parke JT: Neurologic issues of importance to the pediatric cardiologist. In: Garson A, Bricker JT, McNamara DG (eds.) The Science and Practice of Pediatric Cardiology. Philadelphia: Lea and Febiger, 1990;3:2310–2327.

44. Presbitero P, Demarie D, Aruta E, et al.: Results of Total correction of tetralogy of Fallot performed in adults. Ann Thorac Surg 1988;46:297–301.27.

45. Hesz N, Clark EB: Developmental outcome in children with transposition of the great vessels. Arch Dis Child 1988;63:198–200.

46. Somerville J: Congenital heart disease in the adolescent. Arch Dis Child 1989;64:771–773.

47. McNamara DG: The adult with congenital heart disease. In: O'Rourke RA, Crawford MH (eds.) Curr Probl Cardiol. Chicago: Year Book Medical Publishers 1989;14:57–114.

48. Manning JA: Congenital heart disease and the quality of life. In: Engle MA, Perloff JK (eds.) Congenital Heart Disease After Surgery: Benefits, Residua, Sequelae. Yorke Medical Books, 1983;347–361.

49. Jones EL, Conti R, Neill CA, Gott VL, Brawley RK, Haller JA: Long term evaluation of tetralogy patients with pulmonary valvular insufficiency resulting from outflow-patch correction across the pulmonic annulus. Circulation 1973; 17 and 18(suppl III)11–18.

50. Taussig HB, Crocetti A, Eshaghpour E, et al.: Long-time observations on the Blalock-Taussig operation I. Results of first operation. Johns Hopkins Med J 1971;129:243–257.

51. Kirklin JW, Blackstone EH, Shimizaki Y, Maehara T, Pacifico AD, Kirklin JK, Bargeron LM: Survival, functional status, and reoperations after repair of tetralogy of Fallot with pulmonary atresia. J Thorac Cardiovasc Surg 1988;96:102–116.

52. Quattlebaum TG, Varghese PJ, Neill CA, Donahoo JS: Sudden death among postoperative patients with tetralogy of Fallot: a follow-up study of 243 patients for an average of twelve years. Circulation 1976;54:289–293.

53. Zimmerman M, Friedli B, Adamec R, Oberhanski I: Ventricular late potentials and induced ventricular arrhythmia after surgical repair of tetralogy of Fallot. Am J Cardiol 1991;67:873–878.

54. Vaksmann G, el Kohen M, Breviere GM, Rey C, et al.: Incidence and factors favoring

ventricular arrhythmias after surgical repair of tetralogy of Fallot. Arch Mal Coeur 1990;83:659–663.

55. Zahka KG, Horneffer P, Rowe SA, Neill CA, et al.: Long term valvular function after total repair of tetralogy of Fallot. Relation to ventricular arrhythmias. Circulation 1988;78(suppl III):III-14–III-19.

56. Rowe SA, Zahka KG, Manolio TA, Horneffer P, Kidd L: Lung function and pulmonary regurgitation limit exercise capacity in post operative tetralogy of Fallot. J Am Coll Cardiol 1991;17:461–466.

57. Perrault H, Drblik SP, Montigny M, Davignon A, Lamarre A, Chartrand C, Stanley P: Comparison of cardiovascular adjustments to exercise in adolescents 8 to 15 years of age after correction of tetralogy of Fallot, ventricular septal defct or atrial septal defect. Am J Cardiol 1989;64:213–217.

58. Kobayashi J, Nakano S, Matsuda H, Arisawa J, Kawashima Y: Quantitative evaluation of pulmonary regurgitation after repair of tetralogy of Fallot using real time flow imaging system. Jap Circ J 1989;53:721–727.

59. Redington AN, Oldershaw PJ, Shinebourne EA, Rigby ML: A new technique for the assessment of pulmonary regurgitation and its application to the assessment of right ventricular function before and after repair of tetralogy of Fallot. Br Heart J 1988;60:57–65.

60. Stark J: Do we really correct congenital heart defects? J Thorac Cardiovasc Surg 1989;97:1–9.

61. Silverman SL: Growing up in America: white, male and medically limited. Clin Pediatr 1989;28:214–215.

62. Kramer HH, Awiszus D, Sterzel U, van Halteren A, Classen R: Development of personality and intelligence in children with congenital heart disease. J Child Psychol Psychiatry 1989;30:299–308.

63. Boughman JA, Berg KA, Astemborski JA, et al.: Familial risks of congenital heart defect assessed in a population based epidemiologic study. Am J Med Genet 1987;26:839–849.

64. Zellers TM, Driscoll DJ, Michels W: Prevalence of significant congenital heart defects in children of parents with Fallot's tetralogy. Am J Cardiol 1990;65:523–526.

65. Burn J: The etiology of congenital heart disease. In: Anderson RH, Macartney FJ, Shinebourne EA, Tynan M (eds.) Pediatric Cardiology. Edinburgh, Churchill Livingstone 1987;15–63.

26. Quality of life of patients after 'corrective' open heart surgery for congenital heart defects

F.J. MEIJBOOM and J. HESS

The natural history of patients with congenital heart defects is well known. In the era before surgical treatment was feasible, 30% of all children born with a congenital heart defect died within the first year of life. As a result of the development of open heart surgery in the early 1950s, this was bound to change. One of the major problems that was faced was how to bridge the period in which the patient's own heart was necessarily out of function during the open heart procedure. Inflow occlusion combined with moderate total body hypothermia was reported to be successful for closure of a secundum type atrial septal defect by Lewis [1] in September 1952. Attemps to operate on more complex defects, like ventricular septal defect, or infundibular pulmonary stenosis, failed. Cardiopulmonary bypass, using a pump-oxygenator, was successfully applied by Gibbon [2] for the first time in 1953: an atrial septal defect was closed in an 18-year-old girl. Another method of cardiopulmonary bypass was introduced by Warden [3], Lillehei et al. in 1954. They reported that it was possible to operate on patients with major cardiac malformations who were previously considered not to be correctable. These patients underwent open heart surgery using a cross-circulation system between patient and donor. The donor was lying next to the patient in the operating theatre, 'lending' his heart and lungs to the patient for the time of the operation.

The technical refinement of the pump oxygenators, and the improvement of the cardiopulmonary bypass techniques, made direct vision open heart repair of even complicated heart defects, using a heart-lung machine, possible. From the mid to late 1950's in the United States and some five to ten years later in the rest of the Western World, open heart surgery for congenital heart defects became a routine procedure. Morbidity and mortality were reduced significantly. In the following years, fewer and fewer cases were considered to be inoperable, and application-restrictions such as minimum age and minimum bodyweight to perform open heart surgery gradually disappeared. Figure 1 shows the decline in mortality due to congenital heart defects in the first year of life in the Dutch population. The last few years

Paul J. Walter (ed.): Quality of Life after Open Heart Surgery, 293–301.
© 1992 Kluwer Academic Publishers.

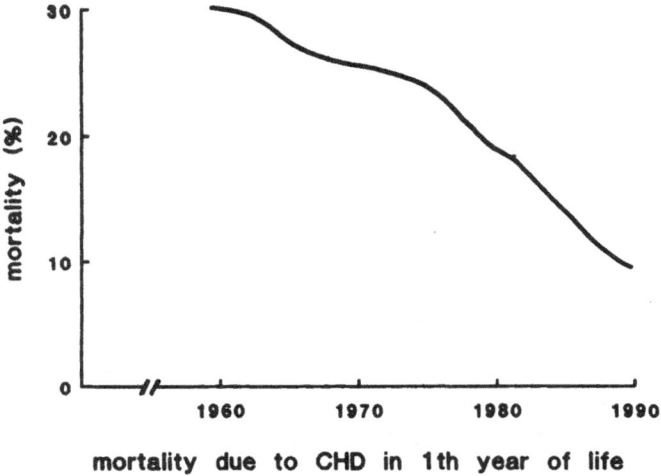

mortality due to CHD in 1th year of life

Figure 1. Mortality due to congenital heart disease in the first year of life.

the mortality is well below 10%. The most spectacular results were achieved in patients with severe cyanotic heart defects.

The natural history of transposition of the great arteries is known: 90% of all patients die within the first year of life, and only 1% will reach adult age. After the introduction of the atrial switch operation, by Mustard [4] in 1963, the survival originally became 80%, and later even over 95% [5].

The natural history of tetralogy of Fallot was only slightly less dramatic; 50% died in the first 5 years of life, and only 5% reached the age of 25 years. Since the introduction of intracardiac repair, 90% of patients reach adult age [6].

Ventricular septal defect is another example in which treatment changed the natural history. Before the onset of cardiovascular surgery, many children with this malformation died in infancy, due to intractable congestive heart failure or pneumonia [7]. In those who survived early infancy, later development of pulmonary vascular obstructive disease ('Eisenmenger's Syndrome') accounted for many late deaths. Once it became possible to close the ventricular septal defect 90% of all ventricular septal defect patients reached adulthood [8].

So the rapid development of surgical techniques resulted in a dramatical improvement of the prognosis of a variety of congenital heart defects, both from the point of mortality as well as morbidity.

Enthusiasm about these results was understandable, and justified. Because of these good results, the word 'correction', or 'total correction' became used to describe almost all open heart operations. The word 'palliation' was reserved mainly for closed heart operations, such as systemic-pulmonary artery shunts and banding of the pulmonary artery. However, the first concerns arose in the late seventies, as thoroughly executed long-term follow-up studies demonstrated considerable morbidity and even mortality a long time after corrective open heart surgery [9].

In the last ten years, growing sceptism could be noticed in most reports dealing with long-term follow-up. Are the results really that good? And are patients – once operated on – free from symptoms for the rest of their lives? Or can they lead a normal life? A challenging and somewhat philosophical overview by Stark, in his article 'Do we really correct congenital heart defects' [10], suggests that, not having internationally accepted definitions, an operation for a congenital heart defect may be considered as 'corrective', if the following criteria are met:

1. normal heart function is achieved and maintained;
2. life expectancy is normal;
3. further medical or surgical treatment is not necessary.

He, very justly, stated that no operation at the time of his writing could be classified as 'corrective', because nobody knows the real life expectancy of the operated group; open heart surgery has existed for only 35 years now! If one is less strict, one can substitute 'normal life expectancy' by 'normal health during the time of the follow-up'. Using Stark's criteria, a repeat assessment of which type of operation can be called 'corrective' may be performed at that time. For example, in the case of transposition of the great arteries, the Mustard repair had its previously mentioned enormous impact on early mortality. However, after ten to fifteen years of follow-up only 60% of patients are free of symptoms and lead a normal life. It became clear that baffle obstruction was present in 10–20% of all patients. Pulmonary venous obstruction was found in 5–10%, and that less than 50% of all patients were in sinus rhythm. Pacemaker implantation occurred regularly, as did reoperations because of baffle obstructions, or pulmonary venous obstruction. Furthermore, concern remains about the ability of the right ventricle to function as the systemic ventricle over a patient's lifetime [11]. It will be clear that the Mustard operation does not fulfill Stark's criteria for correction. Owing to the many complications, alternatives to the Mustard-type repair were tried.

The atrial switch operation according to Senning initially looked promising [12] but, with longer follow-up, similar problems appeared, as after the Mustard-type repair [13]. So no 'correction' here, either.

In a new type of surgical treatment for transposition of the great arteries, the arterial switch procedure, atrial surgery is avoided, and the typical problems seen in Mustard or Senning-type repair do not occur. Late mortality is very rare, and almost all survivors are free of symptoms. At the time of writing, the arterial switch procedure is considered to be corrective [4], but one should be aware of the fact that the follow-up period is still rather short (ten to twelve years maximum). The first complications after arterial switch, sometimes necessitating reoperations, have recently been reported: main pulmonary artery and pulmonary branch stenosis [15], right and left ventricular outflow tract obstruction, aortic valve incompetence, and coronary artery problems [16].

The second example is again tetralogy of Fallot. Of all the operated patients, 90% survive until adulthood. The majority feel healthy, and lead normal, active lives, with normal or only slightly diminished exercise tolerance [17]. In virtually all patients pulmonary incompetence with enlarged right ventricles is seen, but this is usually well tolerated. The problems arise if, next to the volume overload, elevated right ventricular pressure is present, due to residual pulmonary stenosis. These patients normally do have complaints of diminished exercise tolerance, and progression to right-side heart failure is not infrequent.

Ventricular arrhythmias and conduction distrubances are relatively frequent. Unifocal premature ventricular contractions, right bundle branch block alone, or together with left axis deviation (bifascicular block), appear to be benign [18]. Complete atrio-ventricular block often necessitates insertion of a permanent pacemaker. Serious ventricular arrhythmias, like multifocal premature ventricular contractions, ventricular tachycardia or ventricular fibrillation are associated with sudden death [19], especially if significant haemodynamic abnormalities are present (pulmonary incompetence or stenosis, residual ventricular septal defect). The nature and the occurrence of complications make it clear that in tetralogy of Fallot repair, too, the concept of 'total correction' is questionable.

In ventricular septal defects virtually all survivors are in NYHA class I or II. Abnormal response to exercise was found in nearly half of a group of patients studied three to fifteen years postoperatively [20]. Pulmonary hypertension is a key issue in the long-term prognosis in ventricular septal defect. In patients who were operated on before they were two years old, normal pulmonary vascular resistance is found in almost all [21]. In some patients with preoperative, moderately elevated pulmonary vascular resistance, however, a further increase of the resistance was seen postoperatively [22].

Of the seventeen late deaths among 385 patients who survived ventricular septal repair (in the Joint Study on the Natural History of Congenital Heart Defects [7]), most were known to have residual pulmonary hypertension. Another cause of late death in ventricular septal defect is ventricular arrhythmias [23]. So 'correction' of a ventricular septal defect might not be completely corrective in all patients.

Thoroughly executed long-term follow-up studies revealed that there were more or less serious sequelae after almost all open heart operations for congenital heart defects. Stark stated in his article [10] that only ligation of a persistant ductus arteriosus and closure of a secundum-type atrial septai defect could be considered corrective. McNamara and Latson [8] considered primary repair of secundum-type atrial septal defect *probably curative*, but warned of late and unpredictable occurrences of residual defects or sequelae of the operation.

A recent report from the Mayo Clinic [24] has informed us about excellent results for secundum-type atrial septal defect closure. The mean duration of follow-up in patients operated under the age of 25 years was 30 years. Survival was good (75% after 30 years compared with 85% in the normal population) and very few complications were seen. Surprisingly, the frequency of supraventricular arrhythmias in the group that was operated on at an age younger than 12 years was low. In this study information was obtained from patients by written questionnaires or by telephone interviews. Necessarily, it focused on subjective aspects of well-being.

As a result of this study design, it was hard to obtain a reliable picture of the cardiovascular status of the patients who did not have complaints, had not been admitted to hospital, and were not dead. Sequelae that may be present, sometimes even serious ones, but do not result in complaints (many supra-ventricular tachycardias), may therefore be overlooked. Subjective perception of patients' health, as is given in written or telephone patients' interviews, does not necessarily (and often does not at all) correlate with the 'objective' health status (for example: kidney dialysis patients and patients after heart transplantation generally feel happier and healthier than the normal population). In our opinion, it is necessary, if one is to perform a good follow-up study, to really examine the patients oneself and do an extensive cardiological work up. This is the only way to gain a reliable impression of the late complications present.

The Rotterdam Quality of Life study is an example of a study in which patients who underwent open heart surgery for congenital heart disease have been traced, actually seen, and examined. These patients underwent surgery between 1968 and 1980, and were younger than fifteen years of age at the time of the operation. The aim of the study is to evaluate the 'objective' and 'subjective' and well-being, or 'quality of life', of those who had survived until the present time. The evaluation was performed by a psychologist and a pediatric cardiologist. All patients who participated underwent extensive psychological testing, including intelligence tests, questions about school, profession, social coping, etc. The psychological study design is described by Dr L. Utens in chapter 29 of this book.

In the 13 years from 1968 to 1980, 735 patients were operated. Of these 735 patients, 109 died, 27 moved abroad and 23 were untraceable. Of the remaining 576 patients, 499 did eventually participate, which is 80% (corrected for non-survivors). The medical part of the examination included medical history, patients' interviews, physical examination, ECG, echocardiogram (2-D, M-mode, pulsed, CW, and colour-coded Doppler), bicycle ergometry, and Holter 24-hour ambulatory ECG. The study design was approved by a medical ethics committee.

The logistics of such a study should not be underestimated: tracing all the patients is very time consuming; patients were young when they were operated on and lived with their parents. Most of them were adult at the time of the study, and lived on their own. With the help of municipal registers that list all residents (and, if they have moved to another municipality, where they have gone), almost all patients could be traced. Once the patients were traced, they received a letter announcing the study. All were telephoned one to two weeks after they had received the letter, to make an appointment on a day when they could come to Rotterdam. For the patients this meant taking a whole day off from work or school. The medical examination took two or three hours, as did the psychological test. With lunch in between, and travelling to and from Rotterdam, it took patients six to ten hours that day. Lunch and travelling expenses were paid.

Two patients could be seen per day, so it took about $1\frac{1}{2}$ years to see all 499 patients. Per patient 300 to 500 items were checked, so the bulk of information was enormous; all data were stored in a computer: besides the previously-mentioned psychologist and pediatric cardiolgist, the contribution of a secretary is indispensable in such a study.

At the time of the 'quality of life' congress in Antwerp, in May 1991, the study was not yet finished. Only preliminary results of the group that had been operated on for secundum-type atrial septal defect were available. Between 1968 and 1980, 126 patients underwent surgical closure of secundum-type atrial septal defect; 118 were traced – all were alive – and 103 patients participated in the medical part of the study (82%). Of the 103 patients, 75 had a single secundum-type atrial septal defect, 17 patients had a sinus venosus-type defect with partial anomalous pulmonary venous drainage, 9 patients had insignificant pulmonary valve stenosis, and 2 patients had a small open ductus arteriosus. Preoperatively, 46% of the patients had complaints: diminished exercise tolerance in most, but 3% were cyanosed, and 3% had right-sided heart failure. No arrhythmias were reported, but 1 patient had a complete right bundle branch block, and 1 patient had first degree AV-block. Upon cardiac catheterisation, the left to right shunt was calculated on oximetry, and QP/QS ranged from 1:1.2 to 1:4.5 (mean 1:2.3). The age of operation ranged from 0.3 to 14.1 years (mean 7.3 years). Median sternotomy was done in all patients, and all patients were operated on using complete cardiopulmonary bypass. In 56 patients, this was combined with (mild) hypothermia. At follow-up the mean age ranged from 10 to 34 years (mean 22 years). Duration of follow-up was 9 to 20 years (mean 14 years). As stated earlier, all patients traced were alive. Subjective well-being was generally good (87% of all patients 'good' or 'very good'), and almost all were in NYHA class 1, and in Dr Somerville's Ability Index class 1 or

2. A rather frequent complaint was palpitations (28%). Bicycle ergometry showed 85% of the patients to have a normal exercise tolerance. Echocardiography revealed normal intracardiac anatomy without right ventricular enlargement in 75% of the patients. One quarter of all the patients had residual right ventricular enlargement, 2 of whom had a significant residual atrial septal defect. Only 10% of all these patients were regularly seen in an outpatient clinic and only two as a result of specific complaints. All the other had already been discharged from regular outpatient clinic visits a few years after the operation, which is a normal policy in the Netherlands. Generally they feel healthy, have no limitations in exercises, and the majority even have a completely normal intracardiac anatomy.

The Holter 24-hour ambulatory ECG, however, shows a normal pattern in only 37% of the patients! Using Kugler's criteria for sinus node dysfunction 33% of the patients have sinus node dysfunction, 8% have abnormal ventricular ectopic activity, 15% have a complete right bundle branch block, and 7% have a first degree AV-block. No correlation could be found between the complaint 'palpitation' and abnormal findings on the Holter registration.

What is the clinical relevance of these findings? Supraventricular arrhythmias are notorious in the natural history of the (unoperated) secundum-type atrial septal defect. Before the age of 30 years they generally do not induce many problems, but between 30 and 50 years of age, 50% of all patients with atrial septal defects die. In many cases sudden death was reported, most likely caused by (supraventricular) arrhythmias. In almost all studies arrhythmias have been found after repair of secundum atrial septal defects.

Several possible explanations are given concerning the origin of these arrhythmias: natural history unaltered by surgery, direct damage to the sinus node by surgery (e.g., stitches near the sinus node in sinus venosus-type defect), traction in the atrial wall and septum as a result of surgery with (slowly progressing) fibrosis, and damage to the sinus node artery as a result of cannulation technique [25].

The exact role of cardiac surgery is hard to evaluate, because surgical techniques have constantly changed and improved during the 1970s (myocardial preservation technique, cannulation technique). That is why 'technology assessment' – one of the aims of the Rotterdam Quality of Life study – is so difficult. Results from operations for secundum-type atrial septal defect performed ten years apart may not be comparable due to the differences in surgical or supporting techniques.

Will the finding of such a high incidence of arrhythmias in this study, if they turn out to be consistent and are confirmed by other studies, change the policy towards management of secundum-type atrial septal defect? This is unlikely, as long as nobody knows exactly the nature and prognosis of the arrhythmias. On scientific grounds, a prospective, randomized trial on management of secundum-type atrial septal defects would be desirable. On ethical and numerical grounds this is, of course, impossible. The only thing we can do, and must do, is a longer follow-up of the operated patients, and compare the results with the only controls we have, the historical control group. Written questionnaires and telephone interviews years after an operation are better than discharging patients a few years after the operation and never seeing them again; but it is not good enough. One really has to see the patients oneself, and do a thorough cardiological work up, to obtain reliable information about a patient's general and cardiological condition [26].

Fortunately, in most cases the conclusion will be that, despite the fact that the operation was not 'corrective' in the strict sense of the word, the patient is (incomparably) much better off than he would have been without surgery.

References

1. Lewis FJ, Taufic M: Closure of atrial septal defects with aid of hypothermia: experimental accomplishments and the report of one successful case. Surgery 1953;33:52.
2. Gibbon JH jr: Application of a mechanical heart and lung apparatus to cardiac surgery. Minn Med 1954;37:171.
3. Warden HE, Cohen M, Read RC, Lillehei CW: Controlled cross circulation for open intra cardiac surgery. J Thor Surg 1954;28:331.
4. Mustard WT: Successful two-stage correction of transposition of the great vessels. Surgery 1964;55:469.
5. Mohoney L, Turley K, Ebert P, Heymann MA: Long-term results after atrial repair of transposition of the great arteries in early infancy. Circulation 1982;66:253.
6. Poirier RA *et al*: Late results after repair of tetralogy of Fallot. J Thorac Cardiovasc Surg 1977;75:900.
7. Werdman WH, Blount SG, DuShane JW, Gersony WM, Hayes CJ, Nadas AS: Clinical course in ventricular septal defects. Circulation 1977;56:suppl I;I-56–69.
8. McNamara, Latson LA: Long-term follow-up of patients with malformations for which definitive surgical repair has been available for 25 years or more. Am J Cardiol 1972;50:560–568.
9. Somerville J: Congenital heart disease in adults and adolescents. Br Heart J 1986;56(5):395–397.
10. Stark J: Do we really correct congenital heart defects? J Thorac Cardiovasc Surg 1989;97:109.
11. Graham TP *et al*: Abnormalities of right ventricular function following Mustard's operation for transposition of the great arteries. Circulation 1975;52:678.
12. Bender HW: Comparative operative results of the Senning and Mustard procedures for transposition of the great arteries. Circulation 1980;(suppl I)I:197.
13. Deanfield J, Camm J, Macartney F, Cartwright T, Douglas J, Drew J, Leval H de, Stark J: Arrhythmias and late mortality after Mustard and Senning operation for transposition of the great arteries. J Thorac & Cardiovasc Surg 1988;96:569–576.
14. Quaegebeur JM, Rohmer J, Ottenkamp J, Buis T, Kirklin JW, Blackstone EH, Brom AG: The arterial switch operation: An eight year experience. J Thorac Cardiovasc Surg 1986;92:361–384.
15. Martin RP, Ladusans EJ, Parsons JM, Keck E, Radley-Smith R, Yacoub MM: Incidence and site of pulmonary stenosis after anatomical correction of transposition of the great arteries. (abstract) Br Heart J 1988;59:122–123.

16. Sidi D, Planche C, Kachaner J *et al*: Anatomic correction of simple transposition of the great arteries in 50 neonates. Circulation 1987;75:429–435.
17. Wessel HN *et al*: Exercise performance in tetralogy of Fallot after intracardiac repair. J Thorac Cardiovasc Surg 1980;80:582.
18. Neches WH, Park SC, Edgni EA, Jose A: Tetralogy of Fallot and tetralogy of Fallot with pulmonary atresia. In Garson A, Bricker JT, McNamara DG, eds. Pediatric Cardiology 1st edition, Philadelphia: Lea and Febiger, 1990:1073–1100.
19. Gillete PC *et al*: Sudden death after repair of tetralogy of Fallot. Electrocardiographic and electrophysiologic abnormalities. Circulation 1977;56:566.
20. Maron BJ *et al*: Postoperative assessment of patients with ventricular septal defect and pulmonary hypertension. Circulation 1973;48:864.
21. Hallidie-Smith KA *et al*: Effects of surgical closure of ventricular septal defects upon pulmonary vascular disease. Br Heart J 1969;31:246.
22. Ritter DG, McGoon DC: Medical and surgical long-term follow-up of ventricular septal defect with pulmonary vascular obstructive disease. Am J Cardiol 1979;43:346.
23. Blake RS, Chung EE, Wesley H, Hallidie-Smith KA: Conduction defects ventricular arrhythmias and late death after surgical closure of ventricular septal defects. Br Heart J 1982;47:305.
24. Murphy JC, Gersh BJ, McGoon MD, Mair DD, Porter CJ, Elstrup DM, McGoon DC, Puga FJ, Kirklin JW, Danielson GK: Long-term outcome after surgical repair of isolated atrial septal defect. New Engl J Med 1990;323:1645–1650.
25. Bink-Boelkens M, Meuzelaar KJ, Eygelaar A: Arrhythmias after repair of secundair atrial septal defect: the influence of surgical modification. Am Heart J 1988;115:629–633.
26. Sommerville J: 'Grown-up' survivors of congenital heart disease: who knows? Who cares? Br J Hosp Med 1990;43(2):132–136.

27. Lung function in children after heart surgery

MILAN ŠAMÁNEK, A. ZAPLETAL, J. ŠULC and B. HUČÍN

1. Introduction

There are many reasons for an impairment of lung function in patients with congenital cardiac malformation. Cardiomegaly and distended pulmonary arteries occupy a space at the expense of the developing lung [1]. As early as 1887, von Basch found that pulmonary vascular congestion influences the mechanical properties of the lungs [2]. Decreased dynamic compliance was measured in infants with high pulmonary arterial pressure secondary to an increased left-to-right shunt [3]. A significant reduction of lung compliance was found in patients with atrial septal defect and 2- to 4-fold increase in pulmonary blood flow [4]. In addition, many infants with a high pulmonary blood flow suffer from repeated respiratory infections resulting in a long lasting or permanent damage of the lung tissue in some of them. Changes in the structure of pulmonary arteries in pulmonary hypertension can contribute to an increased lung stiffness [5]. A significant increase of pulmonary diffusing capacity has been explained by an increased size of the capillary bed due to an increased pulmonary blood volume in patients with a left-to-right shunt [6,7]. A rich collateral network in cyanotic heart diseases can contribute to an increased lung stiffness, which was demonstrated in patients with transposition of the great arteries [8].

An effective surgical correction of the heart defect terminates the pathologic pulmonary hemodynamics but it can create new impairment of the lung function by disturbing chest wall mechanics and damaging the function of respiratory muscles (including diaphragm).

Lung function was measured in patients after open heart surgery to establish the frequency, nature and extent of abnormalities in lung volumes, airway patency and lung elasticity. Only those without any residual defect, chest wall deformity, or severe scoliosis, clinically classified as excellent were included in this postoperative patients' population.

2. Patients and Method

Lung function tests were carried out in 208 children and adolescents after an open heart surgery for atrial septal defect, ventricular septal defect,

Paul J. Walter (ed.): Quality of Life after Open Heart Surgery, 303–311.

pulmonary stenosis, tetralogy of Fallot or simple transposition of the great arteries. The age at surgery ranged from 3 months to 24 years. The youngest patient at lung function testing was 6 and the oldest 27 years old. The lowest time interval from the operation to the testing of lung function was one year and the longest one was 14 years.

Lung volumes were measured from a spirographic record and in a constant volume body plethysmograph [9]. The indices of airway patency were calculated from the maximal expiratory flow-volume curve [10]. Instantaneous maximum expiratory flow rates were measured per unit of total lung capacity at a defined level of the total expired volume. Peak expiratory flow rate represents the maximum velocity of the expired gas at forced expiration. Maximum expiratory flow rates were expressed per unit of total lung capacity ('specific' maximum expiratory flow rates). Airway resistance was measured simultaneously with thoracic gas volume in a body plethysmograph at the level of functional residual capacity (total airway resistance). It was expressed as its reversal value, called airway conductance, per unit of thoracic gas volume ('specific' airway conductance). Static lung recoil pressure and static lung compliance were measured from the expiratory pressure-volume curve [9].

All measurements were taken in a sitting position. The results were compared with our own data measured in the body height-, sex-, and age-matched healthy population [9]. The value which differed by more than two standard deviations from the mean reference value was labeled as abnormal. The Student's paired t-test was used to evaluate the significance of differences.

3. Results

A disturbance of the lung function – a difference from the mean reference value of more than 2 standard deviations – was found in 135 (64.9%) of 208 patients with the excellent results of intracardiac repair of a congenital heart malformation. The frequency of affected patients and the prevalence of abnormalities in lung volumes, airway patency and lung elasticity varied with the congenital heart defect category.

3.1. *Atrial septal defect*

An isolated ostium secundum type defect in the interatrial septum was closed at surgery without any residual lesion in 74 children (22 boys and 52 girls) at the mean age of 9.9 (SD ± 2.96) years. The youngest age at surgery was 4.0 and the highest one was 14.8 years. The mean age at the measuring of lung function was 15.0 (SD ± 2.46) years. The youngest patient was 9, while the oldest one was 21 years old at testing. The time interval from surgery to the lung function testing was 5.1 (SD ± 2.45) years. It ranged from 1.9 to 11.3 years.

3.1.1. *Frequency of abnormal lung function tests*
A significant abnormality of lung function was found in 35 (47%) patients after surgical closure of atrial septal defect of the ostium secundum type.

The most frequent finding was the increase of static lung recoil pressure – increased lung stiffness – which was present in 24 (32%) patients. A decreased lung recoil pressure was found only in 2 patients. A concomitant deviation of the opposite direction in the static lung compliance was not statistically significant. Next in frequency were signs of the airway obstruction. Peak expiratory flow rate and airway conductance were significantly lower than in healthy children in 13 (18%) patients. An obstruction of peripheral airways – a decreased maximal expiratory flow rates at 25% of vital capacity and at 60% of total lung capacity – was present only in 4 (5%) patients. A decreased vital capacity was measured in 7 (10%) while an abnormal increase was found in 8 (11%) patients. Total lung capacity was decreased in 9 (12%) and increased in 5 (7%) patients. The indices of pulmonary hyperinflation – increased residual volume and functional residual capacity related to the total lung capacity – were present only in 4 (5%) and in 3 (4%) patients, respectively.

3.1.2. *Mean values of lung function tests*
A significant difference of mean values from the reference values was found in the indices of increased lung stiffness (static recoil pressure) and central airway obstruction (specific airway conductance) (Table 1).

3.2. *Ventricular septal defect*

Lung function was measured in 47 patients (20 boys, 27 girls) after an intracardiac repair of ventricular septal defect. In 34 of them the closure of the defect was the first cardiac surgery performed, while in 13 patients the intracardiac repair followed after the banding of main pulmonary artery.

3.3. *Ventricular septal defect after primary intracardiac repair*

The mean age of 34 patients (15 boys, 19 girls) after the closure of ventricular septal defect without previous banding of pulmonary artery was 3.4 (SD ± 2.5) years at the operation (range 0.6 to 10.7 years) and 13.0

Table 1. Abnormal mean values.

Heart defect	Lung function test	% of predicted mean	SD	p <
Atrial septal defect	Static recoil pressure			
	at 100% of TLC	123	31	0.0001
	at 90% of TLC	107	20	0.05
	at 60% of TLC	114	23	0.0001
	Airway conductance	84	32	0.0001
Ventricular septal defect	Static recoil pressure	128	26	0.0001
primary repair	at 100% of TLC	123	20	0.0001
	at 90% of TLC	146	28	0.0001
	at 60% of TLC	86	19	0.05
	Peak expiratory flow	75	22	0.05
	Airway conductance			
Ventricular septal defect	FRC/TLC (%)	111	9	0.001
repair after banding	RV/TLC (%)	122	25	0.05
	Maximal expiratory flow rate			
	at 25% of VC	79	25	0.01
	of 50% of VC	85	21	0.05
	at 60% of TLC	74	26	0.01
	Peak expiratory flow	82	30	0.01
	Airway conductance	69	30	0.01
Tetralogy of Fallot	Residual volume	134	36	0.001
	FRC	113	18	0.001
	FRC/TLC	113	11	0.001
	RV/TLC	132	32	0.001
	Static recoil pressure			
	at 10% of TLC	116	32	0.01
	Static compliance	85	23	0.001
	Maximal expiratory flow rate	85	36	0.01
	at 60% of TLC			
	Airway conductance	77	31	0.001
Simple transposition	Vital capacity	87	13	0.01
	TLC	93	12	0.001
	Residual volume	106	32	0.05
	FRC/TLC	106	19	0.001
	RV/TLC	113	30	0.02
	Static recoil pressure			
	at 100% of TLC	136	30	0.001
	at 90% of TLC	133	24	0.001
	at 60% of TLC	134	42	0.001
	Static compliance	75	21	0.001
	Peak expiratory flow	90	17	0.001
	Airway conductance	81	24	0.001

FRC = functional residual capacity; RV = residual volume; TLC = total lung capacity; VC = vital capacity.

(SD ± 2.8; 8.2 to 20.0) years at the testing of lung function. The mean time interval which elapsed from the surgery to the testing of lung function was 9.6 (SD ± 2.0) years. The longest time interval was 11.7 years, while the shortest one was 3.7 years.

3.3.1. *Frequency of abnormal lung function tests*

A significant disturbance of pulmonary function was detected in 24 (71%) of 34 patients after primary intracardiac repair of a ventricular septal defect.

The most frequent finding was an increase of static recoil pressure of the lungs which was measured in 15 (44%) patients. Next in frequency to the indices of an increased lung stiffness were signs of the lung volume restriction. A decreased total lung capacity was recorded in 9 (27%), and a reduced vital capacity in 8 (24%) patients. Equally frequent was a decrease of peak expiratory flow rate and specific conductance of the airways (in 27% of patients) suggesting an increased airway resistance. The indices of peripheral airway obstruction, however, were present in only 4 patients. The increased ratios of functional residual capacity and residual volume to total lung capacity were foud in 4 patients. These findings can be explained by a decreased total lung capacity (lung volume restriction) and not by pulmonary hyperinflation.

3.3.2. *Mean values of lung function tests*

The mean values of both vital and total lung capacities, functional residual capacity and residual volume did not significantly differ from the reference values. A highly significant increase of the static lung recoil pressure was measured at all levels of total lung capacity (Table 1). The peak expiratory flow rate was decreased to 86 (SD ± 19.2) of the reference value. The decrease of the mean value of the same significance was calculated for specific airway conductance (75 ± 22.7% of normal). We found no signs of obstruction within the peripheral airways. The maximal expiratory flow rates measured at 25% and 50% of vital capacity and at 60% of total lung capacity ranged from 93 to 96% of the predicted value.

3.4. *Ventricular septal defect corrected after previous banding of pulmonary artery*

Banding of pulmonary artery had been performed at the age of 1.2 (SD ± 1.2) years followed by the intracardiac repair at the mean age of 7.1 (SD ± 2.3; 9.0 to 19.7) years. Lung function was measured at the mean age of 16.2 (SD ± 2.3) years. The time interval from the intracardiac repair to the testing of lung function was 9.1 (SD ± 2.6) years. It ranged from 3.4 to 13.6 years.

3.4.1. Frequency of abnormal lung function tests

A significant disturbance of lung function was found in 10 (77%) of 13 patients, as compared with 71% found in patients subjected to open heart surgery without previous palliative procedure.

The predominant lung function abnormality was an airway obstruction. A significantly decreased maximal expiratory flow rate was measured at all levels of the forced expired lung capacity in 5 (38%) of 13 patients. The same frequency of decreased values was found at the testing of peak expiratory flow rate and specific conductance of the airways. Equally frequent was the decrease of vital and total lung capacities, indicating the lung volume restriction. An increase of the static lung recoil pressure (lung stiffness) was not as frequent as in the patients without pulmonary arterial banding. It was found in 4 (31%) patients. An increase of the ratios of functional residual capacity and residual volume to total lung capacity calculated in 3 patients is probably due to a decreased total lung capacity and not due to the hyper-inflation.

3.4.2. Mean values of lung function test

The maximal expiratory flow rates measured at all levels of lung capacity, peak expiratory flow rate and specific airway conductance were significantly lower than in healthy children and young adults (Table 1). In addition to the airway obstruction, an increase of the ratios of functional residual capacity and residual volume to total lung capacity was proved significant. The mean values of lung volumes, static recoil pressure of the lungs and lung compliance did not differ from the predicted values.

3.4.3. Pulmonary stenosis

Lung function was measured in 11 patients treated surgically for isolated pulmonary stenosis aged 10 to 19 (mean 14.7, SD ± 2.8) years. The time interval from surgery to the testing ranged from 3.5 to 7.0 years.

Abnormalities of lung function were found in only one of 11 patients. It consisted in a significant decrease of vital capacity, total lung capacity and functional residual capacity. The mean values of lung volumes and capacities indices of the lung elasticity and airway patency did not differ from the reference values.

3.5. Tetralogy of Fallot

The lung function testing was carried out in 41 patients (25 girls, 16 boys) 1 to 5 years (mean 3.0, SD ± 1.2 years) after open heart surgery for tetralogy of Fallot. The lung function testing was performed at the mean age of 14.2 (SD ± 4.1) years. The age of the youngest patient at the examination of lung function was 6 years. The oldest patient was 27 years old. The mean age at the corrective surgery was 11.2 (SD ± 4.3) years. It ranged from 2 to 24 years. A shunt operation had been performed in 18 of these patients at the mean age of 2.6 (SD ± 1.4) years, prior to intracardiac correction.

3.5.1. *Frequency of abnormal lung function tests*

In total, 34 of 41 (83%) patients had abnormal one or more lung function tests. Frequency of a disturbed lung function in patients after a shunt operation followed by the intracardiac repair was higher than in patients with primary repair (94 to 74%).

The most frequent finding was an increase of the ratios of functional residual capacity to total lung capacity and residual volume to total lung capacity. It was present in 20 (49%) patients. The next in frequency were the restrictive changes. A decreased vital capacity was found in 19 (46%) patients, and a decreased total lung capacity was measured in 10 (25%) patients. An increase of the total lung capacity was present in 2 patients. The third most frequent finding was an increased stiffness of the lungs. An increased static lung recoil pressure was found in 15 (37%) patients. Signs of an obstruction in the peripheral airways (a decreased maximal expiratory flow velocity at low levels of lung volume) were present in 14 (34%) patients. These signs were accompanied in 11 (27%) patients by a decrease of airway conductance.

3.5.2. *Mean values of lung function tests*

Among static lung volumes, only total lung capacity did not differ significantly from the predicted value. Vital capacity was significantly reduced, while residual volume, functional residual capacity and the ratios of functional residual capacity to total lung capacity were significantly higher than in healthy children (Table 1). An increase in the mean value of static lung recoil pressure and the corresponding decrease of static lung compliance document a trend to an increased lung stiffness in patients after intracardiac repair of tetralogy of Fallot (Table 1). Signs of a decreased airway patency were more pronounced in the larger airways than in the peripheral airways.

3.6. *Simple transposition of the great arteries*

Lung function tests were carried out in 35 patients with simple transposition after the Mustard or Senning operation at the mean age of 11.6 (SD ± 2.9) years. The operation was performed at the mean age of 4.4 (SD ± 3.0) years following balloon atrial septostomy which had been performed in the first postnatal days. The shortest time interval from the surgery to the lung function testing was 2.2 years. The mean time interval was 7.2 (SD ± 1.45) years, and the longest one was 11.1 years.

3.6.1. *Frequency of abnormal lung function tests*
One or more singificantly abnormal findings were measured in 31 (88%) patients. Most frequent were the signs of an increased lung stiffness – high elastic lung recoil pressure (in 66%) and a low value of static lung compliance (in 43%). The second most frequent finding was a restriction of lung volumes. A decreased vital capacity was found in 21 (60%) patients and a low value of total lung capacity in 12 (34%) patients. An increased ratio of functional residual capacity to total lung capacity and of residual volume to total lung capacity was measured in 14 (40%) patients. Low velocity of the maximal expiratory flow was present only in 4 patients. Specific alrway conductance was decreased in one of them.

3.6.2. *Mean values of lung function tests*
A highly significant increase was found in the lung stiffness (Table 1). The mean values of static lung recoil pressure were increased and static lung compliance was correspondingly decreased. The mean values of vital capacity and total lung capacity were decreased. The mean value of residual volume and of the ratios of functional residual capacity to total lung capacity and residual volume to total lung capacity were significantly lower than in the healthy reference population. Specific airway conductance was significantly lower than the reference value, however, no signs of the peripheral airway obstruction were found.

4. Conclusions

One or more abnormal lung function tests were found in the majority of patients after successful intracardiac repair of a heart malformation despite their excellent clinical conditions. Frequency, nature and extent of disturbances in lung function vary with the heart malformation form. A higher frequency of lung function pathology was found in patients in whom the intracardiac repair was preceded by palliative surgery. The disturbed lung function can influence unfavorably the long term results of surgery.

References

1. Stanger P, Lucas RV, Edwards JE: Anatomic factors causing respiratory distress in acyanotic cogenital cardiac disease. Pediatrics 1969;43:760–769.
2. von Basch S: Über eine Funktion des Kapillardruckes in den Lungenalveolen. Wiener Med Blätter 1887;465.
3. Bancalari E, Jesse MJ, Gelband H, Garcia O: Lung mechanics in congenital heart disease with increased and decreased pulmonary blood flow. J Pediatr 1977;9:192–195.
4. Ayres SM, Kozam RL, Lukas DS: Mechanics and work of breathing in atrial septal defect. Circulation 1960;22:718–719.

5. Davies H, Williams J, Wood P: Lung stiffness in states of abnormal pulmonary blood flow and pressure. Br Heart J 1962;24:129–138.
6. Bedell GN: Comparison of pulmonary diffusing capacity in normal subjects and in patients with intracardiac septal defects. J Lab Clin Med 1961;57:269–279.
7. Bucci G, Cook CD, Haman JF: Studies of respiratory physiology in children. VI. Lung diffusing capacity of the pulmonary membrane and pulmonary capillary blood volume in congenital heart disease. J Clin Invest 1961;40:1431.
8. Šamánek M, Zapletal A, Šulc J: Disturbances of lung function in transposition of the great arteries. In: Daum S (ed.) Interaction between heart and lung. Stuttgart: Georg Thieme, 1989;111–112.
9. Zapletal A, Šamánek M, Paul T: Lung function in children and adolescents. Basel: Karger, 1987.
10. Mead J, Turner JM, Macklem PT, Little JB: Significance of relationship between lung recoil and maximum expiratory flow. J Appl Physiol 1967;22:95–108.
11. Hrubá B, Šamánek M, Tůma S: Radiocirculography in congenital heart disease in children with intracardiac shunt. Pediat Radiol 1973;1:47–52.

B: Intellectual Functioning

28. Psychointellectual performance after correction of complex congenital heart defects

H. C. KALLFELZ, H. KAEMMERER, I. LUHMER, H. LACHER,
M. ANACKER, and P. WIETZKE

1. Introduction

Almost 40 years ago the era of surgical correction of complex congenital heart defects started in the USA. Many ten thousands of patients with severe cardiac malformations successfully underwent surgery since that time and are alive. Many reports have been written on long-term survival and complications appearing years to decades after the surgical procedure. On the other hand, only a few papers have been published on the psychological and intellectual development and the social situation in adolescence and adulthood following major cardiac surgery.

We therefore performed an investigation on the physical and intellectual performance and the psychological as well as the psychosocial situation of children, adolescents and young adults operated on 8–16 years earlier for complex congenital heart defects in our institution.

2. Patients and methods

In the study were included randomly chosen patients with simple and complex transposition of the great arteries (TGA) and with tetralogy of Fallot (TOF) having been surgically corrected in the years 1973 through 1980. For comparison a group of patients with a less serious defect, namely coarction of the aorta (COA), was studied in the same manner.

The three groups of patients were comparable with respect to age at surgery (Table 1) and to age at evaluation (Figure 1).

All patients were cared for in our department before surgery and continuously in the postoperative period up to the time of this study. One of the three first authors performed the physical examination and evaluated the results of routine ECG. Holter ECG (TGA and TOF patients) chest X-ray, bicycle exercise test and 2–D echocardiography and PW–CW–Color–Doppler study. A personal interview of each patient and, where possible, of

Paul J. Walter (ed.): Quality of Life after Open Heart Surgery, 315–321.
© 1992 Kluwer Academic Publishers.

Table 1. Age at surgery (y/m). Type of heart defects, number of patients studied and their age at surgery.

Heart defect	Range	mean ± SD
TGA (50)	2m–13y7m	2y ± 1y8m
TOF (35)	6m–14y1m	4y2m ± 2y11m
COA(38)	1m–14y7m	2y4m ± 2y8m

his/her parents took place at the last outpatient visit, dealing mainly with the psychosocial and intellectual performance. In addition the patient and/or parents filled in a detailed questionnaire on many different aspects regarding school, professional training, psychological situation, family background and physical performance or limitations.

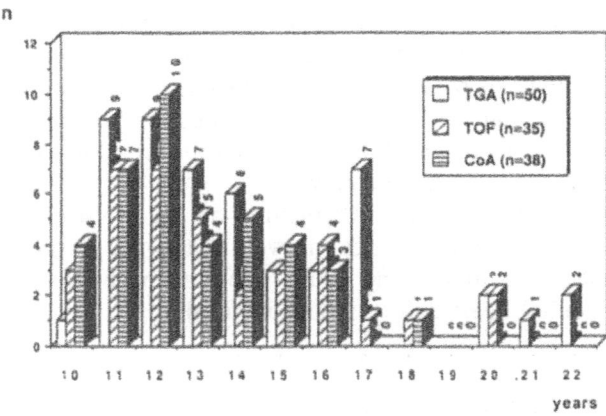

Figure 1. Age distribution of the three groups of patients at the time of the evaluation.

3. Results

3.1. *School career* (Table 2)

Forty-four children of 50 with TGA after inflow correction and repair of additional lesions, where necessary, attended a normal primary school, whereas six other patients primarily had to be taken to a school for subnormal children, with the addition of one more, later on, who had started in a normal school. The average age at which the children were sent to a normal school was 6 years and 9 months, slightly but not significantly older than the average child. When the study was completed eight of the 44 were still in a

Table 2. Types of schools attended by children and adolescents after surgical repair of either TGA, TOF or COA.

	TGA(50)	TOF(35)	COA(38)
Primary School	44 — 8	30 — 5	34 — 13
9 y. Element. School	13	10	14
Middle School	12	12	2
Secondary School	10	3	5
School f. subnorm. Ch.	6 — 7	5 — 5	4 — 4
Repitition of Grades	10	4	12

primary school, 13 were attending or had finished a 9–year elementary schooling, 12 a middle school and 10 a secondary school. Ten children had to repeat one or two grades. Five of the 35 patients with surgically corrected TOF were mentally handicapped and therefore primarily went to a special school. The other 30 children were passing or had already passed through a normal school career; only four of them have had to repeat one grade up to now.

A comparable situation was seen in the patient group after repair of COA, in which 4 patients with a mental handicap primarily were sent to a special school. All other children or adolescents still went to or had finished normal school. However, there was a distinctly higher number of children who had to repeat one or two grades.

3.2. *School performance* (Table 3)

The parents and/or patients were specifically asked for the results in school in average and in detail with respect to main subjects. The results are shown

Table 3. Overall school results in patients after surgical repair of either TGA, TOF or COA.

	TGA (50)	TOF (35)	COA (38)
Excellent	3	2	6
Good	8	5	8
Satisfactory	24	20	12
Sufficient	6	2	6
Poor	1	1	2
Handicapped	7	5	4

Table 4. A high proportion of patients with primarily cyanotic heart defects suffer from a diminished power of concentration.

Heart defect	Yes	No	?
TGA (50)	19	31	–
TOF (35)	14	20	1
COA (38)	10	26	2

in Table 3. It is evident that between 23 and 40% in each patient group achieve excellent to good marks and about 40–65% demonstrate satisfactory results if the primarily handicapped children are excluded.

A more detailed analysis showed that there was an even distribution of strengths and weaknesses with regard to subjects as mathematics and languages.

Since parents repeatedly complained about a serious lack of concentration of their off-spring, particularly in school, we tried to evaluate this issue in greater detail. This resulted in a significantly higher proportion ($\sim$40%) in patients with a primary cyanotic heart defect. (Table 4).

3.3. *Personal assessment*

When asking patients and parents for a personal assessment of the present situation in school or in vocational training the vast majority grouped themselves as feeling normal or even very good. Only around 20% in each group felt somehow impaired or even poor (Table 5). The self-assessment of the children and adolescents with regard to their physical condition resulted in 50 to 60% who feel healthy and fit. There is, however, a remarkable proportion in all three groups (about 30%) who feel some physical impairment. By contrast, almost none assesses him- or herself as unfit and unhealthy. Similarly to the question on the situation in school or training, 10–15% were unable to give a clear answer (Table 6). The answers of three patients were far more positive or optimistic than their real physical condition would warrant.

Table 5. The overwhelming majority in each group assess themselves as being normally or even very well adapted.

Heart defect	Very good	Normal	Impaired	Poor	?
TGA (50)	7	30	5	2	6
TOF (35)	5	18	6	–	6
COA (38)	7	21	4	4	2

Table 6. More than half of the patients assess themselves as being physically normal.

Heart defect	Healthy & fit	Not quite fit	Not healthy, unfit	?
TGA (50)	27	16	1	6
TOF (35)	16	12	–	6
COA (38)	25	10	–	3

3.4. *Psychosocial situation*

The majority of patients claimed to be well informed about the nature of their heart disease and had fully accepted living with it. Only a small proportion in all three patient groups felt really impaired by the cardiac problem and, according to the statements of their parents, sometimes expressed some fear; more often when a diagnostic procedure or a second operation was about to be performed. Almost all children and adolescents, regardless of the underlying lesion, felt socially fully accepted, having school friends and participating normally in all school and other social activities. A few children, however, said that they felt physically less fit than their classmates and either did not take part in sports or tried to deny their handicap. Only 20% in each group stated that they were somehow annoyed by the scar. Surprisingly there was no difference between girls and boys.

Five young adults either were performing vocational training (three) or were fully employed. Only two patients above 18 years of age were unemployed.

4. Discussion

The retrospective study of the intellectual performance and the psychosocial situation of children and adolescents having been operated on for either TGA, TOF or COA revealed that the majority of patients pass through school without major problems and in this respect do not differ significantly from the average population. Kramer et al. [4], in their study of 128 patients with congenital heart disease, found that whether surgically corrected or unoperated, the intellectual performance was significantly lower compared to a normal control group in those children who suffered from physical limitations. In those patients without a physical handicap, however, they detected no significant difference to the control children. These results seem to be quite in accordance with our data, which were derived from patients which had corrective surgery fairly early in their life and, except for those with a neurological handicap, had no overt physical limitation.

With regard to the psychological impact of heart disease and the psychosocial adoption of children and adolescents, most of the investigations that have been performed earlier were associated with patients who had no or late or only palliative operations, or who were considered inoperable [1–3].

This might explain why, in general, the personal situation of patients with congenital heart disease is viewed as being poorer than it actually is. No doubt each patient has individual personal difficulties, as does his/her family, but as long as the patient's physical condition and intellectual ability is not significantly impaired, no definite difference from the average population arises. The ability to cope, both for the family and the patient, seems to increase the earlier in life and the better corrective surgery is performed. This is one more important argument for performing operations for most of the congenital heart diseases as early as is safely feasible. This might probably prevent many of the well-known maladjustments in earlier decades.

5. Summary

A study was performed in children and adolescents with transposition of the great arteries ($n = 50$), tetralogy of Fallot ($n = 35$), and coarction of the aorta ($n = 38$) who had had surgical correction of their cardiac defect 5 to 18 years earlier, the aim being to evaluate their intellectual performance, psychological situation and psychosocial adaptation at the present time. With the exception of 16 patients, who suffered from neurological sequelae acquired prior to surgery or perioperatively, almost all others were performing well at or above average at school. There was, however, some lack of concentration, which was at least one reason for a higher number of children who had to repeat grades. Most of the patients took a full part in social life, had friends, and did not complain of any difficulties with regard to psychosocial adaptation. The results of the investigation yielded a better outcome than previous studies, perhaps due to the fact that the great majority of the patients had had their corrective surgery early in life and had already experienced life as normal individuals, with little or no restriction, before entering school.

References

1. Donovan EF: Psychosocial considerations in congenital heart disease. In: Adams FH, Emmanouilides GC, Riemenschneider TA (eds.): Heart disease in infants, children and adolescents. 4th ed. Baltimore: Williams and Wilkins, 1989.
2. Garson SL, Baer PE: Psychological aspects of heart disease in childhood. In: Garson Jr A, Bricker JT, McNamara DG (eds.): The science and practice of pediatric cardiology. Malvern: Lea and Febiger, 1990.
3. Kahlert G, Hilgenberg F, Jochmus J: Psychosoziale Auswirkungen schwerer Herzkrankheiten bei Kindern und Jugendlichen. sozialpädiatrie 19;9:644–648.

4. Kramer HH, Awiszus D, Sterzel U, van Halteren A, Claßen R: Development of personality and intelligence in children with congenital heart disease. J Child Psychol 1989;30:299–308.
5. Trusler GA, Williams WG, Duncau KF, Hesslein PS, Benson LN, Freedom RM, Izukawa T, Molley P.: Results with the Mustard operation in simple transposition of the great arteries. Ann Surg 1987;206:251–260.

C: Emotional State

29. Psychosocial aspects of congenital heart disease in children, adolescents and adults

ELISABETH M. W. J. UTENS

1. Introduction

From the early days of pediatric cardiac surgery several scientific publications have attempted to describe the impact of congenital heart disease (further called CHD) on family life [1,2]. In the sixties and seventies most of the studies were conducted using non-standardized interviews and observations of afflicted children and their parents. Over the last 25 years advances in cardiovascular surgical techniques have reduced mortality and (pediatric) cardiologists are now faced with a growing population of adolescents and adults with corrected or modified congenital heart defects whose medical and personal needs are relatively unfamiliar and complex [3].

This chapter consists of four parts. In part two a short review will be given of psychosocial aspects described in the literature concerning adolescent and adult patients with CHD in general. Although many adolescents and young adults with CHD appear to be functioning well [4], the focus will be on the potential psychosocial difficulties of CHD, since it is important that these are known to (pediatric) cardiologists. In part three the methodological design of the Rotterdam Follow-Up Study on Quality of Life in CHD patients will be outlined. This study was started in 1989 and is financially supported by the Netherlands Heart Foundation. In part four some clinical findings of this study will be discussed.

2. Physical, emotional, cognitive and social aspects of CHD

2.1. *Physical aspects*

CHD can cause physical retardation, which can result in the inability to participate in athletics or sports. This may lead to a diminished self-esteem and social isolation. Adolescents with cyanotic heart disease may become

Paul J. Walter (ed.): Quality of Life after Open Heart Surgery, 325–331.
© 1992 Kluwer Academic Publishers.

socially isolated because of their growth retardation, their blue skin or clubbed fingers.

2.2. *Emotional aspects*

CHD influences the family relationships. The emotional adjustment of healthy siblings may be affected by disturbed family relationships. The emotional development of the afflicted child may be hampered by parental attitudes, such as pampering and overprotection, and by maternal anxiety [3,5,6]. Maternal anxiety appears to be primarily a function of the presence of CHD itself rather than its severity [7]. At school age and through adolescence, issues such as school activities, friendship and social activities can result in experiences of failure and ostracism. While parents may feel increasingly ambivalent, adolescents with ongoing CHD may experience confusion, depression, loneliness, guilt, rage ('why me?') and a constant fear of sudden death. They may turn to 'acting out' or childish behaviour, withdrawal from contacts, denial and overcompensation as mechanisms to cope with stress [3,5].

Adolescents and young adults with CHD may experience greater uncertainty, vulnerability or feelings of inferiority than their healthy peers, with regard to crucial developmental issues of adolescence, such as: their body concept (the scar); job hunting; courtship/marriage; intercourse and (anti) conception. They may develop a poor body concept and an over-interpretation of body sensations [3]. Many male adolescents are particularly sensitive to being small or skinny. Feelings of shame about the scar may arise when sexual advances are within reach. Conflicts may arise for young adults when potential employers require a medical examination or when they feel restricted because of physical limits. Rejection for the army is considered as a narcissistic blow. Anxieties tend to be greater when courtship, intercourse and sexual arousal for males and (anti-)conception for females come within reach. Young adults are very often afraid that they will pass their congenital defect to their offspring.

2.3. *Cognitive aspects*

As a result of magic associative thinking combined with an egocentric and restricted comprehension of the world, (young) children often consider medical treatment, hospitalization, experienced pain and thoughts about an early death, as punishment for forbidden fantasies and misbehaviour. Such thoughts are reinforced by insufficient education. Adolescents with CHD are often preoccupied with physical and technical information concerning their illness, which they may consider a punishment for forbidden fantasies or sexual activities [3,5].

Research findings dating from the end of the sixties showed that children with CHD scored lower on intelligence tests than normal children. The lower scores were more evident in the first three years of life and in cyanotic children [6]. However, the methods used to measure intelligence levels in young children were inadequate since they relied heavily on gross motor functioning. Because children with CHD may have impaired physical capacity that limits their ability to perform well on such tests, Linde [6] suggests that, in these children, a better estimate of intellectual functioning may be obtained from adaptive and social behaviour.

For older children with CHD – both cyanotic and acyanotic children – IQ scores within the normal range were found [6]. After having reviewed the literature, Kitchen [7] reaches the tentative conclusion that: (1) no consistent relation exists between CHD (regardless of hemodynamic severity) and cognitive functioning; and that (2) hypothermic open heart surgery does not necessarily have long-term effects on intelligence levels. According to Linde [6] and Kitchen [7], intellectual functioning may be harmed by absence from school because of (cardiac) illness, repeated hospital admissions and consequently decreased social contacts, as well as by coexisting brain anomalies. Next, a short review of some social aspects is given.

2.4. *Social aspects*

Maxwell and Gane [1] investigated the impact of CHD upon family life. They found an inability to adjust to or to accept CHD in 14% of 150 families with an afflicted child. Difficulties with feeding, disciplining and sleeping (such as sharing the parental bed, checking at night), spoiling of the afflicted child, feelings of hostility and jealousy in siblings, deterioration of the marital relationship and the belief of the family that the child might die suddenly, were frequently reported. In 1983 Silverman [8] underlined that families of a child with CHD typically responded initially with shock and guilt, manifested by a stated inability to comprehend even the most simple explanations or to cope with child care at home. According to Silverman the crucial factor in the adaptation process appeared to be the state of the child's medical situation.

As for further social aspects: children and adolescents with CHD are often considered by their peers as 'exceptional cases', which may lead to social isolation. For example: in schoolgoing adolescents irregular school attendance, cyanosis and restricted activities underline their peculiarity. And, as Bowen [5] reported, 'rejection by a peer can be devastating'.

3. Rotterdam Follow-Up Study on Quality of Life in children, adolescents and adults with surgical repair of CHD

During the last decades some follow-up studies into psychosocial functioning of adolescents and adults with CHD have been executed, and they have yielded interesting, as well as confusing results. Most of the follow-up studies contained methodological flaws, such as the use of small and heterogeneous diagnostic samples and the use of inadequate and weakly standardized test instruments [9]. In view of these methodological weaknesses one can only conclude that more, and above all more systematized and multidisciplinary research still needs to be done. Relatively little is known about the long-term psychological effects of CHD. A crucial and unsolved question is whether surgical repair of CHD during childhood results in identifiable and predictable effects in adulthood and whether the nature of these psychological effects is influenced by the age of the child at the time of surgical repair.

To investigate this question among others, in 1989 a follow-up study was started in Rotterdam, the Netherlands, to assess the quality of life (in a medical as well as in a psychological sense) at least nine years or longer after surgical correction for CHD in childhood. The main questions of this multidisciplinary study, carried out by a pediatric cardiologist and a clinical psychologist, are as follows:

(a) Are adolescents and adults with operated CHD able to lead a satisfactory and normal life as for their physical exertion, stamina and muscular strength?
(b) To what extent do they suffer residual cardiac symptoms?
(c) Are there problems concerning their intellectual, social and/or emotional functioning?
(d) Is there any relationship between the original cardiologic anomaly and the current somatic condition and psychosocial functioning?

The study involves all patients who underwent (their first) cardiac surgery for CHD between 1968 and 1980 in the University Hospital, Rotterdam, and who were younger than 15 years of age at the time of surgery: a total of 712 patients. Of this original study population, 102 patients had expired before this study was started; a retrospective medical file search has been executed for this group. Of the remaining 610 survivors, 498 patients participated in this study between November 1989 and May 1991.

At the time of restudy their ages were between 9 and 35 years; for 149 participants ages ranged from 9 to 16 years and for 349 participants ages ranged from 16 to 35 years. A total of 112 patients did not participate in this study; 41 patients were lost to follow-up and 71 patients dropped out for emotional or practical reasons. The response rate, corrected for deceased persons and persons lost to follow-up, is 87.5%. Within the study population a distinction is drawn between six diagnostic groups: atrial septal II defect, ventricular septal defect, tetralogy of Fallot, transposition of the great arteries, pulmonary stenosis and a miscellaneous group.

In the following a view is given of the psychosocial variables, which were measured in the study population by means of psychological questionnaires, tests and semi-structured interviews. Most of the psychosocial parameters used have been standardized at a national or international level. The parents of children younger than 16 years of age were also interviewed and requested to fill out several psychological questionnaires with regard to the behaviour of their child. The psychosocial variables under scrutiny are the following:

- Biographical variables: family constellation, socio-economic status and religion of the parents.
- Intermediating variables: life events.
- Emotional variables: psychological well-being, emotional problems, neurotic symptoms, depression, separation-anxiety, recalcitrance, self-esteem, body-image, behavioural problems, overprotection and favouring by parents, expectancies/ideals for the future.
- Intellectual variable: Intelligence Quotient.
- Social variables: school functioning and school achievements, social competence and social inhibitions, leisure-time activities, rejection for the Army, choice of profession, difficulties in getting a job, employment status, sexual relationships, marital status and pregnancies, problems with insurance, medical examinations and financial costs related to CHD.

Since the data gathering for this study has not been completed, it is not possible to describe systematic results based on statistical analyses here. Statistical analyses will be differentiated for the six separate diagnostic groups. In the near future we intend to publish the final results of this study.

In the following some clinical impressions of this study population will be presented, which in our opinion are supplementary to already existing knowledge about adolescents and adults with corrected or modified CHD.

4. Clinical impressions regarding the study population of the Rotterdam Follow-Up Study on Quality of Life in CHD patients

The majority of the study population appears to be functioning well, in a socially adaptive way, and to be leading productive lives. However, many problems are encountered, such as the following.

Some children and adolescents refused to participate in the study because they suffer severe anxieties regarding hospitals; some of them did not even dare to answer questions for the study by telephone. Further, injections were feared by a great number of participants.

Quite a few patients have visited schools for special education because of learning difficulties or behavioural problems. Difficulties in concentrating are mentioned very frequently. Many patients have the feeling that CHD has at some time had a negative influence on their functioning at school.

Children below 16 years of age frequently suffer from separation anxieties; they are afraid to be left alone by their parents or they worry that they will lose their parents, and they suffer from homesickness. A few children and adolescents report severe nightmares about dying suddenly, about being stabbed with a knife in the heart and about being taken to a hospital at high speed by an ambulance with wailing sirens because of a dangerous heart attack. An 11-year old boy with a pacemaker has horrifying dreams that 'he is living on a time bomb'. This boy has great difficulty in separating from his parents, has to be taken to school by them and wants to sit very close to his schoolteachter in the classroom. According to a mother, her 16-year old son, who behaves very shyly and childishly, has had severe nightmares for one year following his cardiac surgery at 5 years of age. 'We had to take him into the parental bed every night, since he woke up screaming and very anxious about dying and being suffocated. He always had to sleep with the lights on and was afraid that we would leave him.' A few adolescents report sleeping difficulties because they are fixated on listening to their heart beat or because they can hear their valves ticking while lying in bed.

Atypical complaints, such as stabbling chest pains, dizziness, shortness of breath, headaches and being tired and exhausted too easily, often occur. However, these complaints could not be related to the cardiac status of the patients.

Some children are severely teased at school because of their physical incapacities or their cardiac condition; e.g. a boy with a pacemaker was called 'robot' and 'horror-man' and jeered at 'that he would get a heart attack and would drop dead anyway.'

Some adolescents experience loneliness and have difficulties in making friends because they feel more mature than their peers as a result of their hospital experiences. Other adolescents share the same difficulties because of their childish behaviour, which resulted from being overprotected and pampered.

Many adolescents and young adults are very ambitious and achievement-oriented as to prove that they are 'no less than their peers', which can be regarded as a denial of their cardiac condition. For example, some report proudly that they work harder and are less absent from work through illness than colleagues.

Some young adults feel they have to make up for years lost due physical incapacities as a result of CHD; they are frequently testing their (physical) limits 'to take from life as much as possible'. They may choose parachuting or mountaineering as hobbies. A few young adults are overly impulsive in spending their money, which they ascribe to being overindulged in their youth.

Many young adults have unanswered questions and serious gaps in their knowledge as to their previous and present cardiac status, their physical restrictions, their prognosis and preventive measures (e.g. prophylaxis against infective endocarditis). Due to misconceptions and deficient knowledge, young adults may overestimate the severity of their cardiac status and consequently unnecessarily restrict themselves. They may also underestimate the severity of their cardiac status, which can have harmful effects on their health. Future research should address these topics, since misconceptions concerning their medical status may limit young adults in establishing adequate goals for the future.

Acknowledgements

Financial support from the Netherlands Heart Foundation for executing the study (JH 8802) described in this chapter is gratefully acknowledged.

References

1. Maxwell GM, Gane S: The impact of congenital heart disease upon the family. Am Heart J 1962;64(4):449–454.
2. Garson A, Benson RS, Ivler L, Patton C: Parental reactions to children with congenital heart disease. Child Psychiatric Hum Dev 1978;9:86–94.
3. Donovan E: The pediatric cardiologist and adolescents with congenital heart disease. Int J Cardiol 1985;9:493–495.
4. Garson SL, Baer PE: Psychological aspects of heart disease in childhood. In: Garson Jr.A, Bricker JT, McNamara DG (eds.) The Science and Practice of Pediatric Cardiology. Philadelphia/London: Lea & Febiger, 1990;2519–2527.
5. Bowen J: Helping children and their families cope with congenital heart disease. Crit Care Quarterly 1985;8(3):65–74.
6. Linde LM: Psychiatric aspects of congenital heart disease. Psychiatr Clin North Am 1982;5(2):399–406.
7. Kitchen LW: Psychological factors in congenital heart disease in children. J Fam Pract 1978;6(4):390–396.
8. Silverman S: Family adaptation to congenital heart disease: adjusting to physical and moral realities. In: Anderson RH et al. (eds.) Pediatr Cardiol 1983;5:317–326.
9. Utens EMWJ, Erdman RAM: Psychosocial aspects of congenital heart disease in adolescents and adults. In: Hess J, Sutherland GR (eds.) Congenital Heart Disease in Adolescents and Adults. Dordrecht/Boston/London: Kluwer Academic Publishers, 1992: in press.

D: Performance of Social Roles

30. Psychosocial development during school period of children operated for transposition of the great arteries

E. STUCKI, F.P. STOCKER, H. HÄMMERLI, V. RÜFENACHT,
M. STUCKI, J.W. WEBER and P. SCHÜPBACH

1. Introduction

During the past decades the progress of cardiac surgery has brought about an impressive and important improvement in the prognosis of many congenital heart malformations. Many patients now survive into adolescence and adulthood, and more and more attention is being given to psychosocial aspects of congenital heart disease in the long-term follow-up.

The purpose of this study was to look into psychosocial problems during school age of children who had been operated on for simple transposition of the great arteries in the preschool period. In addition, we wanted to get an idea of the impact this had on school achievement, on professional training, and later on, on the chosen profession, and to find ways of improvement in case of significant difficulties.

2. Selection of patients and method of investigation

Our aim was to put together a more or less homogeneous and, by that, comparable group of patients with congenital heart disease leading to severe cyanosis from birth onward, and surviving only with the help of surgery. In order to achieve this, we were looking for the following target group: children operated for simple transposition of the great arteries by the Mustard or Senning procedure, born between 1967 and 1977, living in the German-speaking part of Switzerland, and being followed in our institution during the whole period, i.e. from 1967 to 1991. Twenty-three patients corresponded to these criteria, 15 males and 8 females, being equivalent to 100% of the target group. This group, although small, is representative, and without bias.

In 1983/84 the patients and their parents took part in a first extensive psychological and medical examination. In 1990/91 all 23 patients and 21 of the parents were contacted again for the second part of the study, allowing a follow-up of 7–8 years.

Paul J. Walter (ed.): Quality of Life after Open Heart Surgery, 335–344.
© 1992 Kluwer Academic Publishers.

The psychological examination consisted of interviews, questionnaires, and tests aimed at gaining information on intelligence, minimal cerebral dysfunction, emotional adaptation, school achievement, social behaviour, and leisure time activity. The examination was performed in one day and took about 5–6 hours: assessment of intelligence by the WISC-R intelligence test, assessment of form reproduction by Bender Gestalt test (a German version of the BGT called GFT), and of concentration by d-2 test in children older than 9 years, and by DLT test in children younger than 9 years. Assessment of variables of personality by Hanes personality inventory, and by Marburger children's behaviour check-list. In addition, standardized interviews with parents about problems in education, school achievement, social contact, leisure time activity, and influence of the heart disease on family life style, as well as standardized interviews with patients about school and leisure time activities.

The same day, the patients also underwent a physical examination; ECG, X-ray, and ergometry were done, as well as a Holter 24 h ECG.

The second part of the study in 1990/91 consisted in a half-structured interview regarding psychosocial aspects with the participation of all patients and with the 21 parents: school achievement, problems and special therapies during school period, emotional problems and problems of behaviour, subjective impression of quality of life and of physical capacity, and in addition, in those who had finished school, information about professional education and employment. The medical follow-up relied on an interview and on the medical record.

3. Results of the first study: 1983/84

According to the instructions, the results of the psychological tests were expressed as standardized test results; the results of the interviews were evaluated. Depending on the distribution of the variables, the correlations were either compared with the t-tests or evaluated according to the χ^2 test or t-test. The level of significance was set to 5%, two-tailed testing was performed.

3.1. *Characteristics of subjects*

The tested patients (8 girls and 15 boys) were between the age of $6\frac{1}{2}$ and $16\frac{8}{12}$ (mean age $11\frac{9}{12}$). The average number of 2.8 children per family examined was relatively high, and amongst the patients the youngest children (12/23) dominated. Regarding the socioeconomic situation, the families corresponded to the distribution within the Swiss population. There was little representation of one-parent families (1/23) nor of families originating from

Table 1. Quantitative results.

Score	WISC-R Test in 1983/84	
	General population	Patients
55–69	2%	1 = 4%
70–84	14%	5 = 22%
85–115	68%	17 = 74%
116–130	14%	–
131–145	2%	–

a foreign country (1/23), three patients, however, had one parent from a foreign country. Apart from having a heart defect, four patients showed a further physical handicap (2 hemiparesis, 1 cleft lip anomaly, 1 hearing defect).

3.2. Results of the psychological examination

3.2.1. Intelligence (n = 23)
The group of patients did not come off as well as expected by standard distribution (Table 1).

The qualitative evaluation in 3/23 test sheets gave balanced results. Significant differences between the two parts of the test or the sub-test scores occurred in 20/23 of the cases. In the current literature, such deviations are described in connection with partial impairment of performance or MCD, respectively [1].

Significant correlation of the IQ resulted from: the Bender Gestalt test (more intelligent patients performed better: $r = 0.41, p = 0.03$), the attention perseverance test ($r = 0.55, p = 0.003$), and the frequency of problems of behaviour and upbringing recognized by the parents (more intelligent patients are perceived as less difficult: $r = 0.045, p = 0.015$). Significant differences resulted in regard to intelligence and special therapy (patients with special therapy as a group are significantly less intelligent: $t = 2.22, p = 0.036$).

3.2.2. GFT test (n = 23)
The results of the group of patients correspond to the standard distribution which consisted of one third each of cerebral healthy children, children with suspected brain defects, and children with brain damage. We therefore assume that among the group of patients there is an equal distribution of cerebral healthy children and children with brain damage.

As mentioned, there is a significant correlation between GFT and IQ. In addition, the performance of patients receiving special therapy was inferior to that of patients not receiving therapy ($t = 2.08, p = 0.04$).

3.2.3. *Attention-perseverance test* (*n* = 22)

The test was fully completed by 22 patients, the youngest was overstrained and gave up. The mean value and standard deviation of the group of patients are equal to the standard distribution; hence the patients have an average ability to concentrate not only in respect to the quantity but also to the quality of their performance.

The quantitative result gained from the concentration test correlate with the IQ, quantitative and qualitative results with the frequency of problems of upbringing and behaviour.

3.2.4. *Hanes personality inventory* (*n* = 15)

Neuroticism and introversion/extraversion scale: 15 patients filled out the questonnaire, the remaining patients were too young.

Neuroticism: The group as a whole did not significantly differ from the standard test ($x = 4.7$ vs $x = 5$), 2 values highly above average opposing 5 below average and 8 average. The group's extraversion scale as a whole was highly above average ($x = <0$ 7.4 *vs* x = 4.5).

No systematic correlation with other tested variables were observed.

3.2.5. *Marburger behaviour checklist* (*n* = 13)

A questionnaire for parents of 6–12-year-old children: 13 questionnaires were filled out, 10 patients were older than 12 years of age. Seven of the 13 questionnaires gave inconspicuous results, 6 showed elevated results compared to the overall result as well as in at least 3 out of the 5 subscales. The findings regarding 'fear of social contact' and 'unstable self concept' were most frequently elevated; in only 1/13 was an elevated result found in respect of unsocial behaviour.

3.3. *Results of the interviews*

3.3.1. *School situation*

At the time of the examinations, 21 of the 23 patients received schooling. All of them attended a public school (Table 2).

Table 2.

Preschool	2
Primary school	11
Secondary school	7
Special school for learning disabled	3

- 9/21 were older than their classmates:
- due to later entry: 6
- due to repetition during primary school: 2
- due to later entry as well as repetition: 1

The percentage of schoolchildren older than their classmates is 41% and is certainly higher than the average. There is no systematic correlation with other examined variables.

Psychological examinations in connection with school entrance or with difficulties during school was necessary in 8 of the 23 patients. Also this percentage (34%) is higher than the average in Switzerland.

Twelve patients had never received additional tuition or special therapy for speech disorders, dyslexia or psycho-motor disabilities. Nine are receiving or have received one kind of therapy, 2 patients are receiving two kinds of treatment. The number of patients receiving special therapy again is certainly higher than the average in Switzerland. As mentioned, there is a systematic correlation between (not) receiving special therapy and the IQ and the result from the GFT, respectively. In addition, these patients are experienced as more difficult by their parents in respect to their behaviour or upbringing $(\chi^2 = 9.4, p = 0.002)$.

A comparison with the type of school attended by the patients and their siblings is only possible in 10 patients, a comparison with the average numbers in Switzerland is not possible due to the different schoolsystem between the cantons. A comparison with the siblings shows that within the group of patients, the number of scholars attending secondary or grammar school is lower, and that of those attending a school for learning disabled is higher than within the group of siblings.

3.3.2. *Educational problems*

The parents were questioned on characteristics of behaviour of their heart child in comparison with their healthy siblings. They referred to an average range of problems of 1.4 with the emphasis on impairment of incentive (irritability, hyperactivity) and impairment of performance (problems of concentration, variation in performance, lack of perseverance). For two families (8.7%), the problems had become serious enough to seek psychiatric help for their child. As mentioned, significant correlations existed with the IQ and the necessity for special therapy.

In 10 of 21 families with more than one child, the siblings reacted with jealousy, although of short duration, rejection, or problems of behaviour. Only in 3 families, the siblings negative attitude remained, in the other families, the relations soon returned to normal. Rejection or acceptance of the heart child by the siblings do not show any systematic correlation with other examined variables.

3.3.3. *Social behaviour and leisure time activities*

Outside school, most patients had frequent and close contacts with others of their age. 4/23 were regarded by their parents as being rather solitary. 22 of the 23 patients are active in sports, 3 of them doing competition. Other youth groups are not often frequented.

3.3.4. *Perceived limitations*

The often perceived reduced physical performance is partly felt as also having its positive aspects. Without considering this variable, 11/23 patients do not feel any negative implications from their heart defect. The remaining 12 were mainly suffering from physical characteristics (scars, etc.) as well as from not being allowed to do high-performance sports. One patient states that, as a result, he actually has 'great problems'. Another 2 patients used to have 'great problems', it upset the rest 'a little'.

3.4. *Correlation with 'organic history'*

In order to form an idea about the influence of the patients' organic disease on psychosocial results, we correlated the results of psychosocial examination with the following 'organic facts': age at the first palliative procedure, neurological symptoms before palliation, need of additional palliation, lowest oxygen saturation, highest hemoglobin, neurological symptoms between palliation and correction, age at the time of correction, year of the correction, neurological symptoms between correction and study, result of ergometry, neurological symptoms at the time of the study, medical subjective impression of risk before and after correction.

We found a correlation between minimal cerebral dysfunction and a low oxygen saturation as well as the medical subjective impression of risk between birth and correction. Minimal cerebral dysfunction correlates also with neurological symptoms at the first study but does not correlate with the age of correction despite the fact that children operated at a later age, correspond to a selected group.

Thus, the degree as well as the duration of hypoxia seem to be important factors for psychosocial difficulties. The small number of patients allows only to speak of a tendency but report in the literature on more patients endorse this impression [2,3].

3.5. *Summary of the first study*

The examined patients show various particular characteristics which have little consequences regarding leisure time activities and do not create unsolvable problems within the family. However, they demand that various measures be taken for school success. Hence, two groups are distinguished: the group which has an overall better aptitude also showed better performance in the GFT test, as well as in the attention perseverence test, it showed fewer problems of behaviour and upbringing, and it did not receive special therapy. The patients of the second group, as a whole, are less gifted, make more mistakes in the GFT test, are more difficult (as described by their parents), and receive special therapy. The two groups did not differ in respect of neuroticism and the extraversion scale, social behaviour and leisure time activities, acceptance by their colleagues and healthy siblings, as well as the necessity of a delayed entry to school. Such problems were equally frequent in both groups.

4. Results of the second study 1990/91

4.1. *Results regarding school achievement*

Twenty of 23 patients (=87%) are at the end of or have finished normal public schooling; 3 patients needed special schooling for learning disabled, and none had to attend a school for mentally retarded. On average, patients followed a less demanding level of schooling compared to their siblings.

The best prediction of final school achievement was found by an intelligence test during the first examination in 1983/84, as can be seen in Table 3. The results of the intelligence test were 'right' in 19 of 23 and 'false low' in 4 of 23, i.e. the child with the lowest IQ predicting a special school for mentally retarded, could follow a special school for learning disabled, and 3 children with a test value between 70 and 84 predicting special schooling for learning disabled, were able to follow regular schooling.

The frequency of minimal cerebral dysfunction leading to special therapy was the same as in the first study. Therefore we can say that the necessity for special therapy is usually recognized in the preschool or early school period. Special therapy lasts for three or more years. Minimal cerebral dysfunction has no significant influence on final school achievement, probably due to early recognition and special therapy.

Compared to the general population, patients are often older than their class-mates, mostly due to the late beginning of schooling, very often recom-

Table 3. Prediction by intelligence test.

	IQ of examination 1983/84		
	89–115	70–84	50–69
regular school	17	3	–
special school	–	2	1

IQ is a good predictor with rather 'pessimistic' tendency ('right' in 19/23, 'false low' in 4/23).

ended by medical staff. Repetition of school classes is another but less frequent reason.

4.2. *Professional education and profession*

Sixteen out of 23 patients had finished obligatory schooling at the time of the follow-up study. Thus, about two thirds of the total group brings us information on their professional education and employment.

All 16 have regular jobs, none are working in a special institution for disabled, none depend on welfare money or money from the invalid insurance. All but one have found full-time employment.

Twelve of 16 (=75%) had regular professional education. Two patients passed through special reduced training, and 2 are unskilled, without professional training.

The level of professional education corresponds to the general population. In contrary to the level of schooling, professional education does not differ significantly from that of siblings.

Professional education is best predicted by school achievement, regular schooling leading to regular education in all but one, and special schooling leading to special reduced or no professional education.

4.3. *Emotional problems and problems of behaviour during the follow-up period*

As seen in the first study, emotional problems and disturbances in behaviour did not exceed the level of the general population. Only one patient needed psychiatric treatment during the follow-up period.

4.4. *Subjective impression of the patients*

All patients with regular schooling and regular professional education had the subjective impression that their heart disease had no negative influence on schooling and professional education, while 3 of the 4 patients without regular professional education feel that their heart condition may have had a negative influence on schooling and professional achievement.

Eighteen of 23 patients regarded their physical endurance reduced, usually in activities like long distance runs, in sports classes, or bicycle tours. For half of them, this was not percieved as a handicap and did not interfere with every-day life. 5 had the impression that they were physically more exhausted through work than others, 2 of them, therefore, had changed to a physically less demanding job, one to an 80% employment. Four patients regretted that they could not join in sports competitions and championships with equal chances.

At some point in their life, about one third of the group had problems with physical attractiveness and body appearance. For some time, they had been avoiding going to a public swimming pool or wearing shirts unbuttoned. But only one has problems in social relations due to that. Three out of the group have concerns about possible problems in their future lives related to their heart disease.

4.5. *Follow-up of 'organic history'*

During the follow-up period, a pacemaker was implanted in 3 patients, the indication being a pathological Holter ECG and not syncope. Two patients had episodes with supraventricular tachycardia, and 1 patient had to be reoperated for baffle obstruction.

5. Summary and conclusion

The small number of patients is a limitation of this study, on the other hand, the fact that the group represents 100% of the target group is an advantage eliminating biased results. Another advantage lies in the length of the follow-up. In general, the follow-up results confirm and by that enforce the findings of the first study. It can be shown that the psychological examination can be made early and that a good prediction of school and professional career is possible.

The results of this study are very encouraging since 85–90% of all patients can go through regular public schooling, have regular professional education, obtain regular full-time jobs, and are subjectively satisfied with their school and professional achievements.

On the other hand, the study shows that 40–50% of all patients have signs of minimal cerebral dysfunction with a need for special therapy during three or more years. But it must be emphasized that,with early recognition – possible in preschool or early school age – and with adequate treatment, the minimal cerebral dysfunction has no influence on the later professional outcome.

Neurotic development is not a problem in this group of patients compared with the normal population.

Around 80% have the subjective impression of reduced physical endurance with, in general, no significant influence on professional outcome apart from the influence on the choice of profession.

Correlation of psychosocial findings with the 'organic history' reveals the tendency that the degree and the duration of hypoxia is an important factor for difficulties, a fact shown also in the literature.

On the basis of these findings, we propose two main ways of improvement:

(a) Avoidance of cerebral damage as main cause of later psychosocial difficulties by early diagnosis, good pre-operative management, and early and good surgical correction.
(b) Routine psychological examination post-operatively in preschool age for the evaluation of possible minor cerebral dysfunction, and induction of early and consequent support by special therapy if needed.

References

1. Scholtz W: Testpsychologische Untersuchungen bei hirngeschädigten Kindern. In: Zimermann KW (ed.) Fortschritte der Sonderpädagogischen Psychologie, vol 2. Berlin-Charlottenburg: Carl Marhold Verlagsbuchhandlung, 1972.
2. O'Dougherty M, Wright FS, Garmezy N, Loewenson RB, Torres F: Later competence and adaptation in infants who survive severe heart defects. Child Dev 1983;54:1129–42.
3. Newburger JW, Silbert AR, Buckley LP, Fyler DC: Cognitive function and age at repair of transposition of the great arteries in children. New Engl J Med 1984;310:1495–99.

E: General Satisfaction

31. Quality of life after surgical correction of congenital heart disease: the parents' point of view

M. DHONT, E. DE WIT, H. VERHAAREN and D. MATTHYS

1. Introduction

The purpose of the study, started in 1989, by the Department of Pediatric Cardiology of the University Hospital of Gent, was to explore the impact of Congenital Heart Disease (CHD) on daily life and psychosocial functioning of the child and his family, after surgical correction. This issue is illustrated from the parents' point of view.

The multidisciplinary team (pediatric cardiologists, nurses, social workers, clinical and social psychologists) of this department also wanted to draw up a standardized and manageable inquiry for this population.

2. Methods

2.1. *Subjects*

The sample consisted of parents of 29 children from 9 to 12 years old. There were 15 girls and 14 boys.

The distribution of the pathology was as follows:

ASD	7
Ductus botalli	6
ASD + Pulm. sten.	1
Aortic stenosis	1
Coarctatio	1
ASD I	1
VSD	2
VSD + Mitr. Sten. + Pulm. Sten	1
Tetral. Fallot	5
Trans GR. A.	4

All the patients had undergone corrective surgery at least five years earlier.

Paul J. Walter (ed.): Quality of Life after Open Heart Surgery, 347–353.
© 1992 Kluwer Academic Publishers.

One can expect that normal life has been restored after the intervention. The children were at least two years old at the time of the operation.

Most of the time the mother came alone to answer the questionnaire. About a quarter of the parents came together; in 13% of the cases we saw only the father of the child.

2. Instrument

The questionnaire drawn up by the multidisciplinary team included six chapters:

(1) Identification of the child.
(2) Information about the structure of the family.
(3) Perception of the parents on the medical grounds of the heart defect of their child.
(4) Comparison of (3) with the real medical status of the patient, noted in the cardiologic report.
(5) Functional status of the child.
(6) Psychosocial functioning of child and his family.

There were three types of questions: those which can be answered yes or no, those for which alternative answers are given, and open questions.

2.3. *Procedure*

The questionnaire was used as a structured interview. All the interviews were done by the same interviewer. The conversations had an average duration of $1\frac{1}{2}$ hours. Parents were invited to the clinic outside the period of consultation. In this way, undisturbed, parents can be brought into close touch with their thoughts and feelings about their child's illness.

2.4. *Data analysis*

Due to the methodological criteria it was not possible to carry out a statistical analysis. So we had to work with frequencies.

3. Results

3.1. *Perception of the parents on the medical aspects of congenital heart disease in comparison with the real medical data*

The knowledge of the parents was right in 55% of the cases. About one fifth of them had a totally wrong picture of the medical situation and 24% of the parents had a knowledge of the heart defect which was partly correct. *So almost half of the parents didn't know exactly what was wrong with their children.* This percentage is alarming taking into account that parents came regularly to the consultation after the operation. This information surprised the pediatric cardiologists, who invest a great deal of effort in informing the parents about the medical status of their child.

Certainly this is not an isolated observation. Two years ago in Bern (Working Group for Psychosocial problems in Pediatric Cardiology), Dr. Röhmer (Leiden) communicated his consternation about the defective knowledge of his adolescent patients. One may ask if this has to do with the way doctors describe the medical aspects to the parents. Is the language understandable? Does he use illustrations? Is there any time for questions on the parents' side and time to check on the doctor's side?

Other important elements are the attitudes and emotions of the parents during the consultation. Sohni and co-workers [1] pointed out the reduction of the capacity to accept and assimilate informations as a result of emotional stress.

In this perspective we now proceed to link this data with other findings of this study.

3.2. *Possibility to speak about the child with CHD and associated problems with doctors*

More than half (55%) of the parents say it is not possible to speak with the general practitioner about the child. Fifty-eight percent could not discuss these problems with the pediatric cardiologist, and even 72% of the parents cannot speak about it with the pediatrician. These observations are very problematic, since we know that doctors are a very important support system in case of chronic disease.

What gives the parents the impression they cannot speak about the problems of their child?

Further inquiry revealed that it is essential for the parents to speak about their emotions in connection with the disease of their child. The fact that they have no time to express their individual feelings, makes the conversation with the doctors incomplete.

In the literature we find that when parents learn the diagnosis of the chronic disease of their child, they have to deal with emotions of fear, anger, guilt and sorrow. These emotions reappear in every stressful moment, such as an operation and, although in a minor way, during every further consultation. These emotions cause a sort of psychic deafness to further medical information [2,3].

Only when the doctor is aware of and is interested in these feelings, is he able to increase the *Psychological Permeability*.

Repeated information adapted to the individual level of understanding, combined with attention to the feelings of the parents, is the formula for a good and efficient communication between doctors and parents. This guarantees a better understanding and a better knowledge of the medical aspects for the parents and, in an indirect way, for the child.

3.3. *Parental attitudes towards the child*

The defective parental knowledge of the medical status of their child can lead to an *overestimation of the heart defect* in a negative sense. This provokes extra anxiety. This also affects the educational strategies and the attitudes of the parents towards the child.

After corrective operation 44% of the parents still consider their child as a problem-child. They worry about his physical condition, his school, and his professional career. They admit that the child is given extra attention in 18% of the cases. Twenty-three percent of the parents reveal that the amount of attention given to the child has significantly decreased after the operation. Still, 37% of them say they have to protect their child against stress, anger, fatigue, sorrow and excitement [4].

Another remarkable finding is that almost a quarter of the parents *never speak with the child about his heart defect*. These parents say they don't know if the child is aware of his heart defect. Forty-three percent of the parents don't find a reason to talk about it with their child. They do not want to worry the child by this information. Thirty percent have the conviction that the child cannot understand the information anyway, and 27% say that the child doesn't ask anything, so they are convinced that he has no questions about his health. In our practice, however, we see that this is wrong and that the child certainly does have questions, especially because of the visible sign of his problem: the scar. We can imagine that, taking account of the defective knowledge of the parents, they feel too uncertain to explain the medical aspects to the child.

We know also that children have a very good feeling about the anxieties of their parents. By not asking, they try to spare them.

That communication is an overall problem is illustrated by the fact that one fifth of the parents complain that *conversation about the illness of the child with the partner is impossible*. Each of them has to work through his own emotions and has his own coping style. As a consequence there is little energy left to understand and support each other.

3.4. *Impact of CHD on the child*

3.4.1. *Daily routine*
Here the results of the study are very positive: the operated child doesn't differ from other children of this age group. They behave actively and independently.

3.4.7. *School career*
It is a pity we cannot be so positive about the school career. Of the sample, 14% attend special schools. This is much higher than the 5% in normal population. In the same way, 41% of the patients have school retardation. In a normal population only 13% of the children attend classes below their age level. Parents consider that frequent periods of school absence because of sickness and hospitalisations are cause of this fact.

The following remarks can be made:

– One can wonder if many of the CHD patients are not kept at home without reason.
– Overprotection can cause lack of motivation and lack of perseverance in the children. In this way children can be captured in the vicious circle of anxiety to fail.
– Last but not least, we know the lack of flexibility of the Belgian school system which causes a lot of problems for children with chronic illness.

3.4.3. *Self image*
Thirty-one percent of the children are worried about their physical condition. We see the parallel with their parents.

Twenty-four percent feel different from the other children. In this age group (9–12 years) this is a big problem. 'One of the most striking characteristics is the child's need to be the same as other children, to be accepted by peers and to develop a sense of membership with the peer group' [5].

'The approval of peers is particularly important at this time because it helps the child in his efforts to emotionally move outside the family boundaries and re-direct his affective energies to individuals of his own age' [5].

This is also an important aspect in the evolution towards a positive and sane self image.

3.5. *Impact of CHD on the patient's brothers and sisters*

A last paragraph underlines the impact of the CHD on the brothers and sisters of the patient. Half of the parents mentioned the important problems of these children in periods of stress, especially the heart operation. Brothers and sisters feel powerless: not being really active, although emotionally much involved. They are very worried, nervous, anxious, have sleep disturbances and school problems. Literature confirms these data.

4. Conclusion

4.1. *Concerning the data resulting from the interviews*

Parents and child have a great need for appropriate and repeated information about the medical situation. Style and contents are to be adapted in every individual case.

This knowledge has to be checked regularly.

Daily experience in the contact with parents of sick children learns that it is essential to communicate about the parents' emotions. Only in such a context is there psychological permeability for medical information.

Attentiveness to the feelings and coping of each parent is essential. Data of this study reveal that it is important, too, to be concerned about the possibility of the parents to communicate about the child and his problems.

Periods of stress, such as a heart operation, are very difficult for brothers and sisters. The doctor can involve them actively, e.g. by inviting them for the consultation. In this way behaviour problems can be prevented.

Information about the school career of the child is to be gathered frequently. Contact with school direction and teacher as well as contact with the school psychologist is to be taken when the first signs of difficulties appear.

Open communication between all the persons involved results in a positive and sane self-concept of the child with CHD.

4.2. *Concerning the form of the questionnaire*

The questionnaire is adapted and shortened, taking into account the experience of the interviewer, the suggestions of the parents and the remarks of the members of the Working Group for psychosocial problems in pediatric cardiology.

References

1. Sohni H, Geiger A, Schmidt-Redeman B: Psychische Bewältigung kinderkardiologische Eingriffe. Beobachtungen und Empfehlungen. Klin Pediatr 1987;199:80–85.
2. Rothenberg MB: The effect of chronic illness on the family. In: Christ AE, Flomenhaft K (eds.): Psychosocial family inventions in chronic pediatric illness. New York: Plenum Press 1982;163–178.
3. Baldew IM, Baldew-Visser SA: Chronisch zieke kinderen en jongeren. Nijkerk, Intro, 1985.
4. Losekoot G, Kamphuis RP: Kinderen met een hartafwijking. Medische, psychologische en sociale aspecten. Meppel-Amsterdam: Boom, 1988.
5. Weitzman M: School and peer relations. Pediatr Clin, North Am 1984;31(1):59–69.
6. Bos JM: Het gezin met een hartekind. Lisse, Swets & Zeitlinger, 1977.
7. Sabbeth B: Understanding the impact of chronic childhood illness on families. Ped Clin North Am 1984;31(1):47–57.

32. The role of a parents' organization

R.P. KAMPHUIS

1. Introduction

In 1964 the Dutch Heart Foundation (NHS) was founded with, as its main objective, the combating of heart and vascular diseases in the broadest sense, preventive as well as curative. In 1971 some parents applied to this organization with the request to look after the interests of children with congenital heart diseases. This resulted in the formation of a parents' organization (OKHF), managed by some parents and representatives of the NHS, a pediatric cardiologist and a psychologist from one of the centres for pediatric cardiology. A popular women's magazine organized a puzzle competition for its readers to raise money for a well-equipped vacation site in the middle of the country.

Up to the present time the OKHF organizes summer camps in that place, as well as in other surroundings in the Netherlands and abroad. Only children with a relatively severe heart condition and/or psychosocial problems are allowed to take part. Special arrangements were made for parents with young children and for mentally handicapped children. Soon other activities followed: meetings about specific topics like handling the child during his stay in hospital, school problems and giving information to the child about his heart. Weekends were offered for adolescents to discuss topics like job possibilities, free time activities, sexuality and so on. Once a year a general one-day meeting was held for all members, with contributions from pediatric cardiologists, surgeons and representatives of other disciplines who are concerned with cardiac patients. Gradually, individual support and guidance developed as an important service, and the NHS paid for several social workers. Twice a year parents who had lost a child with a congenital heart disease were given the opportunity to meet each other. A group of about 300 adolescents and young adults became active in the organization independently of the parents. Their own periodical is incorporated in the journal for parents 'Cordaad'.

Over the years about 2000 parents and/or adolescents became member

Paul J. Walter (ed.): *Quality of Life after Open Heart Surgery*, 355–362.

of the OKHF. However, not all of them participated in the different activities just named. Moreover, the Board of the OKHF got the impression that many participants took part several times, while others seemed never to do so. So the need was felt to know more about the members, their children and their expectations of the organization.

An investigation was set up with the following questions in mind: what are the characteristics of the members of the OKHF and their children? What do they think about the cardiac status of their children and their functioning in daily life? Are there any problems in this respect? What do they expect from the OKHF? How do they appreciate the OKHF program? Is there any relationship between the cardiac situation of the child as judged by the parents and their behaviour towards the parents' organization?

2. Methods

A semi-structured questionnaire was sent to all 2167 members of the OKHF, 2069 parents and 98 adolescents who are registered independently of their parents. The 52 questions were arranged in 4 categories: demographic data, cardiological data of the child (including physical status and life situation), participation in the OKHF and evaluation of the OKHF activities.

3. Results

About half of the questionnaires were returned (52%), so the data of 1128 respondents (1058 parents, 65 adolescents) could be analyzed.

3.1. *Family data*

On average the parents became a member of the OKHF when the child with the congenital heart disease was 11 years old. At the time of filling in the questionnaire the mean age was 17, as can be seen in Table 1. Half of them are the only or the eldest child in the family (51%), 53% are boys. Most children live at home (76%), 18% live on their own. The others stay in an institution or in a protective environment separated from their family. About a quarter (24%) visits a elementary school, 36% are too young for school (3%), employed (full time 16%, part time 7%) or unable to work (10%). In 8% of the families a child has died as the result of a congenital heart disease. The remainder of the children take part in vocational training or visit high school.

The mean age of the parents was 46 (fathers 47, mothers 45) with a remarkable range (15–89 years), partly due to the age of the adults with a

Table 1. Family data.

Age	Mean	Standard deviation	Range
Father	47	11.1	24–89
Mother	45	10.4	15–87
Child now	17	8.6	0.5–50.2
Child at time membership	11	6.4	0.4–29.4

Child	%	*n*	
Boys	53	456	
Girls	47	405	
·cardiac origin	8	82	
†otherwise	2	17	
Special education:			
– elementary	5	44	
– secondary	3	30	
Unable to work	10	96	

Family problems due to heart disease			
Relational (divorce)	3	38	
Financial:			
– sometimes	26	260	
– often/always	13	130	
Housing conditions			
(adaption necessary)	12	125	

congenital heart disease who responded independently. The oldest patient was 50 years old. The educational level of the parents was slightly higher than in the general population. (Primary school only: 13%, higher education/ university: fathers 20%, mothers 11%.)

Family problems due to the heart disease were reported with regard to the relation of the parents (3%), financial matters (39%) and housing accommodation (12%).

3.2. *Cardiological data*

Most children were treated by a pediatric cardiologist in specified centres (54%) or – at the age of at least 14 years – by a cardiologist for adult patients (32%), often in the same university hospital. Table 2 summarizes important medical data as judged by the respondents.

The next part of the questionnaire concerns the physical consequences of the cardiac state of the child for his daily life (see Table 3). It is important to note that no statistically significant correlation was found between restrictions imposed by the physician (16%) and limitations felt by the respondents (65%), as was observed in other studies as well (Kamphuis 1976, 1984).

Table 2. Cardiological data as judged by the respondents.

Physician in charge		%	
Pediatric cardiologist		54	
Cardiologist		32	
Pediatrician		5	
Other physician		9	

Medical aspects	%	Results	%
Operation performed	75	+	38
		+/−	53
		−	9
		Complaints	67
Operation expected	15		
Might be an operation			
but not for sure	39		
Medication	23		
Spontaneously recovered	4		
Other malformations	24		
Mentally handicapped	15		

Table 3. Experienced consequences of the heart disease.

Restrictions imposed by physician	16%
Felt limitations in physical activities:	
− none	35%
− some	43%
− many	19%
− almost incapable	3%
No sports	21%
Physical complaints	
Fatigueness	26%
Shortness of breath	17%
Perspiration	19%
Insomnia	7%
Problems at school	
Absence through illness	7%
Concentration	12%
Pace	11%
Fatigueness	4%
Subject matter	8%
Classmates	5%
Teacher	2%

Problems at school were reported to a lesser degree, and were no different from figures in the general population.

Most respondents took the view that the congenital heart disease was seemingly serious or worse (78%). About a third (36%) judged the future

Table 4. Appraisal of the severity of the heart disease by parents and adolescents/young adults.

Category	%
Not serious	32
Seemingly serious	32
Serious	23
Very serious	13
Perspectives in comparison with healthy children	
Better	6
The same	58
Less	26
Extremely less	10

of the patient in comparison with healthy children as more gloomy (Table 4). These data are in accordance with the impression of the OKHF that its members are not representative for the general population of patients with congenital heart disease.

3.3. *Participation in the parents' organization*

More than half of the respondents (53%) heard from a pediatric cardiologist about the OKHF, others were referred by a home physician (2%) or their family (12%). Sometimes the attention was drawn to the organization by means of journal, radio or TV (9%). Only 7% considered themselves as an active member, while about 450 parents and adolescents (40%) is taking part in the activities. Their participation ranges from 8% (vacation weeks for families) and 9% (weekends for parents) till 34% (summer camps for children) and 40% (national meeting for parents and adolescents), with asking for personnal advice and guidance somewhat in between (15%).

Individual guidance (61%) and summer camps for children (57%) scored highest in the evaluation of the respondents (see Table 5).

Planning to take part in the future is expressed by about 500 members (44%). In this respect it may be noted that the topics "preparation for an operation" and "contacts with hospital and/or physician" were mentioned by 11 and 14% respectively.

3.4. *Interrelations*

The interpretation of the figures concerning participation and planning to participate is hampered by the fact that most activities of the OKHF only are relevant for specified subgroups. Therefore the clustering of data around several topics of interest for the parents' organization needs further analysis.

Table 5. Participation in activities of the OKHF (in %).

Activity	Participation	Planning to participate	Evaluation '(very) important'
Summer camps for children	34	18	57
Vacation week for families	8	5	35
Journey to foreign country	14	17	35
Thematic weekend for parents	9	8	33
Weekend for adolescents/			
young adults	14	15	47
National meeting	40	23	53
Regional meeting	25	28	53
Meeting parents died children	2	4	45
Individual advice	15	18	61

The choice of these key variables implies some subjectivity. Moreover little is known about the non-responders to the investigation (48%). Therefore the grouping of the data at best can be considered as a description, without any claim to generalization to the population of parents of children with congenital heart diseases at large. Subsequently the introduction, the membership and the importance of the OKHF are put to a χ^2 analysis with all items of the questionnaire.

Only statistically significant relations ($p < 0.05$) with the key variable are indicated in the text.

3.4.1. *Introduction of the OKHF*

In general the severeness of the heart disease plays a role for those who mention the existence of the parents' organization to the parents, with the exception of the home physician. For parents who know about the OKHF through journal, radio of TV, the possibility of an operation of the child is an important incentive (more than 28% of the respondents).

No relation is found between coming into contact with the OKHF and preliminary training of the parents, inoperability of the child, financial problems or treatment centre (there are 8 centres for pediatric cardiology in the Netherlands).

Only 4.3% of the parents report their child to be a member independently of the parents. Most of these children are over 22 years old and live on their own.

3.4.2. *Membership of the OKHF*

On the average the parents join the OKHF when their child was 5 to 6 years old (range 0–29 years). Less than 10% became a member when the child was younger than 4 years of age. A strong statistical significant relationship is found ($p < 0.001$) between preliminary training of fathers and mothers and the period of membership: most of those who are a member for more than 10 years have less than senior high school. More often than not becoming a member is associated with the fact that the child is younger than 10 years of age, has a severe or very severe heart disease and is treated by a pediatric cardiologist. Rarely any support by family or friends is experienced.

No relationship can be observed between membership of the OKHF and getting support from the home physician, the centre for pediatric cardiology or the OKHF. This last finding means that people who had contact with the OKHF not necessarily become a member of this organization.

3.4.3. *The importance of the OKHF*

The appreciation of the parents for the parents' organization keeps pace with the seriousness of the heart disease of their children. Age or level of education of both parents do not relate to their judgement, nor does the extent in which they think their child has physical limitations or a gloomy future.

With regard to parents who have lost a child the period since the loss and the age of the child at that time don't differentiate in their positive evaluation of the OKHF.

Parents with a preliminary training below junior high school stress the importance of contacts between children with a congenital heart disease more often than parents with a higher level of education do. The same point is made for children older than 19 years, and those who have had an operation, or patients with a severe heart disease and/or physical complaints. No relation was found between this variable and the number of children in the family, remaining complaints after an operation, gloomy expectations or the treatment centre.

Especially for parents younger than 40 years the interchange of experiences with other parents matters. The same interest is expressed by 60% of the parents who have lost a child. No statistically significant relation exists with the level of preliminary training of the parents, the seriousness of the heart disease of the child, his expectations or his possible physical complaints. Also the support of friends, the home physician or the centre for pediatric cardiology do not play a role in this respect.

4. Conclusions

The questionnaire is filled in by only 52% of the members of the OKHF, so conclusive remarks should be carefully-worded. Probably the high percentage of non-responders points to the often observed fact in many clubs that a considerable part of the members do not take part in the activities, but do not cancel their membership either.

A relatively small group of parents take part in the activities of the OKHF or is planning to do so. They are active in several respects.

The data give the impression that mostly parents of children with a severe congenital heart disease and/or those who experience their child as physically handicapped become a member of the OKHF, meanly when their child is already 10 or 11 years old. The group of parents of (very) young children is underrepresented considerably. This does raise the question if parents in general are informed about the parents' organization properly and in due time. Otherwise it could be possible that the need for the OKHF develops mostly some time after certain categories of these children visit elementary school and problems appear or can be expected. Further study may be of value to clarify this point.

References

1. Kamphuis RP: Kinderen met aangeboren hartafwijkingen en hun ouders. 's-Gravenhage: JH Pasmans, 1976.
2. Kamphuis RP: Aspects of everyday life. In: Ottenkamp J (ed.) Tricuspid atresia: anatomy, therapy and (long-term) results. 's-Gravenhage: JH Pasmans, 1984.

33. Pediatric heart transplantation: the recipient's perspective

KATHY S. LAWRENCE, F. JAY FRICKER and SUSAN CARDILLO

1. Introduction

Transplantation is the miracle of contemporary medicine. Pediatric heart transplantation has achieved dramatic results. It has given dying children new and active lives. The reality of that activity cannot be questioned. When measured against the New York Heart Association scale, most pediatric transplant patients are categorized in Functional Class I. And for those who have survived several years after transplantation surgery, that active lifestyle is long-lasting. But, what is the quality of life of these pediatric recipients?

Research studies focused on measuring quality of life have tried to answer this question. Standardized testing done at the University of Pittsburgh [3] and the University of Michigan, with patient populations from several institutions [7], have had similar results. In physical activities of daily living, patients improved [3]. Overall self-concept and anxiety were similar to healthy peers. However, transplant recipients between the ages of 8 and 18 lacked social skills and appropriate strategies necessary for successful adaptation [7].

2. Method

After eight years of intense work with these patients, it was evident to the authors that the results of standardized testing conducted in previous research studies did not describe accurately the quality of children's lives following transplantation. Most children had defense mechanisms that this type of testing did not penetrate easily. Therefore, another method of gathering data was utilized.

Pre-adolescent and adolescent transplant recipients were interviewed by a trusted mental health professional. This age group was selected because of the ease with which they articulated their feelings. The interviews were structured to elicit a description of the experience of living with a heart

Paul J. Walter (ed.): Quality of Life after Open Heart Surgery, 363–370.
© 1992 Kluwer Academic Publishers.

transplant. Parents were questioned in separate sessions. Excerpts from the interviews have been reported [4].

Experts studying the psychosocial ramifications of pediatric organ transplantation have called for the return to the case study method of research to more accurately describe the effects of transplantation on the lives of children [8]. They also believe that standardized testing is not capturing the problems these children face. Therefore, for this paper, one adolescent was selected from those interviewed for a paradigm case study presentation. The data was collected from the interview session and from the medical record.

The adolescent to be discussed is Lani Smith (The names of the patient and her family members have been changed.) Lani's case was chosen because she was one of the early pediatric heart transplant patients, and she encountered circumstances that many other children will face as they, too, grow up with transplants. Living with a transplant, Lani matured from early adolescence to young adulthood. She underwent retransplantation and experienced the change in immunosuppression from cyclosporine to FK506.

3. Case study

The case study begins in 1982 in a small town in a midwestern state. Twelve-year-old Lani was living with her mother Judy, stepfather Bob and two half-sisters – ages 15 and 8. Bob was employed by a state agency and Judy worked for a small, family-owned store.

Lani was a slender, pretty brunette with striking blue eyes. She had an active life, enjoying friends, family, school and sports. Her health was perfect until May when she complained of fatigue and gastrointestinal distress. Following a cardiac catheterization, the diagnosis of viral myocarditis was made. In the next three months, Lani's condition deteriorated dramatically. She was hospitalized frequently and time at home was spent in a wheelchair or bed. Bob's supervisor sponsored benefits to raise money for the family. Bob was forced to take time off work to care for the two healthy children. Judy, needing to stay at Lani's bedside, had to quit her job.

In the fall of 1982, Lani was transferred to Children's Hospital of Pittsburgh to be evaluated for a heart transplant. Her condition was precarious, and she required intense medical management. Three weeks after being accepted as a transplant candidate, Lani received the new heart that she so desperately needed and wanted.

While their hopes soared, the family's financial situation plummeted, and bills mounted. The family's medical insurance coverage was limited. They still owed twenty thousand dollars from Lani's previous hospitalizations.

Unfortunately, Lani's post-operative course was plagued with complications – seizures, renal failure, hypertension and rejection. Lani struggled with intense physical therapy to strengthen her debilitated body; and, three months after admission, she was discharged. Even then, Lani continued to be separated from family and friends. She and her mother were required to spend another month in Pittsburgh for Lani's out-patient care. Already in financial distress, the family maintained two households, one in Pittsburgh and another in their hometown. The bills continued to mount.

Over the next two years, Lani and her mother made the costly trip to Pittsburgh ten times for biopsies. Each trip cost approximately $300 for gas, food and lodging. The emotional cost was equally high. Lani worried about rejection and being separated from her family and friends.

As Lani's condition stabilized, she was followed at a metropolitan hospital near her hometown. However, even these trips became a financial burden for the struggling family. Judy could not find an employer who would tolerate the frequent absences necessary to care for Lani.

It also was during this time that cyclosporine was placed on the commercial market. The Smith's were hit with astronomical medication bills – $900 per week. By October 1982, the family was forced to sell their home to pay for medical expenses not covered by third party payers. After essentially missing one year, Lani, 14, returned to school. She no longer belonged in her circle of old friends. Not only had time separated them; but Lani was now 'different' – she had a new heart. Classmates viewed her as a 'transplant', not a fellow student. Her altered appearance made that difficult to forget. Due to frequent episodes of rejection, Lani required continued use of steroids. She gained excessive amounts of weight; her Cushingoid facies were so extreme that striae appeared on her cheeks, a Buffalo hump on her neck. Her linear growth was stunted. The cyclosporine made her hirsute, and gingival hyperplasia covered the beautiful teeth of which she had been so proud. Even her menses was much later than her peers. That fact distanced her farther from the other girls in one more ego-shattering way. In 1983, one doctor augmented the usual description of Lani's normal exercise test by saying, 'Only meds separate her from her peers.' That statement was far from the truth. Other teenagers were afraid of Lani. She never had a 'best friend'. And, although the relationships she made with fellow transplant recipients were important, they were tempered with the knowledge that they may not be long-lasting because these children could die.

Lani's schooling and attempts at re-establishing friendships continued to be interrupted by routine check-ups and biopsies. Additionally, she needed treatments for the side effects of immunosuppression, such as painful excision of overgrowth of gums and surgical drainage of sinuses. Battles continued to keep hypertension, hypercholesterolemia and decreased renal function under control. Lani never had the opportunity to forget about her transplant.

As Lani's peers rejected her, she became closer to her mother. The two were drawn together continually during trips to the hospital. For Lani, the crucial adolescent quest for independence was aborted. Her growing closeness to her mother also increased her stepfather's and half-sisters' jealousy toward Lani. Judy felt her other two daughters had 'lost their mother'. As the years passed, the gulfs between family members grew even larger.

Lani was scheduled to graduate from high school in the summer of 1988. Two weeks before the ceremony, however, the principal told her that she lacked one-quarter credit because of absences for health reasons. Enduring an entire semester of additional class work and the teasing of the other students, Lani graduated one year after the rest of her class.

In the fall of 1988, Lani's transplanted heart showed signs of deteriorating function. Lani was now suffering from restrictive cardiomyopathy secondary to transplant atherosclerosis. She remained asymptomatic, yet the dreaded fear of the need for a second transplant loomed overhead. Several months later, Lani sustained a posterior myocardial infarction and developed second degree heart block. She was flown by helicopter to Pittsburgh. On completion of the evaluation, Lani was placed on the transplant list for a second time. The threat of sudden death was ever present.

Her precarious condition required Lani to stay in Pittsburgh. Judy remained at her side. Lani, now 19, was in competition for adult-sized hearts. The wait extended into four agonizing months. Financial considerations escalated to crisis proportion. Again the family was maintaining two households on a salary that could barely support one. The emotional stress on the separated family reached a crescendo. Bob threatened to divorce Judy.

Eventually, Lani's condition did stabilize. It was recommended that she and her mother return home to await a donor. Nine months after being listed for a second transplant, a suitable organ was found.

Lani's immediate post-operative recovery was uneventful except for sinus node dysfunction and the need for a permanent pacemaker. Some of Lani's spirit seemed to die the day that the pacemaker was implanted. She thought the new heart, for which she had waited so long, was defective. Like other transplant recipients, Lani correlated her own self-worth with the functioning of her new organ [2].

Before discharge, Lani's strength was tested further. She again battled the omnipresent enemy, rejection. Because of her previous transplant, her panel reactive antibody percentage was high. She was treated with intravenous steroids and two courses of painful RATG injections. With each failed treatment, Lani's hope faded. Six weeks after admission, she was discharged from the hospital.

Bills continued to mount. Repeated trips to Pittsburgh were necessary. The only way the family could finance them was by selling their furniture and other valuables. They struggled to find a way to salvage their car; it was needed to travel to Pittsburgh.

Lani tried to normalize her life. She searched for a boyfriend just as other girls her age. However, boys were hesitant to get involved with her, expecting her to die prematurely. Lani's self-esteem continued to diminish.

By September 1989, two months after her second transplant, Lani's left ventricular function had decreased significantly. The doses of immunosuppressive drugs were pushed to the maximum. Lani's mood swings, induced by high doses of steroids, were unbearable. With undaunted focal rejection causing continued loss of graft function and Lani showing evidence of toxicity from the conventional immunosuppressive drugs, she was switched to the experimental FK506.

By January 1990, FK506 had begun to perform its magic. Lani's graft function improved. Off steroids for the first time since the initial transplant, Lani's weight and blood pressure fell within normal ranges. Her physical portrait began to look rosy. Lani's emotional well-being also improved. At last, she had found a boy who truly cared about her. They planned a future together. Just as there seemed to be new hope for Lani, pieces of her life began to fall apart again.

Society continued to 'single out' Lani because of her transplant. Having no financial resources for college, she entered the work force and faced yet additional obstacles. A paycheck for a full-time job would mean the loss of the state financial aid she desperately needed. Furthermore, Lani lacked the stamina to work an entire day. One employer, eager to hire her for the publicity of employing a transplant recipient, soon tired of the restrictions in her work schedule. Lani felt she had failed again.

In May, signs of FK506 toxicity required a drop in the dosage. Lani feared the rejection that threatened to accompany the decrease in medication. Her fear became reality in June when the biopsy showed cellular rejection. The roller coaster ride had started again.

Soon afterward, the family was forced to file for bankruptcy. Guilt enveloped Lani. She felt personally responsible for her family's hopeless situation. One day, staring intensely at her mother, Lani lamented saying, 'You look like a mom who has aged 20 years in the last eight. I'm sorry.'

With each trip to Pittsburgh, Lani felt emotionally torn. She described Pittsburgh as the only place that treated her as 'just another person', not a 'transplant'. Yet she longed to stay home: Lani wanted her life to be 'normal'.

As her rejection episodes were controlled, Lani was given a reprieve. She could stay home for three months. Nevertheless, the financial crises continued unabated and the family conflicts increased. Lani overheard her stepfather yelling at her mother, 'If it were not for your daughter, we would not be in the position we are now.' Distraught by the constant tension in the home, Judy threatened to leave.

In the weeks that followed, Lani was described as 'empty'. In November 1990, after an episode of what, at that time, seemed to be a common cold, Lani died suddenly at home. Lani's death was not the fault of medical science but of society. Several days after her death, one author received a shoe box from Lani's family. It was filled with Lani's prescribed but unused immunosuppressive drugs. Lani had taken her own life.

The story has another addendum. A letter was found after Lani's death.

She implored one author to find a way to ease the pain of other transplant recipients.

These children must be helped.

The tragedy of Lani's case is not unusual. The impact of transplantation is acute on the developing personality of a child. With careful examination, many of the exquisitely painful elements of Lani's story are present in the lives of other transplant recipients, and as they mature, many will encounter the same problems Lani faced each day.

4. Summary

The miracle of transplantation extended Lani's life for eight years. It enabled her to return to an active life, attending school and participating in family activities. However, Lani and her family struggled with the sequelae of transplantation. Lani endured constant medical supervision and innumerable intrusive procedures. She lived with the constant threat of rejection and the burden of an unpredictable future. She was isolated from peers and potential boyfriends; she experienced discrimination at school and at work. The medical intervention divided her family members, both physically and emotionally. It devastated them financially.

5. Conclusion

Lani and her contemporary pediatric transplant recipients are sacrificial lambs. They benefit from the advances of medical science but suffer because of them. It is conceivable, however, that one day transplantation will not cause the heartache that Lani experienced. Until then, each of these patients deserves extraordinary intervention.

6. Recommendations

– For those countries that do not currently have effective systems, ways to cover catastrophic health care costs (i.e. $1 million for Lani's treatment) must be found. In turn, loopholes need to be included to allow transplant recipients to maximize their self-esteem by being productive members of the work force without the threat of jeopardizing their health care coverage.
– The special needs of these children must be advocated in the school system. The children cannot be over-protected nor denied special considerations.
– In the medical management of this population, it is particularly important

to minimize the side effects of medications and limit absences for medical intervention.

- Counseling programs must be funded for these children. Therapists need to maintain regular contact with the recipients to assess their emotional status and assure that a therapeutic relationship can be readily accessed when problems arise [5]. Ironically, only when the turbulence of the intensive clinical treatment has passed do transplant recipients begin to mourn lost capacities and capabilities [1]. Programs designed to enhance the coping skills of these children need to be implemented.
- Support for other members of the recipient's family must be provided. The effectiveness of parental coping is directly proportional to the child's [2]. Counseling also can help ease the marital tension that occurs with medical setbacks [6]. In turn, siblings need to be included in counseling programs.
- The recipients must be treated at medical centers where the professionals have expertise in understanding their special problems [1]. Adolescents use established relationships with caring professionals to help them cope with the stress of living with a transplant.
- Programs need to be designed to encourage interaction with fellow transplant recipients. Such programs help decrease the feeling of isolation. However, support must be available when the death of one recipient makes the others more aware of their own vulnerability.

Pursuing these interventions will help health care providers go beyond the biomedical model to optimize patient survival. May Lani's experiences with heart transplantation serve as the catalyst for change.

References

1. Hengeveld MV, Houtman RB, and Zwaan FE: Psychological aspects of bone marrow transplantation: A retrospective study of 17 long-term survivors. Bone Marrow Transpl 1988;3(1):69–75.
2. Hudson K, Hiott K: Coping with pediatric renal transplantation rejection. Am Nephr Nurs Ass 1986;13(5):261–263.
3. Lawrence KS, Fricker FJ: Pediatric heart transplantation: quality of life. J Heart Transpl 1987;6(6):329–333.
4. Lawrence KS, Fricker FJ, Hangard LJ, Armitage JM, Beerman LB, Pahl E, Cardillo S: Growing up with a transplant – unique adolescent issues. Presented at Loma Linda International Conference on Pediatric Heart Transplantation. Palm Desert, Ca. March 1990.
5. Rappaport BS: Evolution of consultation-liaison services in bone marrow transplantation. General Hospital Psychiatry 1988;10(5):346–351.
6. Reinhart JB, Kemph JP: Renal transplantation in children: another view. Comment in J Am Med Ass 1988;260(22):3327–3328.
7. Uzark K, Sauer S, Lawrence KS, Miller J, Addonizio L, Crowley D: Psychosocial outcomes

following pediatric heart transplantation. Presented at American Heart Association 63rd Scientific Sessions. Dallas, TX. November 1990.
8. Zamberlan K: Quality of life following transplantation. Presented at Children's Hospital of Pittsburgh. Pittsburgh, PA. November 1990.

34. Quality of life of children having undergone heart transplantation

J. KACHANER, J. LE BIDOIS, D. SIDI, J.F PIÉCHAUD and
P. VOUHÉ

1. Introduction

Heart transplantation is now accepted as a reasonable approach to the treatment of patients with end-stage cardiac disease. Since the mid-eighties, this also applies to children [1,2], infants, and even neonates [3,4]. With encouraging early survival rates and spectacular immediate improvement of the functional status of the survivors [5–8], the number of patients belonging to the paediatric age group undergoing heart transplantation has increased tremendously with more than 900 registered cases throughout the world in the last report of the International Registry [9]. First dedicated as 'the last chance procedure' to children with intractable cardiomyopathies or complex congenital heart malformations [10] having often already been unsuccessfully operated on, it appears now as an option among many others. Given the enormous difficulties raised by organ procurement, leading to an increasing delay on the waiting list, some even recommend considering the transplant option for patients whose life expectancy might be estimated to exceed 6 or even 12 months [11].

Is such enthusiasm justified? In other words, should we just address the problem in terms of postoperative mortality rates or actuarial survival curves, and say: "Now we can transplant, just let's do it?" We think that many other factors linked to the heavy long-term postoperative programme and contributing to what can be called the patient's quality of life, are to be seriously taken into account prior to any decision.

Everybody knows now that such a life looks like a steeplechase, full of physical as well as psycho-emotional trials. It starts with the waiting time on the list, and its blend of hope and anxiety. It goes on with the operation itself and the dreadful immediate post-surgical time, since most of the casualties and complications usually occur within the first days and weeks after the graft [12]. This is when many painful, serious treatments and investigations are imposed on the child; and this is also when the parents who dreamt about the operation day as a magic milestone, hardly understand why a

Paul J. Walter (ed.): Quality of Life after Open Heart Surgery, 371–379.

'successful' intervention does not ever mean that the most difficult task has just been accomplished, but remains to come. And finally, as far as long-term is concerned, are we sure that this very 'normal life' which everybody – doctors and media – promised to the child and to the parents, will be as normal as was stated, and that unexpected, additional complications, traps and even late catastrophes will not occur?

We started a paediatric heart and heart-lung transplantation programme in January 1987 [13]. More than four years later, we think we have learned enough to anticipate what the transplanted child's life will be. The main purpose of this work is to present these qualitative data as objectively as possible in order to help anybody involved in deciding whether a young person should have his or her heart replaced by knowing how and to what extent his or her life will be modified.

2. Population

From January 1987 to April 1991, 39 heart transplantations have been undertaken in 13-day to 15-year-old children (median: 33 months). They had either end-stage cardiomyopathies (62%) or congenital heart malformations not amenable to conventional surgery or already but unsuccessfully operated on (38%). The overall mortality, early and late, was 41%, decreasing to 22% in the last 18 cases.

3. The transplantation and the immediate postoperative course

In our experience, the children awaited for a suitable organ from 3 days to 8 months with a mean of 2.8 months. The operation itself does not usually present major difficulties to a well-trained surgical team. Within the first few postoperative days and weeks, however, many problems await the patients.

As a rule, it takes several days for the transplanted heart to recover a normal function, leading to the transient use of vasoactive drugs. The patient is usually weaned from artificial ventilation 24 to 48 hours postoperatively and can be discharged from the intensive care ward at the end of the first week.

Enhanced by a very active immunosuppressive therapy, infections, mainly bacterial, are a major concern at this stage and we lost a 6 year old girl 5 days after an uneventful transplantation from a *pseudomonas* sepsis. This is why continuous efforts have to be made to track such complications by multiplying samples and cultures, and by withdrawing any foreign bodies, including indwelling lines, as soon as oral feeding is possible.

Rejection episodes are the next and tormenting issue. They usually take place from the second or third week after the graft, and may be difficult to

Table 1. Follow-up protocol after heart transplantation.

Outpatient visits	: 2nd month after Htx : once a week 3–6 months after Htx : twice a month thereafter : once a month
Each visit includes	: X-ray, EKG, Echocardiography/Doppler Blod samples for RBC, WBC, platelets ionogram, creatinine cyclosporine level
Endomyocardial biopsy	: routine indications : 1, 3, 6, 12 months additional indications : suspicion of AR control indications : 5–7 days after AR treatment
Renal functional tests	: twice a year

AR = acute rejection.
HTx = heart transplantation.
RBC = red blood cell count.
WBC = white blood cell count.

identify by non-invasive means. We thus strongly recommend checking the transplant tolerance by performing endomyocardial biopsies, even in the very young, as a routine procedure at the end of the first month and whenever there is a clinical suspicion of rejection. The femoral vein approach, which we use under local anesthesia, is easy to use and painless for the child. Rejections do not usually impair the patient's hemodynamic status and are accepted by the parents as a 'normal', expectable event. Treatment includes high-dose, pulsed steroids, as well as polyclonal or monoclonal antibodies in the most severe cases.

Transient and moderate renal failure is nearly constant at that stage, but dialysis or ultrafiltration were uncommon postoperative needs in our experience.

Finally, we think that the patient should be managed in a special, isolated aseptic ward during the first two weeks following surgery, in order to restrict human contacts to those which cannot be avoided: mother and father, and those nurses and doctors who are specifically in charge of the patient. These measures are then alleviated and discontinued at the end of the first month.

4. The medium and long-term course

4.1. *Follow-up, hospitalizations*

After discharge from our centre, the patient is bound to a follow-up protocol (13) which is summarized in Table 1. It can be seen how compelling it is within the first months; mainly the first three months. For the family this means they have to remain in a relatively close neighbourhood to this centre, which again, may mean a number of daily problems for those who used to

Table 2. Immunosuppressive therapy after heart transplantation in children.

Drug	Dose	Duration	Route
Rabbit antithymocyte globulins	5 mg/kg/day	5–7 days	IV (central line)
Methylprednisolone	100 mg/m2/day	5 days	IV
	tapering doses	next 5 days	IV
Cyclosporine	2 mg/kg/day	the 1st day	IV
	increase doses	next days	IV, then oral
	adapt doses to whole blood RIA residual levels (200–400 ng/ml to start with; 100–200 ng/ml at the end of the first year)		
Azathioprine	2 mg/kg/day	ever	oral
Oral steroids	never, except uncontrolled chronic rejection		

live far away. But, as a rule, such as issue could have been anticipated prior to the transplant and might have been reasonably solved as a result of social workers' and psychologist's efforst. Such a programme has two main goals: to track rejections and to avoid drug related complications, mostly infections, which are still the main limitations on a long-term good outcome [14].

Rejection is first suspected on the basis of non-invasive criteria, including clinical behaviour, EKG, X-ray and echocardiographic changes [3,13]. But none of these allows safe conclusion to be drawn and, with increasing experience, we have changed our mind in recommending endomyocardial biopsies as the best standard for asessing the graft tolerance. We indicate it (Table 1): (1) as a routine follow-up procedure, four times a year in the first year; (2) as often as necessary in case of clinical suspicion of rejection; (3) as a control test to assess the result of the treatment of a rejection episode. Since 1989, our survivors underwent a mean of 6 biopsies/patient/year within the first postoperative year, with a maximum of 12 in less than four years in one child.

Drug-related complications are the next matter of concern. Some arise expectedly from immunologic depression, such as infections again, mostly viral after the first month, including severe diseases due to cytomegalovirus (CMV), herpesviruses, Epstein–Barr virus (EBV), and other. Four of our patients were deeply affected, three of whom died from late viral infections (1 CMV and 2 EBV related malignancies). Other complications are due to side-effects of the drugs. As a rule, oral steroids were excluded from our chronic protocol (Table 2) to avoid their well-known deleterious consequences on growth, systemic blood pressure, skeleton, etc. But azathioprine and cyclosporine also carry potential risks: bone-marrow depression for the former; hirsutism, gingival hypertrophy, seizures, and, overall, renal damage for the latter. In addition, some patients need tri-therapy and this carries a further risk of systemic hypertension. This is why each visit to the outpatient clinic should include blood sampling to check haematologic items, renal function, and residual cyclosporine levels.

Hospitalizations should be as limited in number and duration as possible since they remind everybody that the child remains a patient even if he or she looks perfect. Therefore, they are increasingly less well tolerated by both the patients and the parents. Increasing experience and organization allow us to lower the time spent by the child as an in-patient and every check-up should be set up during day-hospital sessions, even if it includes endo-myocardial biopsy. In our series, they did not last more than 15 days/year as a mean for the first year after discharge. Nevertheless, hospital stays remain quite common and are difficult to avoid since we feel much more comfortable this way when looking at a patient presenting, for instance, with an unclear episode of fever possibly related to acute rejection or lymphomatic process.

4.2. *Treatments*

Our immunosuppressive protocol is summarized in Table 2. We use to prescribe a strong initial immunosuppression in order to avoid the occurrence of early acute rejection episodes, at a stage of higher hemodynamic vulnerability. Neither intravenous antithymocyte polyclonal globulines nor methyl-prednisolone raised significant tolerance problems.

We consider cyclosporine as the fundamental basis of the long-term anti-rejection prophylaxis and this means that we are able to avoid chronic steroid therapy in the majority of our cases. Among many minor and/or transient side effects, progressive renal impairment appears to be a real matter of concern for the future. We have obtained pathological data from prospective renal biopsies and found a significant number (3/11 studied patients) of moderate to severe interstitial and tubular lesions no later than 6 months after initiation of cyclosporine therapy, with a good correlation with tubular functional deterioration [15]. In order to minimize or delay such a renal dysfunction, a close follow up of glomerular and tubular functional tests is mandatory as mentioned on Table 1, as well as a careful assessment of the lowest cyclosporine dose providing acceptable residual blood levels of the drug in each individual patient.

Systemic hypertension occurs in almost 75% of the adult and pediatric [7] patients whose immunosuppressive regimen includes three drugs (cyclosporine, azathioprine and prednisone), whereas it was very uncommon in our series, except in the first few postoperative days or weeks. This is possibly the result of a steroid-free, long-term protocol and was also observed by other groups treating their young patients the same way [3,4]. Nevertheless, we must say that some children need a tri-therapy protocol to overcome mild but resistant rejection.

4.3. *Late rejections*

The incidence of late rejections decreases significantly with time but may occur during all of the first year after the graft, and even later. They often have very little clinical expression and can only be identified by routine endomyocardial biopsies, as we have already mentioned. Repeat biopsies obviously weigh on the child's life, even if performed during a day-hospital stay. Only severe acute rejections require hospitalization of the patient to give him or her high pulsed doses of intravenous steroids and/or polyclonal or monoclonal antibodies. Subsevere and mild rejections can be treated by oral steroids at home.

4.4. *Late infectious complications*

Beyond the first month, infections are less likely to occur. The most common affect the upper respiratory tract and the lungs, and are related to viruses, mainly CMV. Seven of our children experienced a late CMV infection, which was lethal in two. They are currently treated with gancyclovir, which is given intravenously to symptomatic patients (fever, pneumonia, diarrhaea) as soon as the virus has been identified in blood or alveolar lavage fluid. Other agents may be involved and lead to serious problems: herpesvirus, pneumocystis, toxoplasm, etc.

4.5. *Late malignancies*

Three of our patients developed a late lymphoproliferative process, clearly related to an EBV infection in two. Two died, 3 weeks and 29 months after successful transplantations from the mediastinal form of the disease. The third one experienced this complication 3 months postoperatively as a cerebral disease together with lung tuberculosis; the condition had a very stormy course but the patient finally recovered almost completely, owing to specific immune therapy. This is why special diagnostic efforts, including bone marrow check, scan and MRI imaging, and surgical biopsies if necessary, should be undertaken to rule out such a life-threatening complication if there is the slightest reason to suspect it. Prolonged, unexplained fever may be one of these reasons and this, again, means a hospital stay.

4.6. *Growth*

The most critical advantage of the long-term cyclosporine/azathioprine protocol over the tritherapy regimen which includes steroids, is to allow a normal growth in weight and height throughout childhood in almost all cases. This was observed in all but two of our patients. But, as we mentioned previously, some cases require tri-therapy which, in turn, has its own side-effects: high blood pressure leading to additional drug therapies, growth retardation and Cushing-like appearance with their psychological consequences.

4.7. *School attendance*

All children in our series aged 3 or more normally attend school. In every case, school attendance could be started again no more than 2 months after the transplantation and absences were relatively uncommon, since all visits to the Transplant Centre were organized so as to take place on holidays.

4.8. *Exercise tolerance*

Children with transplanted hearts may share in all physical activities they want. Since the transplanted heart has lost its nervous connexions, its ability to adapt to exercise is progressive so that we just ask our patients to avoid sports requiring sudden and intense muscular stretching such as judo and related activities.

5. Conclusions

Athough a considerable amount of numeric data have been recently collected, it is still difficult to conclude that heart transplantation is a valid treatment in infants and young children. We know a great deal about survival rates at various terms, nature and incidence of complications, likelihood of hospitalizations/patient/year. Many advances on how to assess and how to manage have been made and many others are expected to appear in the near future. But some exceedingly important questions remain unanswered so far: will accelerated coronary atherosclerosis be a significant issue for the next ten years, as it already is in adults [16]? Is long term cyclosporine therapy going to induce irreversible renal damage? How will these infants and little children, who are supposed to become healthy adolescents, behave with the absolute necessity of taking drugs, and comply for the rest of their life with a rather compelling follow-up programme?

We certainly ought to let the parents of a transplant candidate have all the information we have just described, as simply and objectively as possible, without omitting any early, medium and long-term hazards. This is more to help them face and suffer possible forthcoming bad days following the operation, than to choose between two options, one of which being their child's quick, fatal outcome.

Beyond figures and actuarial curves, we have learned from our experience that there were two groups of transplanted children, approximately divided into two halves. Some will accumulate rejections, complications, complex treatments, side effects, hospital stays, and finally have a poor fate in spite of an enormous amount of medical effort. Others will surprisingly do well by going through all these traps, meet with a limited number of rejections and infectious episodes, and tolerate well a minimal immunosuppressive regimen. We still have no markers to predict into which group any individual patient will fall, but if he or she is lucky enough to belong to the latter, his or her life will be very similar to that of a normal child. Here is the final bet. By and large, we think that a child surviving heart transplantation often has a very good quality of life, good enough to let us go further into our programmes, despite many hazards, many unanswered questions, but with the strong hope of crucial advances coming very soon.

References

1. Pennington DG, Sarafian J, Swartz M: Heart transplantation in children. J Heart Transpl 1985;4:441–445.
2. Starnes VA, Stinson EB, Oyer PE *et al*: Cardia transplantation in children and adolescents. Circulation 1987;76(Suppl V):43–47.
3. Bailey LL, Nehlsen-Canarella SL, Doroshow RW *et al*: Cardiac allotransplantation in newborns as therapy for hypoplastic left heart syndrome. N Engl J Med 1986;315:949–951.
4. Boucek MM, Kanakriyeh MS, Mathis CM, Trimm RF, Bailey LL: Cardiac transplantation in infancy: donors and recipients. J Pediatr 1990;116:171–176.
5. Kachaner J, Le Bidois J, Sidi D, Vouhé P, Neveux JY, Touati G: Transplantations cardiaques et cardio-pulmonaires chez l'enfant. Indications, méthodes et résultats. Arch Fr Pédiatr 1988;45:727–733.
6. Gersony WM: Cardiac transplantation in infants and children. J Pediatr 1990;116:266–268.
7. Starnes VA, Bernstein D, Oyer PE *et al*: Heart transplantation in children. J Hart Transplant 1989;8:20–26.
8. Trento A, Griffith BP, Fricker FJ, Konmos RL, Armitage J, Hardesty RL: Lessons learned in pediatric heart transplantation. Ann Thorac Surg 1989;48:612–623.
9. Kriett JM, Kaye MP: The Registry of the International Society for Heart Transplantation: seventh official report – 1990. J Heart Transplant 1990;9:323–330.
10. Mayer JE, Perry S, O'Brien P *et al*: Orthotopic heart transplantation for complex congenital heart disease. J Thorac Cardiovasc Surg 1990;99:484–492.
11. Addonizio LJ, Hsu DT, Fuzesi L, Smith CR, Rose EA: Optimal timing of pediatric heart transplantation. Circulation 1989;80(Suppl III):84–89.
12. Vouhé PR, Tamisier D, Leca F *et al*: Heart transplantation in children: risk factors of early and late mortality. Europ J Cardiothorac Surg 1991;5:176–182.
13. Le Bidois J, Guarnera S, Sluysmans T *et al*: Aspect pratique de la surveillance des greffes cardiaques et cardio-pulmonaires chez l'enfant. Arch Fr Pédiatr 1988;45:755–759.
14. Braunlin EA, Canter CE, Olivaria MT, Ring WS, Spray TL, Bolman RM. Rejection and infection after pediatric cardiac transplantation. Ann Thorac Surg 1990;49:385–390.

15. Le Bidois J, Niaudet P, Habib R *et al*: Renal function and pathology in infants and children treated with ciclosporine after heart transplantation. IIIrd World Congr Pediatr Cardiol. Bangkok, 28 Nov–1 Dec 1989. Abstr 135–136.
16. Pahl E, Fricker FJ, Armitage J *et al*: Coronary arteriosclerosis in pediatric heart transplant survivors: limitation of long-term survival. J Pediatr 1990;116:177–183.

F: Summary

Quality of life after surgical correction of congenital heart disease

FRANCO P. STOCKER

1. Discussing the quality of life after surgery for congenital heart disease is equal to a quality control for the most pertinent part of work in the field of congenital heart disease since survival with normal and good quality of life in every respect must be the ultimate aim of our efforts. A quality control not only for the surgeons but also for all the others caring for patients with congenital heart disease. Cardiac surgery is, without any doubt, the event which has made the most and fundamental changes in the fate of patients with significant and critical congenital heart disease, and it was a highlight of the session to have Dr. Lillehei presenting a first-hand report of the pioneer days of open-heart surgery in patients with congenital heart disease, as well as the results of his follow-up of the first operated patients. Cardiac surgeons and cardiologists form a team which is probably more linked together than in any other organ speciality. Interventional catheterization which replaces some surgical procedures and which was not discussed, does not separate but consolidates this team even more. As was shown during this session, this team must be helped by a wide spectrum of other specialists such as the intensive care team, neurologists, psychologists and psychiatrists, and social workers, if quality of life is the target.

2. An ideal quality control is hardly possible, particularly in congenital heart disease where surgical correction is increasingly performed in the infant or young child, and where the aim is not only an improved quality of life for 5 to 10, maybe 20 years as in coronary heart disease, but for a normal life span of 70 to 90 years. Ideally, we should compare the natural history (without any intervention) of the different cardiac malformations with a post-operative complete physical, psychological, and social follow-up of 70 to 90 years. We attempt to follow-up our patients as completely and as long as possible, and we are able to show success and tendencies with some probability in a number of lesions where corrective surgery has been available for a relatively long time. However, we must be aware of the fact that we are still

Paul J. Walter (ed.): *Quality of Life after Open Heart Surgery*, 383–386.
© 1992 Kluwer Academic Publishers.

far away from the ideal and that we have to be ready and willing to change our opinion and judgement when further follow-up reveals new facts.

3. The reports of this session give a detailed analysis of physical, psychological, and social findings over a long post-operative period for different lesions covering the spectrum of congenital heart disease from ASD-secundum to complex cyanotic lesions.

It becomes clear that quality of life can be and must be evaluated objectively but it can also be seen in a subjective way by the patient. Ultimately, the subjective impression and satisfaction are the most important and essential issues. Therefore, it is very fortunate that, in general, the subjective satisfaction is in all respects better than the objective results. Care must be taken in order not to diminish the subjective personal satisfaction and wellfeeling, despite some minor objective impairment, by putting too much emphasis on this.

It also becomes clear, and this should be emphasized, that quality of life in psychological and social respect depends mostly and significantly on the physical quality of life, on good cardiac and neurological function. In other words, a successful and good correction is the best guarantee for a good psycho-social quality of life. A successful operation, of course, implies optimal pre-operative diagnosis and management including optimal indication for surgery, optimal surgical work, and optimal post-operative management.

Another important fact needs to be mentioned: in about one quarter of all patients, additional non-cardiac malformations are present, and very often, the quality of life is influenced much more by these, e.g. in trisomy 21.

Also, we have to realize that in children with congenital heart disease, the important role of the parents has to be taken into account. On the one side, we have to consider the quality of life of the parents and the family; on the other side, parents influence to a great extent the quality of life of children with congenital heart disease.

4. How are the results of our quality control in detail? The surgical corrections of different lesions can be divided into three main groups:

4.1. In the first group, there are lesions which can be corrected completely or nearly completely, with a very low mortality and morbidity. Patent ductus arteriosus is probably the only lesion which can be completely cured by surgery. Isolated valvar pulmonic stenosis and isolated ASD-secundum can be corrected almost completely with insignificant morbidity and very low mortality, the impact of long-term evolution of mild pulmonic insufficiency or of ECG abnormalities being yet unclear. Repair of isolated ventricular septal defects, if done before pulmonary-vascular changes take place, also has a very good outlook. Finally, correction of coarctation of the aorta without significant additional lesions may also, be put into the first and very satisfying group of operations. This group makes up around 60% of all surgical corrections if an unbiased count is done. In congresses and symposia, the figures are usually biased as more severe lesions are predominant in famous and large centres and, accordingly, in their reports. The subjective quality of life in this group is normal in 90–95% of the patients putting them in the red region of Dr. Jane Somerville's 'ability index', a scale which is more informative than the New York Heart Association's classification considering the overall quality of life. The remaining patients are in the yellow part, practically none lower. Since only significant lesions are operated, the surgical success in this large group is excellent. Without an operation, these patients would not have a normal life expectancy and, furthermore, would suffer from increasing morbidity. In the future, we must maintain this excellent standard, and this group of corrections must be kept in the hands of highly qualified surgeons and teams, and not become second rated.

4.2. The second group consists of lesions which cannot be corrected completely but where the majority of patients, despite the remaining impairment, can enjoy a good quality of life. Most of them are in the red and yellow part of 'ability index', fortunately, only a small group in the lower parts. The main lesions in this group which consists of 34–36% of all surgical corrections, are aortic stenosis, atrio-ventricular defects, tetralogy of Fallot, and uncomplicated transposition of the great arteries. In this group, improvement is possible and should be attempted: on the one side, improvement in surgical technique, e.g. in transposition of the great arteries by the arterial switch operation; on the other side, by intense multidisciplinary long-term postoperative management including psychological and social help.

4.3. In the third group with complex lesions such as tricuspid atresia, univentricular heart, etc. which, fortunately, is small and makes up only 6–8% of the operations, surgical mortality and post-operative morbidity are significant. We should probably not speak of 'incomplete correction' but rather of 'good palliation'. Despite encouraging short- and middle-term results in respect to quality of life, there is not a long enough follow-up period for a final prognosis.

5. In patients with a low quality of life due to cardiac disease, heart transplantation brings new hope and improvement. Paediatric transplantation is yet too young to give meaningful long-term follow-up information. In patients with congenital heart disease, heart transplantation at present, is done mostly in adolescence and adulthood, a topic of another session.

6. Our general therapeutic aim is two-fold: on the one hand, we would like to achieve a normal life expectancy for every patient with congenital heart disease; on the other hand, we aim at a normal overall quality of life for all survivors. This brings us in an ambivalent position with two extreme attitudes depending on the priority we put on these two points: quality of life for the survivors as the primary aim, or overall survival as the primary aim. If we only accept a normal quality of life for all survivors, we should only operate on patients of group one. On the other side, if overall survival is the most important for us, we have to operate or try to operate on every lesion regardless of the possible poor quality of life of survivors. Medical art must find the right balanced decision for each individual patient.

7. Congenital heart disease is dealt with primarily in the first years of life but, as our patients become adults, their quality of life also depends on the knowledge, experience, and skill of the physicians and the team taking over their care from the paediatric group. Due to cardiac surgery, the number of surviving adults with congenital heart disease, is increasing continuously, and the organization of their optimal care becomes a major task.

8. The great amount of information on the different aspects of quality of life after correction of congenital heart disease which is given in this chapter as well as the extensive and interesting discussions during the meeting, prove the need and importance of such an interdisciplinary approach. Professor Walter has to be congratulated for his initiative and concept in organizing the symposium and editing the book.

PART FOUR

QUALITY OF LIFE AFTER HEART TRANSPLANTATION

A: Physiological State

35. Long-term results: morbidity and mortality of patients after heart transplantation

C. CABROL, I. GANDJBAKHCH, A. PAVIE, V. BORS, Ph. LEGER,
E. VAISSIER, J.P. LEVASSEUR, M. DESRUENNES and
A. CABROL

Quality of life after heart transplantation (HTx) has considerably increased since the use of a potent immunosuppressive agent – cyclosporine (Cy) – which allows this operation to be an acceptable therapy for patients with terminal and irreversible cardiac failure. This explains why the total number of heart transplantations performed is more than 16 000 in the world, almost 4000 in France, and 880 in our own unit in La Pitié. Nevertheless a low percentage of morbidity and mortality still persists due mostly to three main complications: rejection, infection and other complications of immunosuppressive therapy.

Rejection is a constant threat and was observed from 4 to 6 days after transplantation, up to 20 years for the present longest survivors, although a certain tolerance seems to appear with time. In our experience, Cyclosporine A considerably decreased the frequency and the severity of rejection overall (2.3 per cent patient years in the first year after transplantation and 0.8 in the following years). But recently, in the last two years we have again experienced acute, severe and sometimes lethal rejection episodes, like those seen with the conventional therapy. In spite of a careful inquiry, we were unable to explain this phenomenon, which has also been by other groups, and sometimes requires retransplantation.

In most cases, Cyclosporine A suppressed the usual clinical, electrical and hemodynamic symptoms of rejection which were no longer constant, nor relevant in such conditions. So the diagnosis of rejection, which it is so important to counteract as soon as possible to avoid the short and long term consequences of such lesions, remains a current problem in cardiac transplantation. At present the only way to be sure of an ongoing rejection is by histologic diagnosis (which unfortunately is an invasive method) by way of a percutaneous introduction of a cardiac bioptome and the retrieval of a small piece of right ventricular endomyocardium which, under microscopic examination in case of rejection, presents important lymphocyte infiltration and myocyte necrosis.

However many non-invasive methods are under evaluation, such as cyto-

Paul J. Walter (ed.): Quality of Life after Open Heart Surgery, 389–395.
© 1992 Kluwer Academic Publishers.

immunologic monitoring, based on the determination of the absolute concentration of circulatory lymphoblasts and prelymphoblasts, which has been shown to closely correlate with acute cardiac rejection within the first 3 months after transplantation, but has a significant loss of sensitivity in the late post operative course and cannot replace the routine endomyocardial biopsy [1]. Promising preliminary results have been obtained by measurements of urinary polyamines which may provide daily information on the recipient's immunologic status [2] or the experimental [3] and clinical use of magnetic resonance imaging as well as the immunopathology with monoclonal sera [4]. Simpler methods, like the detection of changes in cardiothoracic ratio and cardiac volume on conventional chest X-rays may be helpful [5]. The value of serial and two-dimensional echocardiographic findings, considered as valuable by some groups [6,7], seems to present a correlation with rejection episodes. The early detection of rejection by echo Doppler studies (isovolumic relaxation time and pressure half time) appears to be more interesting. In our experience this is quite satisfactory and is now our routine technique of rejection control [8,9].

This technique appeared both sensitive (90%) and specific (90%). It also allows us to detect a new mode of acute rejection episodes: acute vascular rejection characterized by lymphocyte infiltration localized around small vessels and respecting the myocardium. These lesions gave early modifications of the segmental ventricular contraction and usually corresponded to the severe and sometimes refractory rejection episodes already mentioned above and leading to retransplantation.

Besides acute rejection episodes, one of the most intriguing and dangerous problem in cardiac transplantation is the secondary occurence *of occlusive coronary lesions* (25% of the patients after 5 years post transplantation), the so-called 'accelerated graft arteriosclerosis' which are dependent on the chronic evolution of vascular rejection and were characterized in our experience by 3 stages: early inflammatory arteritis, late obliterative fibrous arteritis, and late atherosclerosis.

Early inflammatory arteritis occurs generally between 3–8 months after transplantation on small coronary arteries. It is characterized by lymphocyte infiltration, arteritis, and sometimes thrombosis. Its etiology is certainly immunological and it represents a rejection lesion potentially reversible [10].

Late obliterative fibrous arteritis occurs usually 2 years post transplantation on large and medium size vessels. The lesions are essentially fibrosis of the intima with, at times, disruption of the media, without an important lymphocyte infiltration. It possibly represents the end stage of the previously described lesions – the inflammatory arteritis – and it is slowly progressive.

The appeareance of late atherosclerosis occurs usually after 2 years post transplantation on the large coronary arteries. The lesions are essentially fibrotic with atheromatous deposits similar to the usual coronary atheroma. They are the same lesions previously described (late obliterative fibrous arteritis) in patients with high risk factors for atheroma which infiltrate these lesions with lipidic plaques. The angiographic aspect is typical, with diffuse multiple distal lesions. These lesions are rapidly progressive. They are silent (without angina) in this denervated heart and detected only by systematic routine coronary angiography. They cannot be treated by coronary artery bypass and require retransplantation [11]. Their frequency, and their severity, is a major threat to transplantation and the matter deserves future research, in which the nutritional status of transplanted patients must be taken in account [12].

Besides graft arteriosclerosis and acute rejection refractory to all medical therapy, another lesion may require *retransplantation:* diffuse myocardial sclerosis sometimes seen after multiple iterative, acute rejection episodes. The survival rate after retransplantation, although different according to the various indications, is, as a whole, satisfactory, averaging forty percent.

For these retransplantations, in half of the cases we could find a suitable donor's heart in time. But in the other half, the hemodynamic deterioration was so rapid and so severe that we had to use some kind of *circulatory support:* standard extracorporeal circulation with a membrane oxygenator and peripheral canulations (ECMO); centrifugal pumps connected with plastic lines to the input and the output of the failing ventricles; external ventricular assist devices, connected the same way to the heart but producing not a continuous flow, like the preceeding supports, but a pulsatile one; and finally a total artificial heart Jarvik 7 put (in contrast to all the other devices already mentioned) inside the thorax after excision and in place of the failing ventricles. External ventricular assist devices and total artificial hearts, which provide a pulsatile flow, are based on the same principle of a blood chamber pneumatically activated through a flexible diaphragm with the aid of an external drive machine.

To avoid either acute or chronic rejection, immunosuppression therapy is required. The ideal *immunosupressive regimen* still has to be found. Most of the teams are using the so called 'triple therapy': moderate dosage of cyclosporine, appropriate doses of azathioprine and steroids in lower dosage. 'Quadruple drug therapy' (addition of antithymocyte globulin for the first 4–6 days and in severe rejection episodes) is also common [13]. To avoid complications related to the use of corticosteroids some teams recommend suppression of maintenance steroids (double drug therapy) but the increase in frequency and severity of rejection episodes is a major inconvenience of this regimen [14]. Furthermore, in the occurrence of severe rejection, all teams rely on the same therapy: high doses of steroids and use of 'rescue' antithymocyte globulin. Recently the introduction of OKT3 monoclonal antibody appeared as a valuable and effective agent in refractory allograft rejection [15] and its prophylactic administration in the first days of transplantation is now recommended [16] instead of antithymocyte globulin; however its side effects (fever, chills, diarrhea and sometime pulmonary oedema) justify precaution in its use and more complete appreciation.

The use of immunosuppressive therapy introduced its own iatrogenic complications, mainly because of depression of immunodefence: *infection*. Secondary and late infections, although lessened by the use of cyclosporine, remain frequent (1.8 per cent patient years) and involved mainly the lung; they are bacterial pneumonia but also fungal infections (candida [17], aspergillus and even more infrequent germs (mucor mycosis [18]). A careful screening of the donor is essential in that respect, to avoid the frequent transmission of diseases like toxoplasmosis and cytomegalovirus (CMV) infection. The treatment of CMV infection can benefit of an early detection by a CMV antigen test [19] and the use of promising new antiviral agent DHPG [20]. Whatever the cause of pulmonary infection may be, its identification is often difficult and may require special investigations, such as transtracheal aspirations, fine needle aspiration biopsy [21] and bronchoalveolar lavage.

Besides pulmonary localisations, extra-pulmonary infections have also been observed: myocarditis, retinitis, cerebral abscesses due to toxoplasmosis; mononucleotic syndrom, hepatitis, pancreatitis and also retinitis due to cytomegalovirus.

Other complications due to immunosuppression were observed, such as chronic nephrotoxicity induced by cyclosporine (55% of our patients). This is demonstrated by the elevation of the serum creatinine level, more pronounced in older patients that in younger, and aggravated by the use of nephrotoxic antibiotics sometimes needed to treat severe infection. These lesions are characterized histologically by a tubular atrophy and interstitial fibrosis without glomerular alteration and can be prevented by using low doses of cyclosporine. If, nevertheless, they do appear, they are potentially reversible by discontinuing cyclosporine and switching to more conventional therapy, but that requires caution [22]. The experimental and clinical use of a new analog of cyclosporine, cyclosporine G, was not really advantageous [23]. A new Japanese drug, FK 506, is under trial.

The systemic hypertension observed in 65% of our patients treated with cyclosporine A also remains a threat; despite extensive studies by our group [24] and others [25] we were unable to find any alteration of the renin angiotensive system, nor of the aldosterone level, and the only abnormal observation was a constant hypervolemia. This systemic hypertension is best treated by administration of calcium channel blockers. Cyclosporine, allowing a lower dosage of steroids, also lowered the frequency of osteoporotic complications but was responsible for hirsutism, hypertrophy of the gingiva, infrequent hepatic dysfunction and tremor.

The immunosuppressive therapy also gave rise in our experience to the possibility of malignancy (1 cancer of the bladder, 1 cancer of the pancreas, 3 lymphomas, 1 Kaposi syndrome, 4 skin tumors).

In the early experience, specially with the intercaval opening of the right atrium, some disturbing AV blocks were observed; the use of a pacemaker with two atrial electrodes, one in the recipient, one in the donor atrium, and a dual chamber pulse generator provided atrioventricular synchrony and a chronotropic response to exercise [26].

The *overall results* of heart transplantation can now be appreciated with a sufficiently long-term follow up. If the survival rate can reach 85 or 90% in recent series in which a strict selection of recipients and donors is maintained, this rate is about 60% in larger series, outrating 500 cases and 7 years of follow up like in the Stanford, Pittsburg and our own experience, results which are quite acceptable in regard to the large acceptance in such series of aged and borderline suitable recipients.

As demonstrated by the latest statistics (up to January 1991) of the World Registry of the International Society of Heart Transplantation, the survival rate appears to depend on a number of variables. First the age: 60% for patients younger than 1 year of age, 71% for patients between 1 and 18 years, 82% for patients older than 18 years at 2 years follow up. So older patients have excellent outcome and that allows transplantation to be proposed to patients 60 or 65 years old and even older in carefully selected cases. The lower survival rate in young patients is explained by the higher mortality observed in patients less than one month of age.

The survival rate after 10 years follow up also improved with time: 20% for patients transplanted before 1979, 40% between 1979 and 1984 and 70% at 5 years since 1985!

The type of immunosuppressive therapy also modified the survival at 5 years: 76% for triple therapy (Cy, Aza, corticoïds) and 68% for other protocols.

Finally, as we have already mentioned, the actuarial survival rate at 5 years after retransplantation is lower (38%) than after primary transplantation (70%).

In our series, 540 patients are presently alive. All live a virtually normal social and familial life. Three of our transplanted women had babies, one of them two siblings. The physiological adaptation of the transplanted heart to exercise is near normal with only a small delay in the onset of the response, allowing many of transplanted patients to practice sport. Full-time employment was resumed by 45% of the patients, and 35% of other patients retired. Quality of life after HTx is excellent, provided patients strictly follow their treatment and has regular controls.

References

1. Fieguth H-G, Haverich A, Schafers H-J, Wahlers T, Herrmann G, Frimpong-Boateng K,

Cremer J, Kremnitz J, Borst HG: Cytoimmunologic monitoring in early and late acute cardiac rejection. J Heart Transplant 1988;7:95–101.

2. Carrier M, Russel DH, Davis TP, Emery RW, Copeland JG: Urinary polyamines as markers of cardiac allograft rejection. A clinical evaluation. J Thorac Cardiovasc Surg 1988;96:806–810.

3. Aherne T, Yee ES, Tscholakoff D, Gollin G, Higgins C, Ebert PA: Diagnosis of acute and chronic cardiac rejection by magnetic resonance imaging: a non-invasive in-vivo study. J Cardiovasc Surg 1988;29:587–590.

4. Chomette G, Auriol M, Louahlia S, Delcourt A, Cabrol C: Immunopathologic du rejet au cours des transplantations cardiaques humaines. Arch Anat Cytol Path 1988;35:250–253.

5. Laczkovics A, Grabenwogen F, Teufelsbauer H, Dock W, Wollenek G, Wolner E: Noninvasive assessment of acute rejection after orthotopic heart transplantation: value of changes in cardiac volume and cardiothoracic ratio. J Cardiovasc Surg 1988;29:582–586.

6. Ciliberto GR, Cataldo G, Gronda E, Mangiavacchi M, Alberrti A, Faletra F, Pezzano A, De Maria R, Bonacina E, Pellegrini A, Rovelli F: Trapianto cardiaco: ruolo dell'ecocardiografia nella diagnosi di rigetto. G. Ital Cardiol 1988;18:184–191.

7. Hosenpud JD, Norman DJ, Cobanoglu MA, Floten HS, Conner RM Starr A: Serial echocardiographic findings early after heart transplantation: evidence for reversible right ventricular dysfunction and myocardial edema. J Heart Transplant 1987;6:343–347.

8. Desruennes M, Corcos T, Lechat P, Rossant P, Leger P, Vaissier E, Pavie A, Gandjbakhchi I, Cabrol A, Cabrol C: Evaluation par échocardiographie-Doppler de la fonction diastolique ventriculaire gauche dans le rejet aigu du greffon après transplantation cardiaque. Arch Mal Coeur 1988;81:193–198.

9. Desruennes M, Corcos T, Cabrol A, Gandjbakhch I, Pavie A, Leger Ph, Eugene M, Bors V, Cabrol C: doppler echocardiography for the diagnosis of acute cardiac allograft rejection. J Am Coll Cardiol 1988;12:63–70.

10. Yowell RL, Hammond EH, Bristow MR, Watson FS, Renlund DG, O'Connell JB: Acute vascular rejection involving the major coronary arteries of a cardiac allograft. J Heart Transplant 1988;7:191–197.

11. Bergdahl LAL, Baldwin JC, Aziz S, Stinson EB, Shumway NE: Retransplantation of the human heart. Il Cuore 1987;4:459–464.

12. Grady KL, Herold LS: Comparison of nutritional status in patients before and after heart transplantation. J Heart Transplant 1988;7:123–127.

13. Reichenspurner H, Odell JA, Cooper DKC, Novitzky D, Human PA, Von Oppell U, Becerra E, Boehm DH, Rose A, Path MRC, Fasol R, Zilla P, Reichart B: Twenty years of heart transplantation at Groote Schuur Hospital.

14. Laufer G, Laczkovics A, Wollenek G, Schreiner W, Wolner E: Results of orthotopic heart transplantation with and without the use of maintenance steroids. Eur J Cardio Thorac Surg, 1988;2:237–243.

15. Sweeney MS, Sinnott JT IV, Cullison JP, Weinstein SS: The use of OKT3 for stubborn heart allograft rejection: an advance in clinical immunotherapy? J Heart Transplant, 1987;6:324–328.

16. Bristow MR, Gilbert EM, Renlund DG, DeWitt CW, Burton NA, O'Connell J: Use of OKT3 monoclonal antibody in heart transplantation: review of the initial experience. J Heart Transplant 1988;7:1–11.

17. Oaks TE, Pae WE, Pennock JL, Myers JL, Pierce WS: Aortic rupture caused by fungal aortitis: successful management after heart transplantation. J Heart Transplant 1988;7:162–164.

18. Studemeister AE, Kozak K, Garrity E, Venezio FR: Survival of a heart transplant recipient after pulmonary cavitary mucormycosis. J Heart Transplant, 1988;7:159–161.

19. Van der Bij W, Van Dijk RB, Van Son WJ, Torensma R, Prenger KB, Prop J, Tegzess AM, The TH: Antigen test for early diagnosis of active cytomegalovirus infection in heart transplant recipients. J Heart Transplant 1988;7:106–110.

20. Watson FS, O'Connell JB, Amber IJ, Renlund DG, Classen D, Hohnston JM, Smith CB,

Bristow MR: Treatment of cytomegalovirus pneumonia in heart transplant recipients with 9 (1,3-dihydroxy-2-propoxymethyo)-guanine (DHPG). J Heart Transplant 1988;7:102–105.

21. De Vivo F, Pond GD, Rhenman B, Icenogle TB, Vasu MA, Copeland JG: Transtracheal aspiration and fine needle aspiration biopsy for the diagnosis of pulmonary infection in heart transplant patients. J Thorac Cardiovasc Surg 1988;96:696–699.

22. Stevens L, Halbrook H, Berron K, Spears C, Hormuth D: Conversion for Cyclosporine to Azathioprine in heart transplant recipients. J Heart Transplant 1988;7:119–122.

23. Grant Hoyt E, Hagberg RC, Billingham ME, Baldwin JC, Jamieson SW, Analysis of the immunosuppressive and nephrotoxic effects of Cyclosporin G. J Heart Transplant, 1988;7:11–18.

24. Rottembourg J, Mattei MF, Cabrol A, Leger P, Aupetit B, Beaufils H, Gluckman JC, Pavie A, Gandjbakhch I, Cabrol C: Renal function and blood pressure in heart transplant recipients treated with Cyclosporine. J Heart Transplant 1985;4:404–408.

25. Oyer PE, Stinson EB, Jamieson SW et al: Cyclosporin A in cardiac allografting: a preliminary experience. Transplant Proc 1983;15:1257–1262.

26. Verani MS, George SE, Leon CA, Whisennand HH, Noon GP, Short HD, III, DeBakey ME, Young JB: Systolic and diastolic ventricular performance at rest and during exercise in heart transplant recipients. J Heart Transplant 1988;7:145–151.

36. Quality of life of patients on LVAD support

NANCY L. ABOU-AWDI and O.H. FRAZIER

1. Introduction

During 1989, 1689 cardiac transplants were performed in the United States
[1]. Although experience has shown that this therapy could benefit an even
greater number of patients, this has not become a reality. An estimated 30–
40% of cardiac transplant candidates die of hemodynamic instability before
a suitable donor becomes available, despite treatment with inotropic agents
and an intraaortic balloon pump (IABP). The IABP augments cardiac output
by only 15–20%, which may not provide adequate perfusion [2]. Low cardiac
output can adversely affect all body systems, especially the kidneys and liver.
To prevent permanent damage to these organs during the waiting period,
more advanced ventricular assist devices are being developed to maintain
circulation in patients who require a bridge. One such device, the Heart-
mate® left ventricular assist device (LVAD) (Thermo Cardiosystems, Inc.,
Woburn, MA), has been used successfully as a bridge to transplant in 12
men since 1988. The device restored adequate perfusion in these patients
and allowed them to undergo rehabilitation, making them the healthiest
candidates for transplantation [3–5].

The Heartmate is an abdominally implanted LVAD, with an external
driveline connected to a console. It has a maximum stroke volume of 83 mL
and a potential output of 10 L/min. A unique characteristic of this pump is
the textured blood-contacting surfaces that promote the formation of a bio-
logic lining [6,7], which may reduce the risk of thromboembolism. In more
than four years of cumulative experience, no device-related thromboembolic
events have occurred.

The 12 patients placed on the Heartmate were all approved transplant
candidates, suffering hemodynamic deterioration despite conventional treatment methods. All patients were on inotropic support; nine were also treated
with the IABP, and two had been treated with the Hemopump® (Johnson
and Johnson Interventional Systems, Rancho Cordova, CA). Twelve of the
patients were supported by the LVAD for more than 30 days (average, 117

Paul J. Walter (ed.): *Quality of Life after Open Heart Surgery*, 397–401.
© 1992 Kluwer Academic Publishers.

days; range, 31–233 days), including one patient who was still on support at 110 days when this study was performed. Eleven patients had undergone successful transplant operations, with the longest survivor having a 3-year follow-up examination.

Quality-of-life measurements are varied and dependent on individual perceptions. Studies to evaluate quality of life usually focus on one treatment. Assessing quality of life in the LVAD population is difficult because duration of support is usually relatively short, and follow-up is complicated by the factors associated with cardiac transplantation. Therefore, this article will focus on quality of life during LVAD support, with emphasis on physiologic and psychosocial status.

2. Quality of life assessment

All patients in this series had signs of end-organ dysfunction prior to LVAD implantation. Before treatment, all patients had serum bilirubin levels indicating hepatic dysfunction, but immediately before transplant, the values were within normal ranges. The average reduction was 65% of pre-implant values. Renal function was assessed by testing urine output, serum blood urea nitrogen, and creatinine levels. Five patients had acute tubular necrosis and were undergoing treatment with either continuous arteriovenous hemofiltration or hemodialysis at the time of implant. At transplant, 10 patients had normal renal function, and the one patient whose renal status failed to improve despite hemodialysis treatment during LVAD support underwent renal transplantation after heart transplantation.

All patients were in New York Heart Association (NYHA) functional class IV at the time of device implantation. The time to improvement in NYHA classification varied, depending on recovery time from device implant and the degree of debilitation or end-organ function at the time of implant. Patients were able to exercise during support, and a physical therapist assessed muscle mass and tone. The intensity of each patient's exercise program increased as physical status improved. Only two patients were unable to walk independently during LVAD support, both of whom had required IABP and Hemopump support prior to treatment with the Heartmate. The remaining patients exercised daily using a stationary bicycle and walking without assistance. Two patients were involved in aggressive programs, which included working out on an incline treadmill, and one started a weight training program. All patients had improved their muscle tone and exercise tolerance during LVAD support and were in NYHA functional class I at the time of cardiac transplantation. Many of the patients stated that they had never been in better shape.

Patients suffering from congestive heart failure are at risk of becoming malnourished [8]. This condition, which increases the risk of morbidity and

Table 1. Cost comparison between conventional and LVAD therapy.*

Treatment	Daily hospital charges ($)	Daily physician charges ($)	Total charges ($)
Conventional	3815	350	4165
LVAD	650	60	710

* Conventional therapy includes inotropic and IABP support. The charges shown were the average cost for treating a stabilized patient.

mortality in surgical patients, is frequently difficult to reverse because of chronic hypoperfusion. Patients supported by the Heartmate LVAD are able to resume oral intake, and improved perfusion effected improved nutritional status [9] in 91% of the patients. At the time of cardiac transplantation, all patients were able to meet or exceed their caloric requirements by oral intake alone. The improved nutritional status of these patients further optimized their transplant candidacy status.

Another important aspect of recovery regarding quality of life is related to the patient's ability to relate to family and friends. Patients awaiting cardiac transplant are encouraged to attend support group meetings. Eight of the LVAD patients participated in these support meetings while they were on support. In addition, the LVAD patients who were mobile visited other LVAD patients who remained in the intensive care unit, providing encouragement and information.

Because of their overall improvement in health, most of the patients were hospitalized for a shorter length of time post-transplant, an average of 18 days. The average stay in our historical transplant group has been 27 days. The duration of hospitalization was longer for the patient who also underwent renal transplantation. An additional benefit of the LVAD has been a reduction in cost for critical care. Whereas the average cost of hospitalization in a critical care unit, at our institution, is more than $4000/day for a conventional non-LVAD patient, the cost for the LVAD patients was greatly reduced (Table 1).

The ability to return to normal activities and to work is considered an improvement in quality of life. A survey of our cardiac transplant patients showed that 69% of those who did not receive LVAD support were either working or capable of returning to work within 1 year of transplantation. In comparison, 92% of the LVAD patients were working or capable of doing so at the time of study (Table 2).

Follow-up was obtained through personal and/or telephone interviews. A modified version of a questionnaire developed by Ruzevich *et al.* [10] was used to assess psychologic response to the LVAD (Table 3). The results may be skewed positively as a result of the patients' successful LVAD support and transplant experience. All patients, without exception, stated they would

Table 2. Comparison of historical and bridge-to-transplant patients returning to work within one year of cardiac transplant.

Status	Non-LVAD No.	(%)	LVAD No.	(%)
Working or capable of returning to work	135	(69)	11	(92)
Retired/disabled	47	(24)	0	(0)
Too sick to work	5	(3)	1	(8)*
Lost to follow-up	10	(5)	0	(0)
Total	197	100%	12	100%

* LVAD treatment was ongoing at the time of study.

Table 3. Psychologic effects.

Patient Questions	Agree (%)	Disagree (%)	Unsure (%)
1. The emotional effects of the assist devices were worse than the physical effects.	92	8	0
2. When I rest quietly or sleep, I sometimes feel or hear the device.	50	50	0
3. While on the device, I frequently thought I would not survive.	25	75	0
4. I have a brighter outlook on life since my illness.	100	0	0
5. I have suffered long-term effects from being on the assist device.	0	100	0
6. I feel I have returned to a normal life-style.	92	0	8
7. It would bother me to visit the intensive care unit and the people who took care of me.	0	100	0
8. I was worried about finances/insurance coverage.	17	83	0
9. I felt I was being treated as an experiment.	0	100	0
10. I would recommend a heart assist device to someone who needed one.	100	0	0
11. If I needed the device again, I would reconsent.	100	0	0
12. I fear I may need the device again.	0	100	0
13. I am afraid I will not live very long.	0	100	0

receive the device again if necessary and would recommend its use for other patients in the same situation.

3. Conclusion

While efforts continue to develop a totally implantable device that does not restrict mobility or cause undue psychologic or physical distress, the Heartmate is a positive technologic step. Our experience shows that it is capable of providing adequate circulatory support without deleterious effects. In addition, the patients treated with the device had reversal of hepatic and renal dysfunction and improved functional ability. They were able to participate in rehabilitative programs, which improved their status as cardiac transplant candidates. Finally, support with the Heartmate enhanced their quality of life.

References

1. United Network for Organ Sharing Registry: Richmond, VA, 1990 statistics.
2. Norman JC, Cooley DA, Igo SR *et al*: Prognostic indices for survival during postcardiotomy intra-aortic balloon pumping. J Thorac Cardiovasc Surg 1977;74:709–720.
3. Frazier OH, Duncan JM, Radovancevic B *et al*: Successful bridge to heart transplantation using a new ventricular assist device. J Heart Lung Transplant 1992 (in press).
4. Abou-Awdi NL: Thermo Cardiosystems left ventricular assist device as a bridge to cardiac transplant. AACN Clinical Issues in Critical Care Nursing 1991;2:545–551.
5. Abou-Awdi NL, Ragsdale O: Futuristic Nursing. RN Magazine l991; May, pp. 42–44.
6. Frazier OH, Nakatani T, McGee MG *et al*. Extended support prior to cardiac transplant using a left ventricular assist device with textured blood contacting surfaces. Artif Organs 1989;13:296.
7. Dasse KA, Chipman D, Sherman CN *et al*: Clinical experience with textured blood contacting surfaces in ventricular assist devices. ASAIO Trans 1987;33:418–425.
8. Berkowitz D, Croll MN, Lifoff W: Malabsorption as a complication of congestive heart failure. Am J Cardiol 1963;11:43–47.
9. Vega JD, Poindexter SM, Radovancevic B *et al*: Nutritional assessment of patients with extended left ventricular assist device support. ASAIO Trans 1990;36:M555–M558.
10. Ruzevich SA, Swartz MT, Reedy JE *et al*: Retrospective analysis of the psychologic effects of mechanical circulatory support. J Heart Lung Transplant 1990;9(3 Pt 1):209–212.

37. Physiological and psychological benefits of exercise rehabilitation after cardiac transplantation

TERENCE KAVANAGH

1. Introduction

The typical heart transplantation recipient is a 44–year old male who, as a result of severe ischaemic heart disease or cardiomyopathy, is in New York Heart Association Class IV cardiac failure [1]. He has experienced months of pre-operative invalidism, suffers from general muscle weakness, and is depressed and fearful. The first step towards recovery is the transplantation procedure itself, with its rapid alleviation of disabling cardiac symptoms and its favourable five- and ten-year actuarial survival rates of 82% and 74%, respectively [1]. However, to take full advantage of the new heart, the patient requires an exercise rehabilitation programme to improve physical fitness, restore self-confidence, and hasten return to full-time employment.

1.1. *Physiological responses to exercise after heart transplantation*

The resting rate of the denervated donor heart is high (approximately 100 bts/min); this is due to the intrinsic rate of its sino-atrial node, now free from vagal inhibition [2,3]. Assuming a normal peripheral demand for blood flow, the resting tachycardia implies a small stroke volume, and therefore during light exercise the Frank–Starling mechanism can produce a substantial increase of cardiac output. During more vigorous activity, any further augmentation in cardiac output depends on circulating catecholamine-induced chronotropic and inotropic responses [4,5]. This explains the attenuated heart rate response to an incremental exercise test, negligible in the first few minutes and then rising more steeply as plasma catecholamines increase (Figure 1). This response is also influenced by the denervated heart's increased sensitivity to circulating catecholamines [6]. Since both norepinephrine and epinephrine plasma clearance rates during recovery are similar in cardiac transplantation patients and normal controls [7] the delayed deceleration of recovery heart rate, in the transplants is likely due to this 'up-

Paul J. Walter (ed.): Quality of Life after Open Heart Surgery, 403–416.
© 1992 Kluwer Academic Publishers.

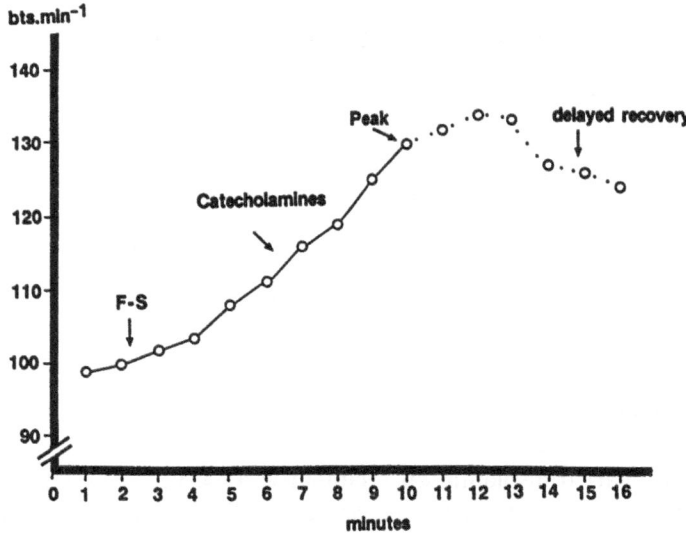

Figure 1. Typical transplanted denervated heart rate response to increasing effort. Note the high resting rate, the delayed rate of acceleration during effort, the delayed deceleration during recovery, and the tendency for the rate to continue to rise after the termination of effort (peak exercise).

regulation' in catecholamine sensitivity. Schell and co-workers [8], have suggested that the persistence of high heart rates during recovery is associated with the elevated blood lactate levels seen in these patients. Peak heart rates are approximately 20–25% lower than those seen in age-matched controls, due to an absence of direct sympathetic innervation of the sino-atrial node [3].

Resting hypertension is a common finding. In recent years, this has been increasingly attributed to the effect of cyclosporine. High dosages may be a factor, and some have suggested that the hypertensive effect is increased by the concomitant use of steroids. The exact pathophysiology remains unclear, but is probably associated with the considerable adverse effects that cyclosporine has been noted to have on renal function [9].

In our experience the peak systolic blood pressure is reduced to approximately 80% of age-matched normal controls [10,11]. This is due to the loss of sympathetic stimulation, with resultant impairment of myocardial contractility. Presumably this impairment only manifests itself after the onset of moderately vigorous effort, since previous workers have shown that contractility, measured at rest, is similar to that in normal subjects. Exercise radionuclide studies by Yusuf and co-workers [12] show patients to have normal systolic function and inotropic reserve during volume loading (leg elevation) and low-level supine exercise (a power output of 15 watts on the cycle ergometer), but some impairment of function at a power output of 45 watts. A further explanation for the reduced peak systolic blood pressure is that chronically elevated levels of serum catecholamines may induce down-regulation of the peripheral arterial alpha receptors [13].

There is evidence of impairment of diastolic function after heart transplantation, possibly the result of increased myocardial stiffness [14]. Factors contributing to this may be (i) myocardial ischaemia from accelerated coronary artery narrowing, (ii) the side-effects of immunosuppressant drugs, or (iii) a prolonged ischaemic time of the donor heart.

The transplantation recipient has a 10% to 50% reduction in lean body mass. This is due to prolonged pre-operative physical inactivity, together with high steroid administration during the immediate post-operative period [10]. Consequently, maximal work output is reduced, and maximal oxygen uptake is only two-thirds of the normal age-matched population.

With regard to cardiopulmonary dynamics, we have found that, at equivalent levels of submaximal effort, oxygen uptake is the same as in normals; minute ventilation, perceived exertion, and the ventilatory equivalent for oxygen are all higher than in normals but the absolute ventilatory threshold is lower, thus implying an earlier onset of anaerobic metabolism. Cardiac output increases linearly, and in normal increments, in response to increase in power output on the cycle ergometer or treadmill, but absolute submaximal values are slightly lower than normal [10].

In summary, then, heart transplantation patients have a typically high resting heart rate, with a normal or near normal resting cardiac output. However, at maximum effort they exhibit a significantly lower work output, heart rate, and systolic blood pressure (and thus double product), as well as a reduced oxygen uptake. Resting and maximal diastolic blood pressure is high compared with normals.

2. The Exercise programme

2.1. *Exercise testing*

This is usually carried out on the treadmill or cycle ergometer. The former is used more frequently in North America and the United Kingdom, the latter in Europe. Common treadmill protocols are modified forms of the Bruce or the Naughton, generally designed to achieve maximum effort in 8 to 10 minutes, with work increments of 1 to 2 Mets (3.5 ml-kg/min to 7 ml-kg/min of oxygen uptake).

In the author's laboratory the test is carried out customarily on the cycle ergometer. Power outputs are increased stepwise by 100 kpm/min every minute (16.7 Watts), or, in severely deconditioned patients, 50 kpm/min every minute (8.3 Watts) until the patient can no longer pedal at the required rate of 60 revolutions per minute. The exercise electrocardiogram is monitored continuously, and the Borg scale of perceived exertion at each stage.

The blood pressure is measured every two minutes, at peak effort, and in recovery. Expired air is analyzed breath by breath for ventilation ($\dot{V}E$), oxygen uptake ($\dot{V}O_2$), carbon dioxide output ($\dot{V}CO_2$), gas exchange ratio (RER), and end tidal oxygen and carbon dioxide partial pressures (PEO_2 and $PECO_2$), by means of a metabolic cart. Peak oxygen consumption is demonstrated by the attainment of an oxygen consumption plateau of less than 140 ml/minute when comparing the final and penultimate power output stages (100 kpm/min).

The ventilatory threshold is determined from a number of variables, which include, in respect to a progressive increase in oxygen uptake, a disproportionate increase in: (i) the ventilatory equivalent for oxygen, (ii) the minute ventilation, (iii) the carbon dioxide output, and (iv) the respiratory exchange ratio. The data are expressed in terms of the oxygen uptake at which the appropriate 'break point' of each plot occurs (Figure 2). The advantage of the 'ventilatory' threshold is that it occurs at approximately 60% of peak oxygen uptake, a level of effort which correlates well with the intensity required for endurance training, and is usually attainable by even those patients insufficiently motivated to exert maximal effort. Our practice is to use disproportionate increase in the ventilatory equivalent for oxygen as our primary measure, with corroboration sought, where indicated, by the previously mentioned variables.

A maximal exercise test, i.e., one in which an oxygen plateau is attained, is a relatively stable measurement in the normal subject. It bears a clear relationship to maximal cardiac output and has a high test-retest correlation. However, because of their severely deconditioned state, only about 50% of cardiac transplantation patients are likely to meet the criteria of an oxygen plateau at the initial test [10]. Corroborative evidence of maximal effort is therefore sought in a respiratory gas exchange ratio greater than 1.10. The indication for stopping a test before the demonstration of a plateau are as recommended by the American College of Sports Medicine [15]. It should be noted that the donor denervated heart cannot manifest an ischaemic state by anginal pain. Particular attention has to be paid therefore to the symptoms of dyspnoea, lightheadedness and faintness, as well as the familiar electrocardiographic signs of increasing ectopy and ST-segmental depression. Because the transplanted heart is invariably healthy, exercise electrocardiographic abnormalities are rare, except during bouts of rejection. On the other hand, the late development of an accelerated form of coronary atherosclerosis is not uncommon, and therefore evidence of ischaemia may eventually be seen in longstanding transplants.

2.2. *Training regimen*

The activity prescribed for physical training will depend upon the experience and preference of the rehabilitation team, recognizing that cardiovascular

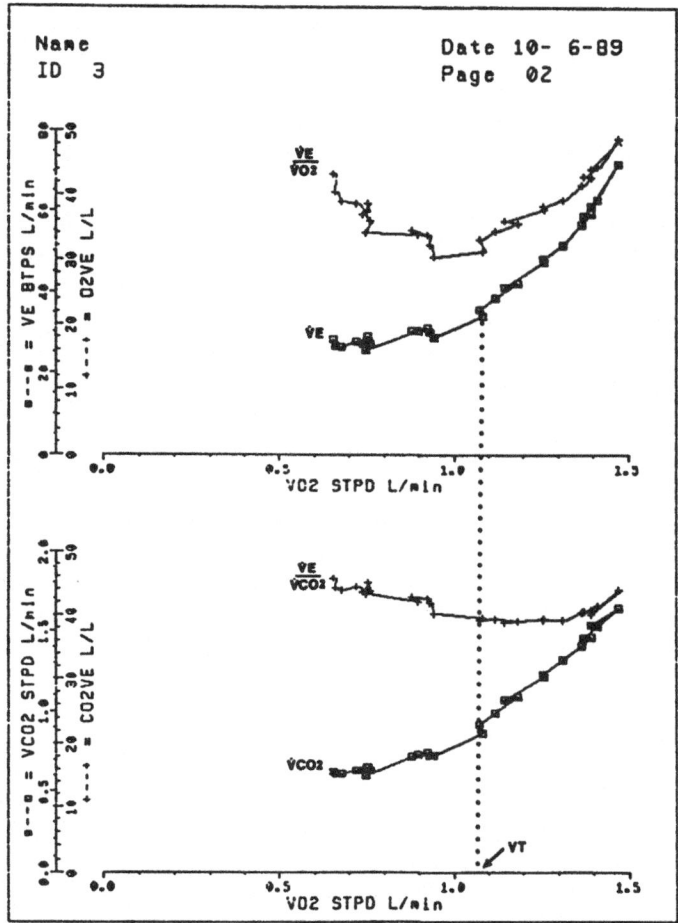

Figure 2. The ventilatory threshold (VT) is identified, relative to oxygen uptake, ($\dot{V}O_2$) at the upward inflection of the curves for the ventilatory equivalent for oxygen (VE/$\dot{V}O_2$); the minute ventilation (VE), and the carbon dioxide output ($\dot{V}CO_2$); note that the ventilatory equivalent for carbon dioxide (VE/$\dot{V}CO_2$) curve is still flat at the VT.

fitness is achieved most consistently by dynamic activity which can be accurately quantified and monitored, and which involves large muscle groups, e.g., walking/jogging, swimming, cycling, circuit training, etc. The customary training activity used by the author is walking, progressing to jogging, with stationary cycling or swimming either on a temporary or a permanent basis for those who have problems ambulating.

The training regimen utilized for cardiac transplantation has been described previously [16]. Essentially, our objective is for patients to progress from walking 1.6 km, five times weekly, to walk/jogging 6.5 km per session for a total weekly distance of 32.5 km. The prescribed pace is based on 60–70% of peak oxygen uptake, coupled with the ventilatory threshold and a perception of effort equivalent to 13–14 on the original Borg scale [17]. After the first four to six weeks, and regardless of the pace attained, the exercise prescription is adjusted to obtain a training session which should last from 30 to 60 minutes.

Because of the atypical heart rate response and the absence of angina as a warning symptom, accurate pacing is emphasized, as well as thorough familiarity with the concept of perceived exertion and correct interpretation of such symptoms of myocardial ischaemia as excessive dyspnoea, unusual fatigue, lightheadedness, and extrasystoles. Rejection episodes or intercurrent infections may interrupt the training programme from time to time, and patients should be advised of this possibility at the outset.

Accelerated coronary atherosclerosis is a serious late complication after cardiac transplantation [18]. By the third post-operative year, some 40% of patients will show angiographic evidence of this condition. Suggested causes are prolonged use of cyclosporine and/or steroids, post-operative attacks of cytomegalovirus infection, or repeated bouts of rejection [19]. The Stanford group found a high association between hypercholesterolemia and graft atherosclerosis, and have advocated aggressive dietary, and if necessary, drug intervention [20]. The rehabilitation programme will, therefore, pay close attention to serum lipid and glucose levels, and will provide the necessary education to those who have problems in these areas.

3. Effects of exercise training

As might be expected, there are only a handful of reports in the literature to date on the effects of training after heart transplantation. The earliest was from Squires and co-workers [21] who trained two orthotopic transplantation recipients for eight weeks. Benefits included a reduction in submaximal systolic blood pressures and perceived exertion ratings, but no significant changes in resting, submaximal, or peak heart rates. Metabolic measurements were not carried out.

Shortly thereafter Savin et al [22] evaluated the effects of a 16-week stationary cycling programme on five orthotopic patients. Training resulted in a 45% increase in peak work output, an 18% increase in peak oxygen uptake, and a 13% reduction in submaximal heart rates.

More recently, Niset [23] followed 62 orthotopic transplants for one year. The physical benefits included a 30 to 40% increase in peak work output and oxygen uptake, as well as an increase in peak heart rate and peak blood pressure. Submaximal heart rates and systolic blood pressures were unchanged.

Keteyian and co-workers [24] have also reported the effects of a 12-week programme on twenty-one orthotopic patients. Significant increases were observed in peak work output, peak oxygen uptake, and peak minute ventilation. There was no change in resting heart rate.

Table 1. Effects of exercise training program on 36 orthotopic cardiac transplantation patients (mean change ± SD).

PHYSICAL CHARACTERISTICS

	BODY MASS (kg)	LEAN MASS (kg)
All patients	+4.0 ± 6.7**	+1.98 ± 3.31**

HEART RATE (beats/min)

	REST	PEAK
All patients	−3.6 ±10.7*	+12.7 ±16.7**
Highly-compliant	−10.5 ±4.9**	+12.1 ±13.2**

*$p<0.05$, **$p<0.001$.

In the longest study published to date, Kavanagh and co-workers [10] from the Toronto Rehabilitation Centre trained thirty-six orthotopic transplants for two years, using the walk/jog programme described above. Compliance was very good, all patients progressing to an average distance of 24 km per week, at an average pace of 8.5 min/km. Eight of the highly-motivated patients achieved 32 km or more a week, at an average pace of 6.5 min/km. (It was one of these eight who entered and finished the 42–km Boston Marathon twelve months after joining the programme and fifteen months after undergoing the transplantation procedure) [25]. There were few episodes of rejection or infection, and these were so minor that they had little effect on the training regimen.

After training there was a 5.5% increase in body mass, of which 3.2% was lean tissue (Table 1). Resting heart rate for all patients was reduced, with the greatest reduction in those who were highly-compliant. Peak heart rate was significantly increased. Nevertheless, the final resting heart rates remained higher, and the final peak heart rates lower, than in a group of age-matched normal subjects (Table 1). Submaximal heart rates were unchanged in the twenty-eight moderately-compliant patients, whereas in the eight highly-compliant patients, the effect was quite large (Figure 3). There was also an overall and significant marked reduction in the rating of perceived exertion, minute ventilation, and diastolic blood pressure (Figure 4) at equivalent work outputs.

The peak work output increased by 49% (65% in the eight highly-compliant), peak oxygen uptake by 27% (54% in the highly-compliant), with all patients exercising to a larger respiratory minute ventilation and a higher maximal heart rate after training. Since changes in respiratory gas exchange ratio and peak rating of perceived exertion were quite small, it is unlikely that greater voluntary effort was responsible for improved peformance. Neither could any of the changes have been due to an improvement in mechan-

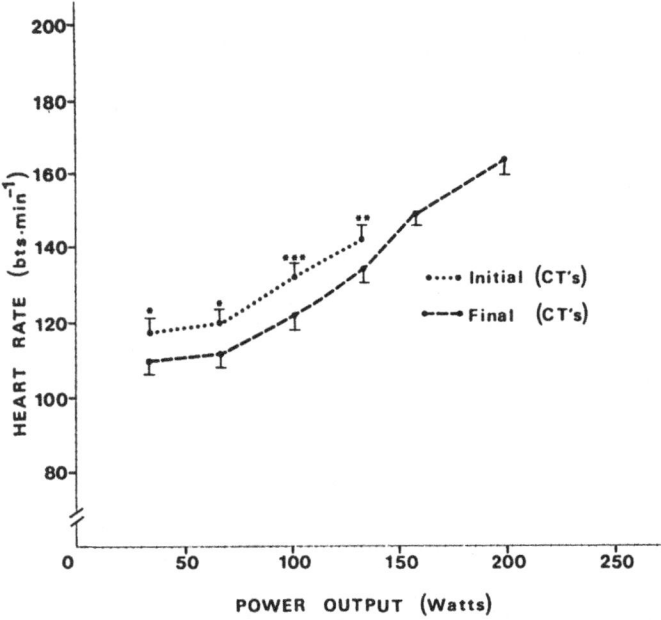

Figure 3. Relationship of heart rate to power output in highly-compliant cardiac transplantation patients (CTs), before and after conditioning. *$p < 0.05$; **$p < 0.01$; ***$p < 0.001$.

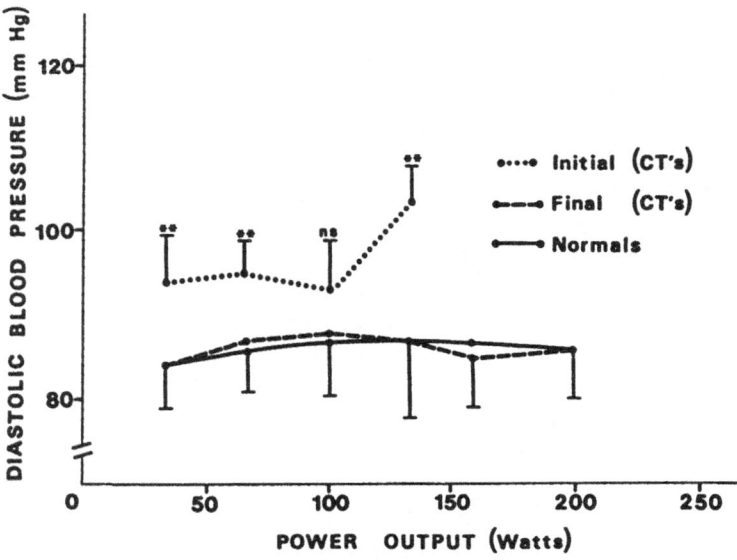

Figure 4. Relationship of diastolic blood pressure responses to power output before and after conditioning. *$p < 0.05$; **$p < 0.01$; ***$p < 0.001$.

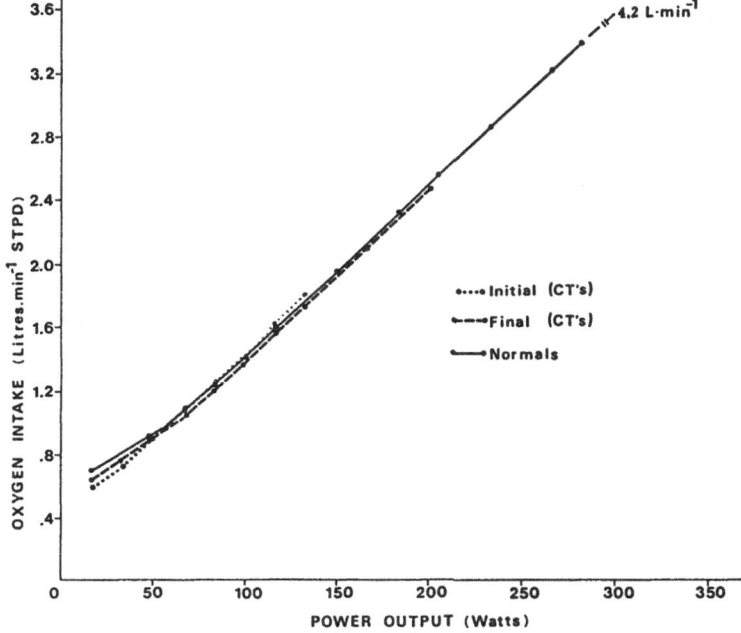

Figure 5. Relationship of oxygen uptake to power output in a group of cardiac transplantation patients (CTs) and age-matched controls. $*p < 0.05$; $**p < 0.01$; $***p < 0.001$.

ical efficiency on the ergometer, since the relationship of oxygen uptake to power output was unchanged (Figure 5).

The reduction in resting and submaximal heart rates seen in those who attained the greatest training distances was thought to be due to a drop in effort-induced levels of serum norepinephrine, and/or down regulation in the sensitivity of cardiac beta-adrenoreceptors. Both of these changes have been shown to occur in animals and humans exposed to vigorous training [26–29]. The entire group's increase in peak exercise heart rate was likely due to a strengthening of leg muscles. This peripheral adaptation would account for the improved power output, and because of a later onset of anaerobiosis, reduced perception of effort and minute ventilation during submaximal exercise. Submaximal cardiac outputs, measured by the CO_2 rebreathing technique, did not change with training in relation to oxygen uptake (Figure 6). This suggests peripheral, rather than central improvement, although one might infer that the reduction in submaximal diastolic blood pressures towards normal values is an indication of improved myocardial compliance.

Currently the heterotopic procedure comprises less than 1% of all heart transplantations, and this explains the paucity of reports on the rehabilitation of this group. Sieurat and his co-workers [30] trained eight heterotopic recipients and demonstrated an increase in peak work output and peak heart

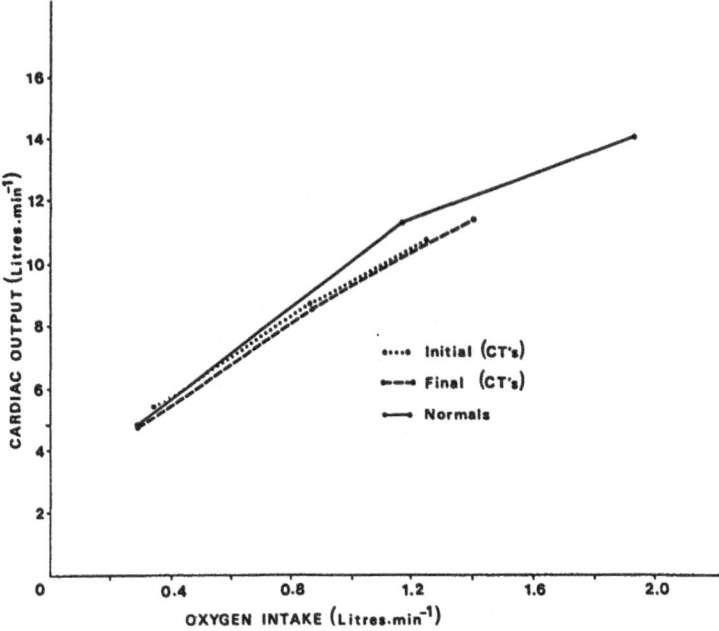

Figure 6. Relationship of cardiac output responses to V̇O₂ before and after conditioning.

rate. The author reported on ten male heterotopes who followed a walk/jog training programme for 18 months [31]. After training, lean body mass increased by 4%, peak work output by 33%, peak oxygen uptake by 23%, and absolute ventilatory threshold by 16%. Resting rate in the donor heart did not change significantly, but the resting rate of the recipient heart fell significantly by 14 bts/min. Submaximal recipient heart rate showed a training bradycardia, and demonstrated less exercise-induced ventricular ectopy than at initial testing. Donor submaximal heart rates were unchanged.

4. Psychosocial aspects

4.1. *Psychological changes*

Information on the psychological effects of heart transplantation remains scant. Buxton *et al.* has used the Nottingham Health Profile to study the quality of life in twenty-nine United Kingdom patients before and after surgery [32]. In all dimensions (physical mobility, energy, pain, emotional reaction, sleep habits, and social isolation) there was a very marked improvement by 3 months; the trend was continuing, although less pronounced at the end of one year [32]. Other workers have noted the high levels of anxiety and depression, the poor sense of well-being, and the negative body image frequently encountered in patients awaiting a new heart. The post-transplantation months can also be highly stressful [33]. In a group of Australian heart recipients, a greater proportion (43%) were more anxious at one year than at discharge (19%) [34]. Causes for their concern included financial problems and being a burden on their family (50%), fear that over-exertion would harm the new heart (43%), excessive weight gain (36%), and inability to exercise (29%).

These findings suggest that a comprehensive rehabilitation programme should have a major role to play in terms of psychosocial benefit, but to date no perspective randomized controlled trial to investigate this possibility has been carried out. Conclusions must therefore be drawn from observation reports.

Degré has carried out psychological assessment on 100 transplantation patients who took part in the structured exercise programme for one year [35]. Acceptance of the new heart and improved quality of life was apparent in the early phases of the programme, but psychosocial items such as anxiety, coping ability, social interaction, and mental alertness, took longer to recover. Ultimately, however, there was a complete return to normality in all areas and in almost all patients.

Kavanagh *et al.* [36] have investigated the influence of a 2-year exercise training programme upon the psychological status of 39 male patients. Although the average time elapsing between surgery and entry to the programme was 8 months, initial testing showed significant depression as well as high levels of anxiety. Training resulted in a significant reduction in depression, and this correlated well with increase in fitness as measured by changes in peak oxygen uptake. Anxiety was also significantly lessened, although this was associated not so much with improved fitness as with the passage of time from the transplantation procedure.

4.2. *Return to work*

Given the high cost of the transplantation procedure and the average age of the recipients, return to work is a highly-desirable goal. In those who have not been entered into a formal rehabilitation programme, the proportion obtaining work after surgery has been variously reported as being anywhere between 32% and 64% [37]. The reasons for failure to find employment are rarely medical, and include age, pre-illness employment pattern, type of work, and availability of disability payments. Degré's experience with a group attending the rehabilitation programme was that 71% of those who were working six months before surgery had returned to work [35]. Age seemed to be a factor in that the return rate was 82% for those under 45, 76% for those between 46 and 55, and 10% for those over 55 years. The high proportion of patients returning to work, i.e., 71%, suggests that a comprehensive rehabilitation programme is of value. In our own experience, 69% of patients attending our rehabilitation programme returned to work, 8% took early retirement, and only 3% were finally unemployed for medical reasons [38].

5. Conclusions

The routine use of a comprehensive exercise rehabilitation programme following cardiac transplantation is fully justified on physiological, psychological, and vocational grounds. It is a safe and effective way to maximize the benefits of surgery. There is, of course, still considerable scope for further research. Questions which remain to be answered include the precise nature of the training adaptations and the contribution made by central and peripheral factors. It is also tempting to speculate on the favourable effects of a rehabilitation programme, which includes not only exercise training, but also dietary advice, weight control, on: (i) the incidence and severity of post-transplant coronary atherosclerosis, (ii) the extent and degree of post-transplantation hypertension, and (iii) the incidence of bouts of intercurrent infection and rejection in the immunosuppressed patient.

6. Summary

The post-cardiac transplantation patient is frequently debilitated as a result of 'end-stage' heart disease and typically demonstrates muscle wasting, with a reduced work capacity, maximum heart rate and peak oxygen uptake. At submaximal effort perceived exertion and ventilation are higher, and the absolute ventilatory threshold lower, than in normals.

A number of published studies have now shown that an exercise rehabilitation programme can induce a good training effect, although possibly not complete restoration of physiological function. The prescription of exercise must take into account the denervated heart's peculiar response to effort, and rely more on perceived exertion and metabolic measurements for defining intensity of training rather than target training heart rates.

Changes in mood and personality have also been noted in these patients, and while these may improve spontaneously with the passage of time, there is some evidence that a rehabilitation programme can help in this regard.

References

1. Heck CF, Shumway SJ, Kaye MP: The registry of the international society for heart transplantation: sixth official report – 1989. J Heart Transplant 1989;8:271–276.
2. Jose A, Collision D: The normal range and determinants of the instrinsic heart rate in man. Cardiovasc Res 1970;4:160.
3. de Marneffe M, Jacobs P, Haardt R, Englert M: Variations of normal sinus node function in relation to age: role of autonomic influence. Eur Heart J 1986;7:662.
4. Donald DE, Ferguson DA, Milburn SE: Effect of beta adrenergic blockade on racing performance of greyhounds with normal and with denervated hearts. Circ Res 1968;22:127.
5. Cannom DS, Rider AK, Stinson EB, et al.: Electrophysiologic studies in the denervated transplanted human heart. Am J Cardiol 1975;36:859.
6. Yusuf S, Theodoropoulos S, Mathias CJ, Dhalla N, Wittes J, Mitchell A, Yacoub M: Increased sensitivity to the denervated transplanted human heart to isoprenaline both before and after beta-adrenergic blockade. Circulation 1987;75:696–704.
7. Banner NR, Patel N, Cox AP, Patton HE, Lachno DR, Yacoub M: Altered sympathoadrenal response to dynamic exercise in cardiac transplant recipients. Cardiovasc Res 1989;23:965–972.
8. Schell J, Meyer M, Liscia P, et al.: Role of catecholamines in the control of heart rate during exercise after cardiac transplantation. Poster presentation at '1990: Up-dating on Cardiopulmonary Rehabilitation', Milan, Italy, September 26–29, 1990.
9. Starling RC, Cody RJ: Cardiac transplant hypertension. Am J Cardiol 1990;65:106–111.
10. Kavanagh T, Yacoub M, Mertens DJ, Kennedy J, Campbell RB, Sawyer P: Cardiorespiratory responses to exercise training after orthotopic cardiac transplantation. Circulation 1988;77(1):162–171.
11. Banner NR, Lloyd MH, Hamilton RD, Innes JA, Guz A, Yacoub M: Cardiopulmonary response to dynamic exercise after heart and combined heart-lung transplantation. Br Heart J 1989;61:21–23.
12. Yusuf S, Aikenhead J, Theodoropoulos S, Shalla N, Wittes J, Yacoub M: Mechanism of cardiac output during dynamic exercise in cardiac transplant patients. J Am Coll Cardiol 1986;7:225A (abstr.).
13. Borow KM, Neumann A, Arensman F, Yacoub M: Clinical evidence for differential sensitivity of alpha and beta adrenergic receptors after cardiac transplantation. Circulation 1985;72(Suppl III):111–129.
14. Hausdorf G, Banner NR, Mitchell A, Khaghani A, Martin M, Yacoub M: Diastolic function after cardiac and heart-lung transplantation. Br Heart J 1989;62:123–132.
15. Hanson P: Clinical exercise testing: In: Blair SN, Painter P, Pate RR, Smith LK, Taylor CMB (eds.) Resource Manual for Guidelines for Exercise Testing and Prescription. Philadelphia: Lea & Febiger, 1988.
16. Kavanagh T: The healthy heart program, 3rd ed. Toronto: Key Porter Books Ltd., 1985.
17. Borg G: Physical performance and perceived exertion. Sweden: Lund, 1962, Gleerup, p. 1.
18. Billingham ME: Cardiac transplant atherosclerosis. Transplant Proc 1987;19(Suppl 5):19.
19. Gao SZ, Schroeder JS, Hunt S, Stinson EB: Retransplantation for severe accelerated coronary artery disease in heart transplant recipients. Am J Cardiol 1988;62:876–881.
20. Kuo PC, Kirshenbaum JM, Gordon J, et al.: Lovastatin therapy for hypercholesterolemia in cardiac transplant recipients. Am J Cardiol 1989;64:631–635.
21. Squires RW, Arthur PR, Gau GT, Muri A, Lambert WB: Exercise after cardiac transplantation: a report of two cases. J Cardiac Rehab 1983;3:570.
22. Savin WM, Gordon E, Green S, et al.: Comparison of exercise training effects in cardiac denervated and innervated humans. (abstr.) J Am Coll Cardiol 1983;1(2):722.
23. Niset G, Coustry-Degré C, Degré S: Psychosocial and physical rehabilitation after heart transplantation: 1 year follow-up. Cardiology 1988;75:311–317.

24. Keteyian SJ, Ehrman JK, Fedel FJ, Rhoads KL: Rehabilitation following heart transplantation. Med Sci Sports Exerc 1989;21:S55.
25. Kavanagh T, Yacoub MH, Campbell R, Mertens D: Marathon running after cardiac transplantation: a case history. J Cardiopulmonary Rehabil 1986;6:16.
26. Hartley LH, Mason JW, Hogan RP, *et al.*: Multiple hormonal responses to graded exercise in relation to physical training. J Appl Physiol 1972;33:602.
27. Sylvestre-Gervais L, Nadeau A, Nguyen MH, Tancrede G, Rousseau-Migneron S: Effects of physical training on beta-adrenergic receptors in rat myocardial tissue. Cardiovasc Res 1982;16:530.
28. Butler J, O'Brien M, O'Malley K, Kelly JG: Relationship of beta-adrenoreceptor density to fitness in athletes. Nature 1982;298:60.
29. Butler J, Kelly JG, O'Malley K, Pidgeon F: Beta-adrenoreceptor adaptation to acute exercise. J Physiol 1983;344:113.
30. Sieurat PP, Roquebrune JP, Grinneiser D, *et al.*: Monitoring and rehabilitation of heterotopic cardiac transplantation patients during the period of convalescence. Archives Mal Coeur 1986;79:210–216.
31. Kavanagh T, Yacoub MH, Mertens DJ, Campbell RB, Sawyer P: Exercise rehabilitation after heterotopic cardiac transplantation. J Cardiopulmonary Rehabil 1989;9:303–310.
32. Buxton M, Acheson R, Caine N, Gibson S, O'Brien B: Costs and benefits of the heart transplant programmes at Harefield and Papworth Hospitals. HMSO (London) 1985; 91–106.
33. Mai FM, McKenzie FN, Kostuk WJ: Psychiatric aspects of heart transplantation: preoperative evaluation and postoperative sequelae. Br Med J 1986;292:311–313.
34. Jones BM, Chang VP, Esmore D, *et al.*: Psychological adjustment after cardiac transplantation. Med J Aust 1988;149:118–122.
35. Degré S: Rehabilitation and psycho-social factors after heart transplantation. Presented at the XIth Congress of the European Society of Cardiology. Nice, France, September 10–14, 1989.
36. Kavanagh T, Tuck JA, Yacoub M, Shephard RJ, Kennedy J, Mertens DJ: The influence of a rehabilitation exercise program on mood and personality following cardiac transplantation (in preparation).
37. Harvison A, Jones BM, McBride M, *et al.*: Rehabilitation after heart transplantation: the Australian experience. J Heart Transplant 1988;7:337–341.
38. Kavanagh T, Yacoub M, Tuck JA: Receptiveness and compliance of cardiac transplant patients to an exercise rehabilitation program., Circulation 1986;74(Suppl II):10.

B: Intellectual Functioning

38. Neuropsychological function before and after cardiac transplantation

R. A. BORNSTEIN, R. C. STARLING and P. D. MYEROWITZ

1. Introduction

A number of studies have demonstrated neuropsychological impairment in patients with cardiac disease who are evaluated in relation to open heart surgery or coronary artery bypass surgery [1–3]. Several studies [4–6] have revealed a high rate of neurological complications in cardiac transplant patients but there has been relatively little investigation of neuropsychological deficits in these patients before or after transplantation. One study [7] evaluated 54 patients with heterogeneous cardiac disease. On an extensive neuropsychological test battery, there was a high prevalence of impaired performance suggesting diffuse cerebral dysfunction. Following transplantation, there were no differences related to the nature of cardiac disease, but there was some evidence that patients over 50 years of age had slightly greater neuropsychological deficit. There were significant improvements on a number of measures, although the magnitude of improvement was interpreted as being of limited practical significance. The improvement in function was unrelated to post-operative emotional status, length of time on cardiopulmonary bypass, and interval between transplantation and post-operative follow-up.

Another study [8] examined a consecutive series of 55 patients who were candidates for cardiac transplantation. In that study, there was a trend for greater impairment in patients with ischemic versus dilated cardiomyopathy. There was a relatively high incidence of elevated scores on the depression scale of the MMPI which was correlated with a summary measure of neuropsychological impairment. However, the magnitude of the correlation was insufficient to account for the extent of the observed neuropsychological deficits. The nature and pattern of the deficits observed in the two studies were very similar with the most frequent and significant deficits on measures of memory, executive function, and motor skills. These studies indicate a high prevalence of impaired neuropsychological function in patients prior to cardiac transplantation, but do not provide any clear indication regarding

Paul J. Walter (ed.): Quality of Life after Open Heart Surgery, 419–424.

the etiology of those deficits. It is possible that the deficits are attributable to diminished cerebral perfusion secondary to a reduction in cardiac output. However, it is also possible that previous neurological events, emotional factors, medication effects, or general malaise associated with the severe state of medical illness could contribute to these deficits. The present study was conducted to examine the relation between pre-operative cardiovascular function and neuropsychological performance. In addition, post-operative changes were examined in a subgroup of the original sample.

2. Methods

2.1. Subjects

The sample included a total of 62 subjects who were admitted to the hospital for cardiac transplantation evaluation. The etiology of cardiac disease was variable, but the primary diagnostic groups were dilated and ischemic cardio-myopathy. The demographic and cardiovascular characteristics of the sample are presented in Table 1. All subjects underwent a thorough neuropsycholog-ical evaluation during their hospitalization. The test battery included the Wechsler Adult Intelligence Scale-Revised, the Wechsler Memory Scale-Revised, Halstead–Reitan Neuropsychological Test Battery, Wisconsin Card Sorting Test, Verbal Concept Attainment Test, Verbal Fluency Test, Grooved Pegboard Test, and the Minnesota Multiphasic Personality Inven-tory. Some subjects were too ill or fatigued to complete the entire test battery. The tests most frequently omitted were the Halstead Category Test and Tactual Performance Test from the Halstead-Reitan Battery.

Table 1. Demographic and pre-operative cardiovascular measures.

	Mean	S.D.	Range
Age	44.9	10.7	23–64
Education	12.4	2.7	7–4
Right atrium pressure (mm Hg)	8.8	6.4	1–28
Pulmonary capillary wedge pressure (mm Hg)	22.3	10.5	3–42
Stroke/volume index (ml/m^2)	28.1	10.4	14–52
Cardiac index (liters/m^2)	2.3	0.7	1.3–5.0
Left ventricle ejection fraction (%)	23.1	11.9	6–61

2.2. *Post-operative study*

Of the original sample, 30 subjects were still alive or had known locations for potential contact. All subjects were sent a letter inviting them to participate in a follow-up study of neuropsychological function. Of the 30 potentially available patients, 15 had undergone transplantation, and 15 were not transplanted. A total of 9 patients (6 transplanted and 3 non-transplanted) thus far have undergone follow-up neuropsychological evaluations. The follow-up neuropsychological examination was an abbreviated version of the initial assessment and included the Wechsler Memory Scale-Revised, Trail Making Test, Finger Tapping Test, Grooved Pegboard Test, Seashore Rhythm Test, Wechsler Adult Intelligence Scale-Revised, Wisconsin Card Sorting Test, and the MMPI.

3. Results

The relationship between neuropsychological performance and cardiovascular function was examined by computing Pearson correlation coefficients. Because of the relationship between age and neuropsychological performance, it was necessary to control the effects of age in these analyses. Therefore, partial correlation coefficients were computed statistically controlling for the effects of age. The results of these analyses are presented in Table 2 which demonstrates a number of consistent relationships between neuropsychological impairment and measures of cardiovascular function. In particular, it can be seen that higher right atrium pressure is associated with worse neuropsychological performance on several measures. In contrast, higher stroke/volume index and cardiac index was associated with better

Table 2. Correlation between neuropsychological performance and cardiovascular function.[1]

	R atrium pressure	P-C wedge pressure	Cardiac index	Stroke/volume index	LV ejection fraction
Verbal IQ	-0.32^a				
VCAT	$-0.25a$			0.32^a	
Vis rep.	-0.38^b	-0.35		0.41^b	
Trail making A	-0.26^a				
Trail making B	-0.38^b				
Pegboard R	-0.48^b		0.32^a	0.36^a	
TPT-memory			0.52^b	0.45^a	
Impairment index	0.33^b	0.21	0.01	-0.21	0.17

Abbreviations: VCAT, a Verbal Concept Attainment Test; Vis rep, Visual Reproduction from Wechsler Memory; Pegboard, Grooved Pegboard, Grooved Pegboard Right Hand; TPT, Tactual Performance Test
[1] Partial correlations controlling for age.
[a] $p < 0.05$,   [b] $p < 0.01$.

Table 3. Mean percentage change in neuropsychological performance.

	Transplanted $\bar{X}(n\text{-}6)$	Non-Transplanted $\bar{X}(n\text{-}3)$
WCST-PE[1]	48.7	23.8
Seashore	9.2	−6.8
Trail making A	−4.5	1.8
Trail making B	6.7	−4.5
Pegboard R	−4.1	−6.8
Pegboard L	−0.7	10.8
Tapping R	14.0	−13.0
Tapping L	6.6	−10.2
Logical memory	4.3	1.3
Visual reproduction	14.4	−10.1
MMPI–D	−10.5	−23.5
MMPI–Pt	5.2	−11.4
MMPI–Ma	−3.7	−5.1

Wisconsin Card Sorting Test, Perseverative Errors.

neuropsychological performance. Pulmonary-capillary wedge pressure and left ventricle ejection fraction were not related to neuropsychological performance. These data suggest that the neuropsychological impairment observed on the pre-operative examination appears to be related to diminished cardiac output. This suggests that cerebral hypoperfusion secondary to impaired cardiac output may be one of the-mechanisms underlying the preoperative neuropsychological deficit.

It was also of interest to examine the extent of post-operative change in the subgroup of patients examined at follow-up. The mean duration between the two neuropsychological examinations was approximately 36 months (range = 29–46) and the mean duration between surgery and post-operative examination in those patients who underwent surgery was 25 months (range = 5–38). Change in neuropsychological performance was computed for each variable using the following formula: (time$_1$ − time$_2$)/time$_1$ × 100). This formula generated a change score which expresses follow-up neuropsychological performance as a percentage of initial performance. The mean percent change for the neuropsychological and personality measures for the transplanted and non-transplanted subjects are presented in Table 3. It can be seen that on some tests such as the Wechsler Adult Intelligence Scale-Revised and Grooved Pegboard Test there were minimal changes which were consistent in both groups. In contrast, there were a number of tests in which the transplanted patients demonstrated substantially greater improvements than the non-transplanted patients. On a number of measures including the Wechsler Memory Scale Logical Memory and Visual Reproduction subtests, Trail Making Test, and Seashore Rhythm Test, the non-transplanted group shows some deterioration whereas the transplanted patients obtained substantial improvement.

It might be argued that the relative improvement in the transplanted patients could be attributable to emotional factors. Patients who receive transplants might be expected to undergo some relief and improved outlook on life. However, review of Table 3 indicates that both the transplanted and non-transplanted patients in fact demonstrate greater degrees of depression at follow-up in comparison to their initial evaluation. The increase in depression is somewhat greater for the non-transplanted patients. In contrast, the two groups differ in the change on the Pt scale of the MMPI which is typically regarded as a measure of chronic tension and anxiety. Table 3 indicates that the transplanted patients were somewhat improved, whereas the non-transplanted patients were somewhat worse in comparison to their initial evaluations.

4. Discussion

These data extend the findings of the previous study [8] by indicating the relationship between diminished cardiac output and neuropsychological impairment at pre-surgical evaluation. The association between neuropsychological impairment and cardiovascular function cannot be attributed to age because this was statistically controlled. In addition, the magnitude of the correlations between neuropsychological performance and cardiovascular function was much stronger than the modest relationships observed with emotional factors on initial examination. These data suggest that cerebral hypoperfusion secondary to diminished cardiac output appears to contribute to neuropsychological impairment in candidates for cardiac transplantation. Increased right atrial pressure and stroke/volume index were related to performance on neuropsychological measures. These data are consistent with previous reports that increased right atrial pressure is a prognostic indicator for heart failure and worse survival [9]. Also consistent with the previous report, ejection fraction was not a good indicator of functional status.

These data also suggest that the neuropsychological deficit identified pre-operatively may be reversible to some degree following cardiac transplantation. Although the sample size of patients seen in follow-up is too small to permit firm conclusions, these initial data are supportive of post-operative improvements in function. On several measures, the transplanted patients demonstrated significant improvement in function, whereas the non-transplanted patients are unchanged or somewhat worse than their pre-operative performance. The post-operative improvements do not appear to be attributable to improved emotional status since the transplanted patients were more depressed on follow-up than they were at initial evaluation. These preliminary data on improved cognitive function following transplantation require elaboration with larger patient groups. In addition, the mechanism underlying this improvement requires elucidation. In particular, the relationship between change in cardiac function and neuropsychological improvement should be investigated.

References

1. Becker R, Katz J, Polonius MJ, Speidel H: Psychopathological and neurological dysfunctions following open-heart surgery. New York: Springer-Verlag, 1982.
2. Willner AE, Rodewald G: Impact of cardiac surgery on the quality of life. New York: Plenum Press, 1990.
3. Sotaniemi KA, Juolasmaa A, Eero MA, Hokkanen T: Neuropsychologic outcome after open-heart surgery. Arch Neuro 1981;38:2–8.
4. Ang LC, Gillett JM, Kaufmann JCE: Neuropathology of heart transplantation. Can J Neurol Sci 1989;16:291–298.
5. Schober R, Herman MN: Neuropathology in cardiac transplantation: survey of 31 cases. Lancet 1973;1:962–994.
6. Montero CG, Martinez AJ: Neuropathological of heart transplantation: 23 cases. Neurol 1986;36:1149–1154.
7. Scahll RR, Petrucci RJ, Brozena SC, Cavarocchi NC, Jessup M: Cognitive function in patients with symptomatic dilated cardiomyopathy before and after cardiac transplantation. J Am Coll Cardiol 1989;14:1666–1672.
8. Bornstein RA, Hammer D, Starling R, Stang J, Lewis R, Magorien R: Neuropsychological impairment in candidates for cardiac transplantation. In: Willner AE, Rodewald G (eds.) Impact of cardiac surgery on the quality of life. New York: Plenum Press, 1990;231–235.
9. Unverferth DV, Magorien RD, Moeschberger ML, Baker PB, Fetters JK, Leier CV: Factors influencing the one year mortality of dilated cardiomyopathy. Am J Cardiol 1984;54:147–152.

C: Emotional State

39. Long-term follow-up of the emotional adjustment of patients after heart transplantation

BRETT JONES, FRANCES TAYLOR, K. DOWNS and P. SPRATT

1. Introduction

Heart transplantation is now an established treatment of end stage cardiac disease. As an indication of the viability of this treatment the International Society For Heart Transplantation Registry in 1990 received data on 13 000 cases from more than 230 transplant centres and reported a five year actuarial survival of 72% [1]. However survival figures are only part of the picture and it needs to be concurrently established that long term survival is associated with an improved quality of life.

A poor quality of life can involve considerable cost to the patient, his family and the wider community through illness, stress and the necessity for social support. Also with the long term use of immunosuppressants there is the increased risk of complications such as lymphoma and osteoporosis [2]. For these reasons we thought it important to measure ongoing quality of life.

Quality of life is seen not as a unitary concept, but as an amalgam of functioning in four different domains, being psychological status, social functioning, occupational functioning and physical status [3].

In the Heart Transplant Unit at St Vincent's Hospital, Sydney, Australia, we have attempted to measure all these domains by assessing patients before and at a number of points after transplantation and in this manner establishing ongoing data on recipients quality of life.

In an earlier study we reported on the psychological adjustment and quality of life of 38 patients up to one year after transplantation [4]. Patients were seen before transplantation, at first discharge and at 4, 8 and 12 months after transplantation. The study quantitated patients' anxiety, depression, body image and subjective quality of life by way of standardised self assessment questionnaires. The patient's satisfaction with relationships and rehabilitation at 12 months was also reported. The results showed that anxiety increased before transplantation in most patients, that some patients showed mild symptoms of depression and other patients showed a deterioration in the

Paul J. Walter (ed.): Quality of Life after Open Heart Surgery, 427–437.
© 1992 Kluwer Academic Publishers.

quality of their lives and a negative body image. After transplantation significant improvements occurred in all parameters that was maintained at follow-up.

Since that report there has been a growing body of literature reporting favourable results on these measures after transplantation [5–8]. Only one study has challenged the belief that heart transplantation results in improved quality of life [9].

In the following article we report on a number of studies that have assessed psychological, social, occupational, physical and cognitive status before and after transplantation.

2. Assessment

Sociodemographic data (age, sex, marital status, employment status) were obtained by interview. The interviews were semi-structured, lasted an hour and were conducted by the psychologist or the social worker. Psychological and quality of life data were collected in face to face interviews before transplant, and at first follow-up. Thereafter, questionnaires were mailed to the patients.

2.1. *Study 1: Psychological adjustment/quality of life*

Psychological adjustment was measured using the Beck Depression [10] Inventory, and the Spielberger State Trait Anxiety Inventory [11].

Well-being was measured using the Campbell Well-Being Scale [3]. Marital satisfaction was also assessed from the Campbell scale.

At five year follow-up the Nottingham Health Profile was added [12]. This profile gives measures on a number of scales with specific reference to patients with cardiac disease. The Profile was not available when the study commenced in 1984.

2.1.1. *Return to work*
Information on return to work was obtained by questionnaire on follow up.

2.1.2. *Body mass index*
Body mass index was compiled from information on height and weight from the patients medical records.

Medical data (diagnosis, rejection and infectious episodes, complications, immunosuppressant medication and body mass index) were obtained by reference to patients' flow charts.

2.2. *Study 2: Cognitive status*

Cognitive Status was assessed using the sub tests of Digit Span, Arithmetic, Vocabulary, Block Design and Digit Symbol from the Weschsler Adult Intelligence Scale (*R*) [13]; the logical and visual memory sections of the Wechsler Memory Scale Form I [14] and the Trails Tests [15].

3. Subjects and methods

Subjects included in these studies were transplanted between February 1984 and February 1990. Patients were excluded from the studies on psychological adjustment and cognitive statu if they were either not English speaking or if they were younger than 15 years of age.

In the first study on psychological adjustment 38 patients were originally assessed and followed for one year after transplantation. By the time of final follow-up, six patients had died and five were non compliant. This left 27 patients who were assessed before transplantation, at first discharge from hospital, then at 4, 8 and 12 months and finally at a mean of 4.2 years after transplantation.

In the second study 43 patients had their cognitive status measured before transplantation and repeat measures were taken at four months after transplantation.

Return to work data was obtained on 154 patients transplanted between February 1984 and February 1990. Body Mass Index was compiled on 118 patients as a measure of dietary compliance.

The influence of medical and demographic variables on psychological outcome and quality of life was also assessed.

4. Statistical analysis

The difference in scores that pertained to emotional states and cognitive studies at each test time were compared by student t-tests. The standard significance level of 0.05 wa divided by the number of tests to account for chance significance (Bonferroni). Pearsons correlational coefficient and Spearman rho was used to assess the relationship between medical and demographic data and emotional state.

5. Results

5.1. *Study 1*

5.1.1. *Subjects*
Of the 27 patients, 21 were male and 6 were female. The average age was 44.6 years and ranged from 31 years to 59 years. Twenty were married and seven were single. Twelve patients had cardiomyopathy, and twelve had ischaemic heart disease. Three patients had valvular disease. They had an average of 1.4 treatable rejection episodes each overall, the range was from 0 to 5. They had a mean of 0.5 treatable infection cpisodes each, the range from 0 to 2. None of the group had any treatable complications. Eleven were treated with triple therapy (cyclosporin, prednisone, azathioprine), four were treated with double therapy (cyclosporin and azathioprine) and two started on double therapy and converted to triple therapy. The remaining ten patients were treated with cyclosporin, prednisone and A.T.G.

5.1.2. *Depression*
The Beck Inventory categorizes patients as depressed or not depressed. The higher the score the greatcr the degree of depression. Patients with end stage heart disease could score in the depressed range on the basis of their physical symptoms (lethargy, weight loss, inability to work). For this reason we set a cut-off of 13, based on item analysis and face validity before patients were classified as depressed. On this basis 37 scored in the depressed range before transplantation. After transplantation one patient scored in the depresed range-at 8 months follow-up, one at 12 months and one at 4 year follow-up. The mean scores at all points of follow up were significantly lower than before transplantation. There was no significant difference between mean scores at any point of follow-up (Figure 1).

5.1.3. *Anxiety*
The Spielberger State Anxiety Inventory measures state (specific reactive) and trait (general) anxiety on a continuum from low to high anxiety. The higher the score the higher the anxiety. Trait anxiety was measured before transplantation. At follow up only state anxiety was measured. In the original study anxiety declined significantly after transplantation and this trend was maintained at follow up. There was no significant difference between mean anxiety scores at any point of follow up. Analysing individual scores all patients reported lower anxiety at first follow up. At four months 23% had higher scores than at first discharge and at 8 months 34% of patients reported a higher score than at 4 months. At 12 months follow up, 31% of patients had a higher score than at 8 months whereas at final follow up only 11% had a higher score than at 1 year follow up (Figure 2).

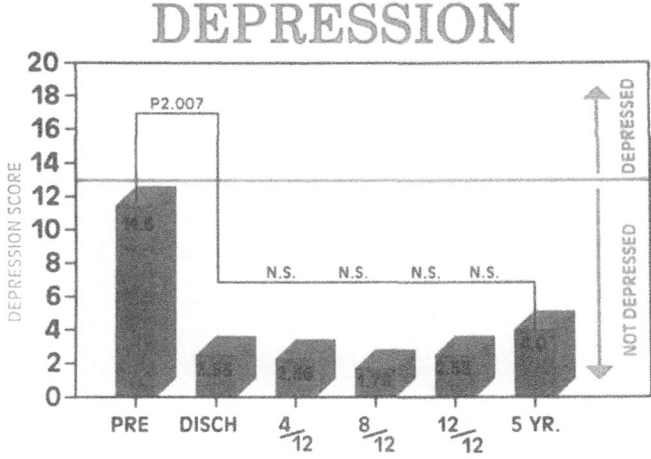

Figure 1.

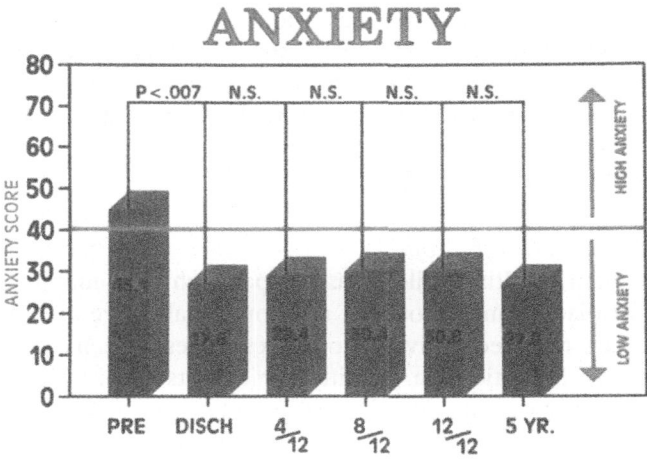

Figure 2.

5.1.4. *Well-being*

The Campbell Well Being Scale provides a subjective measure of well-being. Scores can range between 2.1 (low well-being) and 14.7 (high well-being) with a normal score of 11.77 ± 2.21. The patients rated their satisfaction with their day to day life on a seven point scale with the end points being 'completely satisfied' and 'completely dissatisfied'. Their perception of life

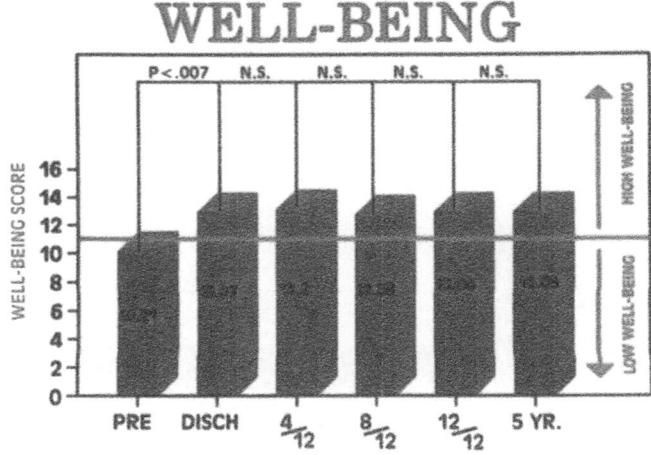

Figure 3.

in general was rated on a series of seven point scales with end points such as 'boring' and 'interesting' or 'easy' and 'hard'. From these results we computed a single score of well-being for each patient. Mean well being scores were higher at each point of follow up than before transplantation. There was no significant difference between mean scores at one and four year follow up. At all points of follow-up, the mean score was higher than for the normal population (Figure 3).

5.1.5. *Nottingham health profile*

The Nottingham Health Profile measures pain, physical mobility, sleep, energy, social isolation and emotional reaction. In all there are 38 statements and patients are required to give yes or no responses to each of the statements which relate to limitations in activities or aspects of distress. A weight is applied to each statement enabling a score ranging from 0 to 100 to be calculated for each dimension. The higher the score the more the patient was experiencing either discomfort or limitations. The scale also asks patients if they are experiencing any problems with their work, social, home or sex lives, holidays and interests and hobbies. Comparison with earlier data was not possible since the data was not available. However, we compared transplant patients' scores with a standardisation sample of general practice patients of comparable age. Transplant patients scored better on 3 out of 6 measures and at the lower end of the range, indicating little discomfort or distress. Two patients reported difficulties with work (one because of an industrial accident); two reported difficulties with their home life and two reported interference to interests and hobbies. Another two reported diffi-

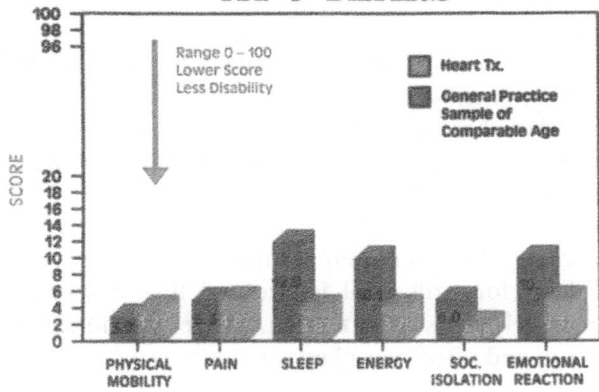

Figure 4.

culties with their social life and five reported difficulties with their sex lives (Figure 4).

5.1.6. *Satisfaction with marriage/relationship*
Of those who were married or in a relationship 95% or 19 were either completely or nearly completely satisfied with their marriage or relationship at five year follow up.

5.1.7. *Influence of variables*
Correlational analysis of the relationships between age, sex, marital status and return to work with psychological and quality of life variables did not reveal any significant trends.

Also there were no significant relationships between diagnosis, infections and rejection episodes, immunosuppressant treatment and psychological outcome.

5.2. *Study 2*

5.2.1. *Subjects*
Of the 43 patients in this study, 36 were male and 7 were female. The average age was 44.3 and ranged from 18 years to 63 years. Thirty four were married and nine were single. Fifteen had ischaemic heart disease, 25 had cardiomyopathy and 3 had valvular disease. Twenty-four had Cyclosporin, prednisone,

azathioprine and ATG for immunosuppression, 14 had cyclosporin, prednisone, azathioprine and OKT3, and 5 had cyclosporin, azathioprine and ATG.

5.2.2. *Wechsler adult intelligence-scale (R)*

(1) *Vocabulary:* The vocabulary test measures word knowledge and is a
measure of verbal intelligence. To some extent it is a measure of pre-morbid
functioning, although influenced by educational attainment. The mean vocabulary score was 9.4 (range 5–19). AS a group they were therefore pre
morbidly of average intelligence.

(2) *Digit Span:* This test requires patients to report on single presentation,
a series of digits forwards until failure and then a series backwards until
failure. It is largely a test of attention. There was no significant difference
in scores before and after transplantation.

(3) *Arithmetic:* This is a test of mental calculatory ability. Patients showed
a significant improvement in their performance after transplantation.

(4) *Block Design:* This is a test of problem solving ability and psychomotor speed. The scores showed little difference in performance before and
after transplantation.

(5) *Digit Symbol:* This test is a test of psychomotor speed and copying
ability. The scores showed a significant improvement after transplantation.

Wechsler Memory Scale: Significant improvement was noted on the scores
of the visual memory section of this test.

Trail Tests: These tests are tests of planning ability and psychomotor
speed. Part A requires subjects to connect a series of numbers in consecutive
order and Part B requires subjects to connect consecutive numbers and
letters, alternating from number to letter. Both tests were timed. There was
no difference in scores on Part A, but Part B was completed significantly
faster after transplantation (Table 1).

5.2.3. *Return to work:*

Subjects: Return to work data was compiled on 154 patients (130 who were
male and 24 who were female). They had a mean age of 43 years, ranging
from 11 years to 65 years.

Sixty-three percent had returned to full time employment or previous
lifestyles, 8% had retired and 29% were in receipt of a government pension.

Results: Body Mass Index: Body Mass Index was calculated for 118 patients
(101 males, 17 females, average age 43.7 years) at one year after trans-

Table 1. Means and standard deviations cognitive tests pre and post.

Test	Mean		Std. dev.		Sign
	Pre	Post	Pre	Post	
Digit span	10.7	10.9	2.9	2.8	N.S.
Arith	9.6	10.3	2.7	2.6	$p < 0.02$
Block design	9.6	9.9	2.5	2.3	N.S.
Digit symbol	7.7	8.2	1.7	2.1	$p < 0.01$
Logical memory	10.2	10.6	3.9	3.7	N.S.
Visual memory	8.6	10.1	3.6	3.1	$p < 0.01$
Trails A	41.0	39.6	14.7	15.5	N.S.
Trails B	101.3	90.6	42.2	31.5	$p < 0.05$

Table 2. Body mass index percentage in each range at follow-up.

	1 Year	2 Years	3 Years	4 Years
Below average	5.0	4.0	6.0	4.0
Average	55.0	54.0	46.0	35.0
Above average	36.0	30.0	29.0	35.0
Obese	4.0	12.0	19.0	26.0

plantation. Data was available on 84 of these patients at two year follow-up; 48 at three year follow-up and 26 at four year follow-up. The results showed a trend for some patients to become either overweight or obese over time (Table 2).

6. Discussion

The main feature of the results in this series of studies, has been the absence of any evidence of mood disorder and the good quality of life enjoyed by this sample of cardiac transplant patients, in some cases up to five years after transplantation.

On measure of mood disorder patients' depression scores improved after transplantation and more significantly showed no evidence of depressive symptomatology at any of the five points of follow-up. Anxiety which was elevated before transplantation, as a reaction to the patients physical condition and impending transplantation declined after transplantation and the improvement was maintained at all points of follow-up.

These scores were of added significance when it was considered that some of the patients may not have expccted to be alive, given the information provided to them at the time of transplantation.

Well-being scores improved after transplantation and at all points of follow-up showed a higher level of well being than for the normal population.

The results on the Nottingham Health Profile whilst only being available for the five year follow-up were at the lower end of the scale indicating good health on all measures. The scores were similar to those found by Caine *et al.* in a prospective study of quality of life before and after transplantation using the Nottingham Scale and therefore gives some validity to our findings [16].

A search of the literature failed to find any studies on patients' cognitive status before and after transplantation. We measured patients' attention, concentration, short term memory and motor speed. Whereas we found no difference before and after transplantation, on the digit span (repeating a series of numbers forwards and a different series backwards), and a non verbal problem solving test, performance on tests of short term memory, psychomotor speed and mental arithmatic showed significant improvement. This may have been either because of improved blood and oxygen supply to the brain or a general improvement in well-being. The changed scores were considered important in terms of patients' quality of life and maybe a factor in increasing the probability that patients would return to work.

Return to work figures were difficult to compare because of different cultural, economic and health insurance policies that exist between countries. However, the percentage of our patients who have returned to either full time work or previous lifestyles compares favourably with published studies from other English speaking countries [17]. The number of our patients re-entering the work force has declined over time as our programme has expanded to include patients 55 and over who are less likely to either seek employment or be suitably re-employed.

These studies have not found any significant relationship between medical and demographic variables and psychological outcome. However, early results on predictive studies relating psychological and demographic variables to outcome suggest such a relationship may exist. We have found significant relationships between marriage and survival, pre-existing anxiety scores and survival, age and intelligence and management problems, a psychiatric history and management problems and socioeconomic status and return to work [18]. Also in another study we found significant differences on quality of life measures between patients on double and triple therapy [19].

The thorn in the side of what were otherwise highly favourable results was patients' poor dietary compliance and the trend towards patients becoming overweight and obese with time. This has the potential to compromise the patients' quality of life because of increased immunosuppression and the resulting health risks.

References

1. Kriett JM, Kaye MP: The Registry of the International Society for Heart Transplantation: Seventh Official Report – 1990. J Heart Transplant 1990;9:323–330.

2. Oyer PE, Stinson EB, Jamieson SW, *et al.*: One year experience with cyclosporin A in clinical heart transplantation. J Heart Transplant 1982;4:285–91.

3. Campbell A, Converse PE, Rodgers WL: The quality of American life. New York: Russell Sage Foundation, 1976.

4. Jones BM, Chang VP, Esmore D, *et al.*: Psychological adjustment after cardiac transplantation. Med J Aust 1988;149:118–122.

5. Mai FM, McKenzie FN, Kostuk WJ: Psychosocial adjustment and quality of life following heart transplantation. Canadian J Psychiatry 1990;35:223–7

6. Shapiro PA: Life after heart transplantation. Prog Cardiovascular Dis 1990;32:405–18.

7. Lough ME, Lindsay AM, Shin JA, Stotts NA: Life satisfaction following heart transplantation. J Heart Transplantation 1985;4:443–449.

8. Samuelson RG, Hunt SA, Shroeder JS: Functional and social rehabilitation of heart transplant recipients under age thirty. Scand J Thor Cardiovasc Surg 1984;18:97–103.

9. Walden JA, Stevenson LW, Dracup K, *et al.*: Heart transplantation may not improve quality of life for patients with stable heart failure. Heart Lung 1989;18:197–505.

10. Beck AT, Ward CH, Mendelson M *et al.*: An inventory for measuring depression. Arch Gen Psychiatry 1961;4:561–571.

11. Spielberger CD, Gorsuch RL, Lushene RE: State trait anxiety manual. Palo Alto, Calif: Consulting Pychological Press 1970.

12. Hunt SM, McKenna SP, McEwen J: The Nottingham Health Profile.

13. Wechsler D: The Wechsler Adult Intelligence Scale – Revised New York: The Psychological Corporation 1981.

14. Wechsler D, Stone CP: Wechsler Memory Scale. New York: The Psychological Corporation 1973.

15. Fromm-Auch, Yaudall: The Trail Making Test – Adult Form. J Clinical Neuropsychology 1983;5:221–38.

16. Caine N, Sharples LD, English JAH, Wallwork J: Prospective study comparing quality of life before and after heart transplantation. Transplantation Proceedings 1990;22:1437–39.

17. Wallwork J *et al.*: A comparison of the quality of life of cardiac transplant patients and coronary artery bypass graft patients before and after surgery. Quality Life Cardiovasc Care 1985.

18. Jones BM, Taylor F, Downs K, Spratt P: The relationship of psychosocial assessment to survival, rejection and infection episodes, management problems and return to work in heart transplantation recipients (in press).

19. Jones BM, Taylor TJ, Wright O, *et al.*: Quality of life after heart transplantation in patients assigned to double or triple therapy. J Heart Transplant 1990;9:392–96.

40. The emotional state of the individual after heart transplantation

FRANCOIS M. MAI and F. NEIL MCKENZIE

1. Introduction

Over the last decade, heart transplantation has become the treatment of choice for end stage cardiac disease. By 1990, more than twelve thousand examples of this dramatic surgical procedure had been carried out worldwide [1]. Although the sense of euphoria and wonder persist, there is now a more sober awareness of the need to deal with the many practical, psychological, social and ethical problems which may accompany the operation.

At University Hospital in London, Canada 275 heart transplants have been carried out on 265 patients since 1981. Of these, 191 (72.08%) were men and the age range was 20 months to 64 years. Seventy-one (25.82%) have died, 46 (16.73) in the early (<90 day) period.

A liaison psychiatrist has been involved with the transplant team since its inception and has played an active part in evaluating referrals and in dealing with pre- and post-transplant psychiatric problems [2–5]. We found that psychiatric problems were common. In the majority of cases, they were secondary to the patients' serious medical problems; hence they were not contraindications to surgery. However, in a small proportion of patients, there was a premorbid history of serious psychiatric disorder which might preclude surgery. We advise against surgery in patients with a history of schizophrenia, intellectual retardation or irreversible brain disease. The decision is more difficult in patients with personality disorders or substance abuse, as these patients may have impaired compliance which may in turn interfere with postoperative course and survival. Initially, such individuals were refused surgery, but our criteria have become progressively more liberal as we have gained experience.

In this chapter, we will review some of the emotional, social and psychiatric problems which may follow heart transplant surgery. These will be discussed under three headings based on the time after surgery: the early postoperative phase (1–10 days); the late postoperative phase (11–90 days); the phase of rehabilitation (>90 days).

Paul J. Walter (ed.): Quality of Life after Open Heart Surgery, 439–444.
© 1992 Kluwer Academic Publishers.

2. Early postoperative phase

The most important psychiatric problem during this phase is a postoperative delirium and this occurred in 18% of cases in our series [3]. This study was based on a retrospective chart review, hence could well have underestimated the true prevalence. In most cases the delirium was mild and transient, but in two it was severe and required large doses of neuroleptics to control the agitation. Studies using a different methodology have found a prevalence of postoperative delirium of 34.3% [6] and 25.9% [7].

Once the patient has recovered from surgery, a major process of psychological adaptation must take place. He needs to adjust to the presence of a vital foreign organ retrieved from a (usually) anonymous person who died. The recipient may have various ideas, feelings and fantasies about this situation and these may include fear, anxiety and guilt. He may benefit from the opportunity to ventilate these feelings. Other patients become euphoric or they are unable to verbalize their feelings to the point of denial [4,8]. When mild, these features can be regarded as adaptive coping techniques; they help the patient make the required psychological adjustment, including those associated with the changed body image which accompanies the improved health status. Denial and euphoria may reach pathological intensity and be characterized as hypomania. Neuroleptics may be required to control the restlessness and agitation.

The uncertainty in physical health and prognosis may alter family relationships. This is a stressful period for family members. They request and require frequent progress reports, and are apprehensive about the possibility of infection or rejection. They may express this anxiety in somatic symptoms such as headaches, insomnia or stomach complaints. This may even lead them to request a medical consultation or attend the emergency department. These difficulties need to be handled appropriately and sensitively by the treatment team. On occasion, a conjoint family interview is necessary to ensure that each member has the same understanding regarding the treatment plan, and that communication within the family is adequate. Family members' tendency to be apprehensive, frustrated or overprotective must also be dealt with patiently and appropriately.

A unique aspect of cardiac transplantation is the recipients' experience of having and now 'owning' a cadaver organ essential for the maintenance of his/her life. Although this is an intangible factor and difficult to quantify it is nevertheless an extraordinary situation with potentially a powerful psychosocial effect. It has been described in terms of a fear of the effects that the graft may have on personality [7] or a difficulty in verbalizing feelings about the graft or the donor [4]. A further aspect of this situation is the bond which is created between the recipient and the family of the donor. Gutkind [9] in a fascinating anecdotal report described the problems and challenges of meetings between a transplant recipient and the family of the donor. Individual reactions to such communication vary widely, and personal contact is probably undesirable unless it is explicitly desired by both parties. Desire to express gratitude is understandably common amongst recipients, and one of our patients (in whom the donor was anonymous) has contracted to publish a 'gratitude' notice in the newspaper each year on the anniversary of her operation.

3. Late postoperative phase

A wide variation in late postoperative psychosocial problems has been described. Most commonly, these are anxiety and mood disturbances, but family dysfunction and problems related to noncompliance may occur at this point. Anxiety, in fact, may be unchanged after surgery, and may even increase in a substantial minority of patients [7].

Although mood disorders do not generally develop de novo after surgery, an individual who has a past history of an affective disorder may develop another attack. The process of adaptation to surgery can act as a major stress which precipitates a relapse in such predisposed individuals.

Family problems also may continue into the late postoperative period. Where surgery has been successful, the great majority adapt successfully to the improved health status [8,10,11]. If there has been preexisting family dysfunction, this may continue postoperatively particularly if the patient has continuing physical disabilities which impair rehabilitation [12]. A relatively high occurrence of difficulties in the psychosexual area has been found which may affect up to 50% of individuals [11,13,14]. This may occur even in the context of apparently healthy marital relationships. The reason for this is not clear, but it is possible that either altered endocrine function or subtly changed marital relationships or both may be involved.

Perhaps the most important problems which may develop during the late postoperative period are those associated with compliance. These may have been present, though unrecognized during the preoperative evaluation. Following surgery the patient may start smoking again, or may show poor motivation for participating in physical therapy programs, or serum cyclosporin levels may indicate that this drug is not being taken as prescribed. Other indicators of poor compliance such as alcohol or drug abuse usually start later during the period of rehabilitation. Problems related to impaired compliance are likely easier to deal with if they have been anticipated. Unlike the patient awaiting a kidney transplant where parameters related to weight change, serum potassium and serum phosphate levels are available to assess compliance, the patient awaiting a heart transplant does not present readily available biological indices related to compliance. The presence of poor compliance therefore requires a careful clinical evaluation. In our unit, we have employed a simple 3-point scale where compliance was rated by the observer as 'good', 'fair' or 'poor' based on the extent to which the patient complied with treatment instructions concerning diet, fluid intake, medication, smoking and alcohol use. In the setting of the renal unit, such clinical ratings have been found to correlate well with biological parameters [15]. We found that there was a significant association between impaired preoperative compliance and both pre- and postoperative psychiatric diagnosis. It seems probable, therefore, that the presence of psychopathology in some way impairs the capacity of an individual to follow a medical regimen [14]. We also found an association between impaired compliance and poorer surgical outcome, hence it is of prognostic importance to identify and manage this problem as soon as it appears.

4. Rehabilitation

Long-term outcome and quality of life is likely the key test of the efficacy (including cost-effectiveness) of a heart transplant program. It clearly is a costly procedure in terms of resources and personnel; however, these layouts are justified if a high percentage of subjects resume a relatively normal life. This in turn, may help to increase the proportion of recipients who return to full-time employment by improving rehabilitative techniques and approaches.

Quality of life is a complex concept which includes as many as 15 different dimensions [16]. It includes such factors as mental and physical health, interpersonal relations, physical and recreational activity and employment status. Because of the economic implications and the relative ease with which it can be measured, return to work has been the most extensively studied of these criteria. The number of subjects who return to full-time work after transplant surgery has been variously estimated as 32% [17], 61% [13], 64% [8] and 55% [14]. It appears that comparatively higher numbers of recipients return to near normal levels of physical activity: 77% [11] and 95% [14]. Physical medicine specialists, and health professionals such as physiotherapists, psychologists, occupational therapists and social workers all may have an active role to play to maximize the rehabilitation potential of each recipient.

5. Discussion and conclusions

It is clear from this review that psychiatric and psychosocial problems may occur at any stage in the surgical process, and influence both the patients' adjustment and surgical outcome. Psychiatric contraindications to surgery are becoming progressively more limited, hence many patients with personality disorders, drug or alcohol problems, impaired compliance or poor social support systems will have surgery. These problems may affect surgical outcome and the success or otherwise of rehabilitation programs. Although there is no clear evidence as yet that psychiatric intervention improves prognosis, it is appropriate that it be offered to those with psychiatric or behaviour problems.

Postoperative delirium has been noted in at least 18% of patients. The etiology is not always clear, but may be related to personal, pharmacological and environmental factors. In the majority it is mild and transient, but it may be severe and life threatening in a minority of cases.

The most common psychiatric problems after surgery are mood disturbances. Anxiety, depression and rarely hypomania have been described. Although there is generally an improvement in family relationships, a minority show deterioration which may lead to separation and divorce. Psychosexual difficulties are common even it those subjects in whom there is no overt marital dysharmony.

Investigation of the longer term quality of life of recipients shows that the majority of survivors have a good outcome. At least 75% and possibly as many as 95% return to normal activity levels and about 50% resume their previous employment on a full time basis. This represents a curious discrepancy, because one would have expected that if an individual resumed normal physical activity, he would likely also be able to return to full-time employment. That this is not so suggests that factors other than level of physical activity determine whether or not a patient returns to work. These could be related to individual motivation, emotional attitude, social relationships and work-related variables amongst others. Prospective studies need to be designed to evaluate these variables in more detail.

Heart transplantation is a major psychological and physiological stress which makes substantial demands on the adaptive processes of the patient and his family. Psychosocial dysfunction may occur at any point in the process and influence surgical outcome. Dealing with these dysfuctional syndromes promptly and effectively improves both the quality of care in transplant programs and the quality of life of recipients.

References

1. Kriet JM, Kaye MP: The registry of the international society for heart transplantation. J Heart Transpl 1990;9:323 330.
2. Mai FM, McKenzie FN, Kostuk WJ: Liaison psychiatry in the heart transplant unit. Psychosom Med 1984;46:80–81.
3. Mai FM, McKenzie FN, Kostuk WJ: Psychiatric aspects of heart transplantation: Preoperative evaluation and postoperative sequelae. Brit Med J 1986;292:311–313.
4. Mai FM: Graft and donor denial in heart transplant recipients. Am J Psychiat 1986;143:159–161.
5. Mai FM: Psychiatric problems in heart transplant recipients. Hosp Ther 1988;13:48–58.
6. Freeman AM, Folks DG, et al: Cardiac transplantation: clinical correlates of psychiatric outcome. Psychosomatics 1988;29:47–54.

7. Kuhn WF, Myers B, Brennan AF, et al: Psychopathology in heart transplant candidates. J Heart Transplant 1988;7:223–226.

8. Jones BM, Chang VP, Esmore D, et al: Psychological adjustment after cardiac transplantation. Med J. Aust 1988;149:118–122.

9. Gutkind L: Transplant proceedings 1988;20(Suppl. 1):1092–1099.

10. Lough ME, Lindsay AM, et al: Impact of symptom frequency and symptom distress on self-reported quality of life in heart transplant recipients. Heart & Lung 1987;16:193–200.

11. Harrison A, Jones B, McBride M, et al: Rehabilitation of heart transplantation: The Australian Experience. J Heart Transplant 1988;7:337–341.

12. McAleer MJ, Copeland J: Psychological aspects of heart transplantation. Heart Transplant 1985;4:232–233.

13. Bedrgeret A, Dureau G, et al: Qualite de vie et reinsertion social apres transplantation cardique. Presse Med 1987;16(44):2207–2210.

14. Mai FM, McKenzie FN, Kostuk WJ: Psychosocial adjustment and quality of life following heart transplantation. Canad J Psychiat 1990;35:223–227.

15. Cumming K, Becker M: Construct validity comparisons of three methods for measuring patient compliance. Health Service Res 1984;19:103–116.

16. Evans DR, Burns JE, et al: The quality of life questionaire: a multidimensional measure. Am J Comm Psychol 1985;13:305–322.

17. Meister N, McAleer MJ, Meister JS, et al: Returning to work after heart transplantation. J Heart Transplant 1986;5:154–161.

41. Psychological well-being of heart transplant patients – cross-sectional and longitudinal results

M. BULLINGER, C.E. ANGERMANN and B.M. KEMKES

1. Introduction

During the past years, clinical endpoints for heart transplantation such as survival and post-operative complications have been supplemented by functional and psychosocial outcomes [1]. Subsumed under the term quality of life, these criteria include expert-rated as well patient-based assessments of physical state, psychological well-being, social relationships and everyday life functions [2,3]. Specifically, investigations address employment situation [4], psychopathology [5] sexuality [6], psychological adjustment [7] as well as general rehabilitative aspects [8,9]. While in most older studies ad hoc physician rating scales prevail, newer studies use psychometrically tested questionnaires for patient self-ratings. In general, studies addressing quality of life are cross-sectional investigations of HTX-survivors predominantly performed the United States [10] an only rarely in Europe [11]. Apart from these large surveys indicating a good quality of life after HTX per se and as compared to other chronic conditions [12], only scarce information is available from longitudinal studies assessing pre-operative as well as long-term post operative states in relation to HTX.

Thus only limited knowledge exists on European patients' self-perceived quality of life as assessed over time and with methodologically sound measures. The present study was performed to approach these issues with both a cross-sectional and longitudinal design and addressed the following research questions.

(a) How is the psychological well-being of HTX survivors as compared to a healthy group, and what is the course of well-being of patients scheduled for HTX before surgery well as in the short- and long-term postoperative phase?

(b) What are the correlates of quality of life as an indicator of psychological well-being among HTX recipients?

Paul J. Walter (ed.): Quality of Life after Open Heart Surgery, 445–455.

(c) Which subgroups of patients can be distinguished with regard to a high post-operative quality of life?

2. Methods

Included in the study were heart-transplantation (HTX) patients of the Department of Cardiovascular Surgery receiving pre- and post-operative care at the Department of Internal Medicine at the University of Munich. Based on a fixed deadline, all adult German-speaking survivors of HTX since the start of heart transplantation at Munich University were included in the cross-sectional (part A) study, while all newly scheduled patients awaiting HTX were included in the longitudinal (part B) study.

Part A patients were asked once to answer a set of quality of life questionnaires at home or while awaiting a routine clinical check-up. Part B patients completed the identical set of questionnaires prior to HTX, three and six weeks as well as six and twelve months after surgery. The questionnaires were also filled out by an age-matched healthy comparison group. According to a multifactorial approach to the quality of life concept, the set of questionnaires pertained not only to a global quality of life rating, but also to self-rated physical state, social relationships, everyday-life functions and psychological well-being [13,14]. The latter component was assessed via four methodologically sound instruments:

1. The 35-item German short form of the Profile of Mood States (POMS:15,16), assessing short term (1 day to 1 week) fluctuations in affect with the subscales depression, fatigue, vigor and irritability.
2. The 22-item Psychological General Well-being Index (PGWB:16,17) assessing longer term emotional changes (past month) with regard to anxiety, depression, control, well-being, health and vitality.
3. The 10-item Affect-Balance Scale (ABS:18) assessing independently positive affect and negative affect as well as their combination in terms of affect balance.
4. The 1-item Anamnestic Comparative Self Assessment Scale (ACSA:19) requiring the patient to rate the present time of his/her life with regard to the prior best and worst time.

Other quality of life measures not primarily focused on in the present paper included a life satisfaction scale, a symptom checklist, an everyday-life questionnaire and a list of life domains being affected by surgery [20]. Sociodemographic (e.g. education, employment status) and clinical data (e.g. NYHA-status, symptoms of cardiovascular dysfunction and post-operative complications such as hypertension, diabetes, neurological symptoms, renal dysfunction as well as symptoms pertaining to skin, bone, lung and gall) were available for patients in both study parts.

All data were obtained upon informed consent, collected with the help of a doctoral student and analysed with the BMDP-statistical program package [21]. Descriptive statistics were used to obtain frequencies as well as distribution characteristics on single items and questionnaire subscales. Differences between groups and over time were analysed by means of t-tests. Spearman correlation coefficients were used to assess relationships between variables.

3. Results

Patient characteristics: In the cross-sectional part A of the study, 41 (36 males, 5 females) of the total sample of 43 german-speaking HTX survivors completed the questionnaire (95% response rate). Patient mean age was 42.7 ± 9.5 years, time since transplantation was 24 ± 17 months, indications for HTX were dilated cardiomyopathy (CMP: 70.7%), coronary artery disease (CAD: 24.4%) and valvular heart disease (4.9%). At the time of inquiry, 56.1% of the patients were retired for health reasons, while only 21.9% worked full-time. Most patients were married (85.3%), had completed a professional education (83.8%) and were white collar workers (52.7%). The majority of patients (97.5%) were in NYHA class I (2 patients in class II). Post transplant coronary disease was present in 19.5% and impaired cardiac function in 7.3% of the patients. Only 12% of patients had not experienced any postoperative complications.

During the 16 month recruitment period for the longitudinal part B of the study, 32 adult German speaking patients scheduled for HTX were approached for participation. One patient explicitly refused to participate and two others did not answer any questionnaires during the study. Four patients died during surgery and three patients during the first three post-operative weeks. Of these, three had not completed the pretransplant questionnaires so that quality of life data were available for 22 of the 32 patients. Since two patients died four and eight months post-operatively and several patients failed or were not approached to respond to the questionnaires, the sample size varied at different measure-points. Mean age of the 22 male and three female patients was 48 ± 8 years, indication for surgery was primarily cardiomyopathy (60%) but also coronary artery disease (33.3%). Patients' preoperative NYHA status was III (53.3%) or IV (40.0%). Frequent complaints in over 50% of the patients included high grades of dyspnea, orthopnea, fatigue, weakness and inappetence, while pronounced palpitations, ancle edemas and chest pain were less frequent (under 20%). The majority of the patients were married (87.7%), had a qualifying professional degree (87.7%) and were white (56.3%) or blue collar workers (31.3%). Before HTX, the patients were mostly retired for health reasons (56.3%) or on sick leave (31.3%).

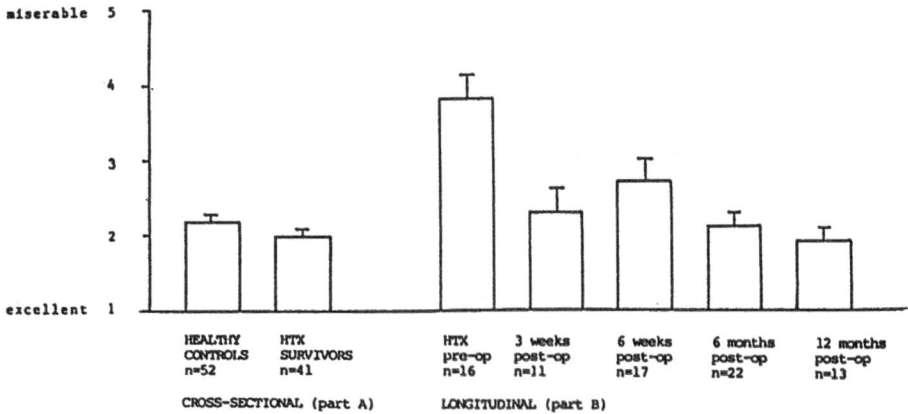

Figure 1. Global quality of life rating (mean and sem).

3.1. *Psychological well-being across groups and over time*

As depicted in Figure 1, HTX-survivors from part A of the study not only did not differ from but slightly exceeded the global quality of life ratings of their healthy counterparts on the 5-point scale from 1 (excellent) to 5 (miserable). After high pre-operative levels indicating a poor quality of life, longitudinal part B patients showed a gradual decrease towards a better ratings. According to *t*-test results the global quality of life differed from pre-operative scores both at 6 months ($p = 0.03$) and 12 months ($p = 0.01$) after surgery.

In the Anamnestic Comparative Self Assessment Scale (ACSA: see Table 1,), HTX survivors described the present time of their life as fulfilling as did the healthy comparisons. Longitudinal data show, that this positive evaluation was present in all post-operative phases, while prior to surgery a clearly negative evaluation prevailed. The increase in ACSA scores from pre- to post-operative scores at months 6 and 12 was highly significant ($p = 0.001$).

In the Affect-Balance Scale (ABS: see Table 1), scores of healthy persons and HTX survivors (part A) were comparable. In the longitudinal part B patients, positive affect dropped slightly from pre-operative to three weeks post-operative levels, then increased substantially at week 6 followed by a decrease at month 6 with a subsequent increase one year after surgery. Negative affect decreased and affect-balance increased continuously from the pre- to the 12 months postoperative measure-point. Compared to before

Table 1. Anamnestic comparative self-assessment scale (ASCA) and affect balance scale (ABS).

		Cross-Sectional (part A)		Longitudinal (part B)				
		Healthy controls $n = 52$	HTX survivors $n = 41$	HTX pre-op $n = 16$	3 weeks post-op $n = 11$	6 weeks post-op $n = 17$	6 months post-op $n = 22$	12 months post-op $n = 13$
ASCA	X	7.82	7.57	1.87	8.20	6.94	7.23	8.46
0–10*+	sem	0.51	0.48	0.52	0.73	0.73	0.71	0.48
ABS								
pos. affect	X	0.91	0.95	0.78	0.50	1.41	0.68	1.15
0–5*+	sem	0.19	0.15	0.21	0.22	0.37	0.33	0.27
neg. affect	X	1.20	1.15	3.19	2.20	1.58	1.48	1.38
0–5*	sem	0.20	0.24	0.45	0.63	0.51	0.41	0.42
af. balance	X	3.91	4.25	2.79	3.30	4.83	4.23	4.28
0–10*+	sem	0.32	0.21	0.42	0.57	0.52	0.28	0.50

* Range of scores; + high scores indicate positive well-being.

Table 2. Psychological general well-being index (PGWB).

		Cross-Sectional (part A)		Longitudinal (part B)				
PGWB		Healthy controls $n = 52$	HTX survivors $n = 41$	HTX pre-op $n = 16$	3 weeks post-op $n = 11$	6 weeks post-op $n = 17$	6 months post-op $n = 22$	12 months post-op $n = 13$
Anxiety	X	16.1	18.8	16.4	17.9	18.0	19.1	19.2
0–25*+	sem	0.7	0.6	1.09	1.69	1.11	0.89	0.90
Depression	X	12.01	13.0	10.3	12.2	12.4	13.12	13.3
0–15*+	sem	0.6	0.4	0.93	0.85	0.56	0.50	0.52
Well-being	X	12.1	13.4	7.8	12.1	13.3	13.9	14.1
0–20*+	sem	0.9	0.5	1.07	1.41	0.72	0.91	0.99
Self-control	X	11.3	12.1	11.1	12.2	11.7	12.2	12.9
0–15*+	sem	0.4	0.3	0.79	0.69	0.49	0.59	0.38
Health	X	11.5	10.5	5.8	8.54	9.7	10.9	12.0
0–15*+	sem	0.5	0.4	0.95	1.15	0.70	0.63	0.61
Vitality	X	12.8	13.9	9.1	12.3	13.2	14.0	14.6
0–20*+	sem	0.6	0.6	1.16	1.32	0.81	0.75	0.80

* Range of scores; + high scores indicate positive well-being (i.e. lack of anxiety and depression).

surgery, the decrease in negative affect was significant at month 6 ($p = 0.03$) and month 12 ($p = 0.02$) as was the increase in affect balance at both measure points ($p = 0.01$).

In the subscales of the Psychological General Well-being Index (PGWB: see Table 2), part A survivors did not differ substantially from the healthy comparison group, but from the pre-operative part B patients in terms of increased well-being, health and vitality. Less pronounced were differences in anxiety, depression and self-control. Over time, part B patients showed

Table 3. Profile of mood states (POMS).

POMS		Cross-Sectional (part A)		Longitudinal (part B)				
		Healthy controls $n = 52$	HTX survivors $n = 41$	HTX pre-op $n = 16$	3 weeks post-op $n = 11$	6 weeks post-op $n = 17$	6 months post-op $n = 22$	12 months post-op $n = 13$
Depression	X	6.4	4.4	9.8	0.6	5.6	3.0	3.1
0–56*	sem	1.2	1.3	1.81	0.29	1.91	0.74	1.49
Vigor	X	16.4	13.7	6.2	7.3	9.53	11.23	11.9
0–28+	sem	0.8	0.8	1.46	1.35	1.39	1.24	1.66
Fatigue	X	8.6	4.7	9.5	4.2	5.82	4.18	2.69
0–28*	sem	0.8	0.8	1.82	1.26	1.08	0.91	0.77
Irritability	X	6.1	3.6	3.3	0.8	2.23	3.63	3.69
0–28*	sem	0.8	0.7	0.90	0.51	0.62	0.89	0.92

* Range of scores; + high scores indicate positive well-being.

an increase of ratings in all subscales, most clearly from the pre- to 3-weeks-post-operative level of well-being.

According to *t*-test results, 6-month post-operative levels of anxiety did not differ significantly from pre-operative levels and the increase in self-control failed to reach significance ($p = 0.06$). In contrast, significant positive changes from pre- to post-operative levels were found for depression ($p = 0.008$), well-being (0.003), health ($p = 0.003$) and vitality ($p = 0.001$). One year after surgery, the same pattern of significant differences to pre-operative data was maintained.

In the depression, fatigue and irritability subscales of the Profile of Mood States (POMS: see Table 3) HTX survivors from part A showed lower scores (i.e. better mood) than their healthy counterparts. The longitudinal data from part B indicate, however, that such well-being is only achieved after a vivid course of mood changes from before to one year after surgery: preoperative levels of depression, fatigue and lack of vigor exceeded the cross-sectional level more than twofold, while irritability levels were comparable across groups. Within the longitudinal group, vigor levels rose continuously over time while there was a dramatic drop in depression as well as in fatigue and irritability three weeks after HTX with an subsequent increase at week 6 and month 6. One year after surgery the POMS scores approached those of the cross-sectional part A patients. *t*-Test results for comparisons between pre- and 6-months postoperative data indicated a significant increase in vigor ($p = 0.02$) and decrease in fatigue ($p = 0.03$), while decreased depression failed to reach significance ($p = 0.06$) and irritability levels remained essentially unchanged. One year after surgery, no significant differences to the six month postoperative data were identified, indicating a stability of mood levels.

3.2. *Correlates of quality of life*

Using the five-point quality of life rating as global indicator of psychological well-being, correlations with psychosocial and clinical data were calculated. In the HTX-survivor group (part A), high global quality of life was correlated with PGWB-well-being ($r = 0.55$) everyday-life function ($r = 0.53$), POMS-vigor ($r = 0.47$), PGWB-vitality ($r = 0.46$) and symptom score ($r = -0.36$). Clinical variables such as time since transplantation, number of post-operative complications as well as age were unrelated to the quality of life rating.

In part B patients prior to surgery, however, clinical variables correlated with high global quality of life, the latter being negatively associated with high grades in NYHA-status ($r = -0.60$) and physical symptoms as orthopnea ($r = -0.59$), nykturia ($r = -0.56$) and angina pectoris ($r = -0.56$). Among the psychosocial variables, relationships to the global rating were found for the physical symptom score ($r = -0.73$), POMS-fatigue ($r = -0.66$) and POMS-depression ($r = -0.65$), ABS-positive affect ($r = 0.63$) and every-day life function ($r = 0.62$) as well as for PGBW-health ($r = 0.62$) and PGWB-anxiety scores ($r = -0.57$). A similar pattern of correlations was present six months after surgery. Here, high global quality of life correlated with POMS-fatigue ($r = -0.65$), everyday-life function ($r = 0.65$) and the PGWB subscores health ($r = 0.63$), vitality ($r = 0.63$) and well-being ($r = 0.62$). In addition to the symptom score ($r = -0.57$), correlations were also identified for clinical data on energy loss ($r = -0.77$), length of hospital stay ($r = -0.61$), angina ($r = -0.52$) and inappetence ($r = -0.52$). In contrast, preoperative correlates of 6-months global quality of life failed to yield substantial relationships to clinical data. High preoperative, POMS-irritability ($r = 0.91$) and PGWB-anxiety ($r = 0.64$) as well as a high symptom score ($r = 0.58$) however appeared to be predictors of a low postoperative quality of life.

3.3. *Subgroup analyses*

In HTX-survivors (part A), significantly impaired global quality of life was found in patients with abnormal vs. normal left ventricular function as well as in patients with transplant coronary disease vs. no disease and in retired vs. employed patients ($p = 0.01$). Other clinical criteria such as short vs. long time span since transplantation, high vs. low number of complications and preoperative diagnosis (coronary artery disease versus dilated cardiomyopathy) did not affect quality of life. For part B patients, preoperative cardiac diagnosis appeared to have an impact on 6-months post-operative state in that CAD patients (vs. dil. CMP) showed a higher global quality of life ($p = 0.04$), increased POMS-vigor ($p = 0.01$) and PGWB-vitality ($p = 0.04$) and a lower symptom score ($p = 0.01$). Again, dichotomization of patient groups in terms of age, NYHA status and number of complications did not yield significant differences with regard to the postoperative psychological state. Employment (in 20%) as compared to retirement for health and age reasons (in 57%) 6 months after surgery positively affected global quality of life ($p = 0.04$) as well as PGWB-well-being ($p = 0.02$) and POMS-depression scores ($p = 0.02$).

4. Discussion

The results of both the cross-sectional as well as the longitudinal part of the present study indicate a high level of psychological well-being of postoperative HTX-patients both with regard to the range of scales as well as to scores of a healthy comparison group. Such a good emotional outcome after HTX has been repeatedly reported in cross-sectional studies. Lough *et al.* [22] reported 'good' to 'excellent' quality of life judgements in 89% of respondents. Similar results were published by Evans *et al.* [11] in the National Heart Transplantation Study with regard to 'life satisfaction', 'well-being' and 'psychological affect', although HTX patients rated these domains as slightly less favorable than healthy controls. Two Australian studies by Jones *et al.* [23] and Harvison *et al.* [24] found even higher scores for Campbells Index of Well-being in HTX patients in comparison with healthy subjects. Thus, the positive outcome of the cross-sectional part A of the study corresponds to the literature. Methodologically, the study in its cross-sectional part is representative of the total sample of HTX patients transplanted at Munich University within the study deadlines (95% response rate). However, the shortcomings of cross-sectional surveys such as sample selection biases and neglect of time effects also apply to part A of the study. Therefore, the longitudinal part B of the study was added. The lack of published longitudinal data on HTX-patients' well-being, however, makes the comparative discussion of the part B results more difficult.

It is not surprising that according to these part B results, patients perceive their preoperative psychological state more negatively than their postoperative state as number and intensity of symptoms decrease and physical capacity increases after HTX. Changes are apparent not only from the time course of the examined variables, but also from the statistical comparisons of 6- and 12-month postoperative well-being indicators to the situation before surgery. This improvement, however, is not consistent across all variables. On a descriptive level, three patterns of change over time can be identified: an almost continuous increase, a dramatic change from before to 3 weeks after the operation with a subsequent steady state at a preoperative level as well as a varied time course with substantial fluctuations during recovery. Although, because of the small sample size, statistical repeated measures analysis was not performed, these patterns of change suggest that specific components of well-being may be differently affected by HTX. Psychological well-being, as a component of quality of life, in itself appears to be a multifacetted construct. By using global (quality of life rating, ACSA scale) as well as profile-type indicators with increasing degree of situational specificity (ABS, PGWB, POMS), a more focussed view on affective changes over time was possible in part B as compared to part A of the present study.

In the longitudinal part, methodological problems arose less with regard to patients' motivation to cooperate than with organizational failures to completely follow individual patients over a one-year course. Missing data thus limited the use statistical methods as well as the conclusions to be drawn from the data. The explorative analyses performed, however, yield potentially relevant suggestions for identifying the emotional potentials and problems of patients during their HTX-experience.

As concerns the determinants of quality of life, both study parts revealed the strong association between psychological well-being and global quality of life. Since the correlation coefficients explained about 25% of the variance, these concepts are neither unrelated (i.e. invalid) nor identical (i.e. redundant) and both merit assessment.

While clinical variables did not correlate highly with quality of life in the cross-sectional part A of the study, they did both at the pre-operative and the 6-months post-operative measure point. Thus, the actual physical state of the patients is associated with their quality of life before surgery and during recovery, but seems to loose its impact in long term survivors.

However, as subgroup analyses show, this is not true for the basic medical condition of the patients. Quality of life was high in cross-sectional patients with good cardiovascular function and in longitudinal patients suffering pre-operatively from CAD as compared to CMP. The latter finding might reflect the younger age and better employment status of CMP patients. In both study parts, employed as compared to non-working patients experienced a higher quality of life. This finding stresses the importance of professional rehabilitation which seems to be achieved in the majority of US-American and Australian HTX survivors [4,11,22,24]. In Germany, HTX-patients willing to work often face a hiring discrimination for health reasons or are offered jobs that earn less than their pension. Apart from employment status, other sociodemographic information such as age education or social network did not differentiate patients with regard to indicators of quality of life and well-being.

In conclusion, the data obtained in both study parts might be relevant for improved patient information and care. In terms of information, patient knowledge about the psychological outcome of HTX as well as about the fluctuations in well-being to be expected different time-spans might be helpful for improved adaptation and recovery [25]. In terms of patient care, individuals with emotional problems might profit from specific psychosocial support from professionals and family [26,27]. Since such interventions need a solid empirical foundation, further longitudinal studies on HTX patients' well-being are necessary.

On the basis of a state-of-the-art assessment of quality of life, which includes use of standardized and tested measures, studies should focus not only on the natural course of HTX-recovery, but also on the type of medical treatment after operation. An excellent example for such a strategy is a recent randomized trial of double vs. triple drug therapy using 11 indicators of quality of life a set of which addressed psychological well-being [23]. An elegant solution to integrating such multiple psychosocial outcomes to a single index for use in survival analysis was provided by O'Brien *et al.* [28]. Thus as a response to recent clinical advances in HTX [29], psychosocial endpoints should be incorporated to evaluate the benefits for the patients and to further identify areas and ways to improve patient well-being by both medical and psychological interventions.

Acknowledgement

This work was supported by the Biomedical Centre for Therapeutic Studies, Munich.

References

1. Hunt SA, Rider AK, Stinson EB, et al: Does cardiac transplantation prolong life and improve its quality? Circulation 1976;54(suppl 3):5660.
2. Wenger NK, Mattson ME, Furberg CD, Ellinson J (eds.): Assessment of quality of life in clinical trials of cardiovascular therapies. New York: Le Jacq Publishers, 1984.
3. Bullinger M, Ludwig M, Steinbüchel N von (eds): Lebensqualität bei kardiovaskulären Erkrankungen. Göttingen: Hogrefe Verlag, 1991.
4. Meister ND, McAleer J, Meister JS, Riley JE, Copeland JG: Returning to work after heart transplantation. J Heart Transplant 1986;5:154–161.
5. Kuhn WF, Brennan AF, Lacefield PK, Brohm J, Sekton VD, Gray LA: Psychiatric distress during stages of the heart-transplant protocol. J Heart Transplant 1990;9:25–29.
6. Mulligan T, Sheehan H, Hanrahan J: Sexual function after heart transplantation. J Heart Lung Transplant 1991;10:125–128.
7. Christopherson LK: Cardiac transplantation: a psychological perspective. Circulation 1987;75:57–62.
8. Christopherson LK, Griepp RB, Stinson EB: Rehabilitation after cardiac transplantation. JAMA 1976;236:2082–2084.
9. Meyendorf R, Dassing M, Scherer J, Klinner W, Kemkes B, Reichart B. Predictive and rehabilitative aspects in patients with heart transplantation. Herz 1989;14:308–321.
10. Evans RW, Manninen DL, Maier A, Garrison Jr LP, Hart LG: The quality of life of kidney and heart transplant recipients. Transplant Proc 1985;17:1579–1582.
11. Buxton MJ, Acheson R, Caine N, Gibson S, O'Brien BJ: Costs and benefits of the heart

transplant programmes at Harefield and Papworth hospitals. DHSS Research Report 12, London: HMSO, 1985.

12. Steward AL, Greenfield S, Hays RD, et al: Functional status and well-being of patients with chronic conditons JAMA 1989;262:907–913.
13. Bullinger M: Definition, conceptualization and implication of quality of life – a methodologists view. Theoret Surg 1991;6:143–148.
14. Bullinger M, Hasford J: Evaluating quality of life measures for german clinical trials. Contr Clin Trials 1991;12:915–1055.
15. McNair D, Lors M, Droppleman LF: EITS manual for the Profile of Mood States. Educational and Industrial Testing Service, San Diego, 1971.
16. Bullinger M, Heinisch M, Ludwig M, Geier S: Scales for the assessment of well-being. Psychometric evaluation of the Profile of Mood States (POMS) and the Psychological General Well-Being Index (PWGB). Z diff diag Psychologie 1990;11:53–61
17. Du Puy HJ: The Psychological General Well-Being (PGWB) Index. In: Wenger NK, Mattson ME, Furberg CD, Ellinson J (eds.): Assessment of quality of life in clinical trials of cardiovascular therapies. Le Jacq Publishers, New York 1984;170–183.
18. Bernheim J, Avonts G, De Schampheleire D, Gelissen I, Sauer AM: Anamnestic comparative self assessment (ACSA) to correlate medical and psychosocial variables with subjective quality of life of cancer patients. Proceedings of the American Society of Clinical Oncology; 1985;4:248–256.
19. Bradburn N: The structure of psychological well-being. Chicago: Aldine, 1969.
20. Angermann CE, Bullinger M, Spes CH, Zellner M, Kemkes BM, Theisen K: Quality of life in long-term survivors of heart transplantation. Europ J Cardiol, submitted.
21. Dixon WJ, Brown MB, Engeman L, et al: BMDP Statistical Software. Berkeley: University of California Press, 1983.
22. Lough ME, Lindsey AM, Shinn JA, Stotts NA: Life satisfaction following heart transplantation. Heart Transplant 1985;4:446–449.
23. Jones BM, Taylor FJ, Wright OM, et al: Quality of life after heart transplantation in patients assigned to double- or triple-drug therapy. J Heart Transplant 1990;9:392–396.
24. Harvison A, Jones BM, McBride M, Taylor F, Wright O, Chang VP: Rehabilitation after heart transplantation: The Australian experience. J Heart Transplant 1987;7:337–341.
25. Gunderson L: Teaching the transplant recipient. Heart Transplant 1985;4:226–227.
26. Rogers KR: Nature of spousal supportive behaviors that influence heart transplant patient compliance. Heart Transplant 1987;6:90–95.
27. Gier MD, Levick MD, Blazina PJ: Stress reduction with heart transplantation patients and their families: a multidisciplinary approach. Heart Transplant 1988;7:342–347.
28. O'Brien BI, Buxton MJ, Ferguson BA: Measuring the effectiveness of heart transplant programmes: quality of life data and their relationship to survival analysis. J Chron Dis 1987;40(suppl I):37S–153S.
29. Edward BS: Recent advances in cardiac transplantation. Current Opinion in Cardiology 1990;5:295–299.

42. Psychosocial outcome after heart transplantation

G. MAGNI and G. BORGHERINI

1. Introduction

With the rapid progress that has been made in the field of heart transplantation over the last 30 years, there has been a corresponding growth in our awareness of the importance of psychological factors in all stages of treatment.

An increasing number of centers are undertaking clinical heart transplantation programs whose focus is not only upon the length of survival, but also upon the quality of life. However, little research has been done on the possible relationship between long-term outcome and psychological variables evaluated before surgery. In the literature there are few prospective studies [1,2]. Mai et al. [1] found a high prevalence of preoperative anxiety and depression. Of 22 patients evaluated at follow-up after transplant three showed symptoms of considerable anxiety while only one patient became depressed. It was also possible to find that subjects with higher scores on the somatic scale of the general health questionnaire (GHQ) showed increased postoperative mortality.

Jones et al. [2] studied 14 of 38 recipients one year after transplant with follow-up evaluations also at discharge from hospital and at four and eight months after surgery. The study aimed to evaluate the recipients' anxiety, depression, body image and subjective quality of life by means of standardized self-assessment questionnaires. Before the tranplantation, 53% of patients reported an increase in anxiety and 24% of patients recorderd scores that indicated mild-to-moderate levels of depression. Thirty-seven percent of patients showed a deterioration in their quality of life and 34% of patients had a negative body image. After the transplantation, significant improvements occured in all parameters, and were maintained at the follow-ups.

We report here a prospective study on the long-term (one-year) outcome after transplantation, in which different psychosocial variables were evaluated.

Paul J. Walter (ed.): Quality of Life after Open Heart Surgery, 457–465.

2. Subjects and methods

We have studied all consecutive patients evaluated preoperatively in the Department of Cardiovascular Surgery of the Padova University between May 1987 and May 1990. Of the 47 patients so identified who underwent transplantation during this period, seven patients were too young (15 years of age or younger), and four patients were not assessed because the interviewer was on leave at the time. In total 36 patients were assessed before transplantation. Five patients died during the waiting period, 5 transplanted patients died before discharge from hospital. All 26 surviving subjects returned for the one-year follow-up study.

This paper presents the results for these 26 recipients who have been assessed before transplantation, then followed-up at discharge from hospital and at three and 12 months after transplantation.

During the study period many more patients underwent transplantation in the same unit (>100) but the majority of them did not enter in the study protocol because their preoperative evaluation took place in other Italian Cardiovascular Departments and therefore patients were not suitable for our prospective study. The population of 26 patients included 24 men and 2 women. Fifteen (58%) had dilatative cardiomyopathy, 7 (28%) had ischaemic heart disease, 2 valvular disease, 1 restrictive cardiomiopathy and 1 heart tumor. After transplant, patients remained hospitalized for a period of about one month (mean 29.4 ± 9.7 days).

Most of the patients (84%) are between 40 and 60 years old, only 10% are less than 30 years old, the mean age is 47.1 years (S.D. 12.1). Of the 26 subjects, 23 patients were married and 3 were single. They had a mean of 8 years of education (range 3–15 years). Their occupations were: pensioners, 9 patients; professional occupations, 6 patients; employees, 4 patients; blue collar workers, 3 patients; self-employed workers, 3 patients; students, 1 patient.

The data were collected by means of interviews (conducted by the same interviewer [G.B]), standardized self-rating questionnaires and, lastly a systematic examination of clinical records cards.

The clinical and medical data collected included age, sex, marital status, occupation, type of cardiac disease, severity of the disease according to the New York Heart Association (NYHA) functional classification, type and number of rejections during one year after transplantation. Feelings about such aspects of transplantation as emotional reaction to the graft were also investigated.

Each patient completed three semi-structured interviews lasting a total of two to three hours during the pre-surgery evaluative period.

Emotional status and psychiatric aspects were measured by the Illness Behaviour Questionnaire (IBQ) [3], the Symptom Distress Checklist (SCL-90) [4], and the Schedule for Affective Disorders and Schizophrenia Lifetime version (SADS-L) [5]. The IBQ provides relevant information for the delineation of patient attitudes, ideas and emotions in relation to disease. It is composed of seven subscales including general hypochondriasis, disease conviction, denial, irritability, etc. (see Table 2). The SCL-90 evaluates the psychological distress experienced by the subject. It is divided into a series of subscales, including somatization, obsessiveness-compulsiveness, depression, anxiety, psychoticism, etc. (see Table 1). The Schedule for Affective Disorders and Schizophrenia is a standardized psychiatric interview which allows to perform psychiatric diagnoses based on the Research Diagnostic Criteria (RDC). After transplantation, when patients were in the Intensive Care Unit, the same psychiatrist evaluated, during a four days period, the presence of acute psychopathology (post-cardiotomy delirium). Statistical analysis was performed with the paired *t*-test, where appropriate.

3. Results

Before transplantation psychiatric diagnoses according to the Research Diagnostic Criteria were as follows: generalized anxiety disorder, 9 (35%); major depression, 5 (19%); minor depression, 1(4%); panic disorder, 1(4%); alcoholism, 1(4%); 15 patients had no diagnosis (58%). Two patients had a double diagnosis and two a triple diagnosis.

Only 8% of the sample (2 patients) presented post-cardiotomy delirium in the immediate post-transplantation period.

The mean scores for psychological distress (Table 1) before and immediately after the operation (before discharge from hospital) showed a significant reduction in scores obtained on several subscales, in particular depression, anxiety, interpersonal sensitivity, and psychoticism as well as in the overall score for the whole test. Marked reductions were found for several subscales of SCL-90 between the mean scores before and three months after transplant and before and one year after transplant.

The percentage of patients with moderate psychological distress (scores of 1 or higher) before transplant (Figure 1) was particulary high for the following subscales: sleep disturbances (50%), somatization (38%), depression and anxiety (27% each). At the one-year follow-up the percentages for the same subscales had dropped to about 4%. The percentage of patients with sleep disturbances remained relatively high (23%).

Table 2 shows the data for the IBQ; there was no significant difference between the preoperative and post-operative scores, except for the subscale measuring disease conviction, which significantly decreased immediately after transplant. Two subscales significantly improved (affective inhibition and disease conviction) three months after surgery while all subscales except denial and psychological vs somatic perception of illness significantly improved one year after transplant.

Table 1. Mean SCL-90 scores before transplantation and at each assessment after transplantation (No. Patients = 26).

	Pretransplant	Discharge	t	P	Pretransplant	3 Months	t	P	Pretransplant	1 year	t	P
1. Somatization	0.8 ± 0.45	0.71 ± 0.47	0.8	NS	0.8 ± 0.45	0.33 ± 0.29	5	<0.0005	0.8 ± 0.45	0.31 ± 0.27	5.6	<0.0005
2. Obsessiveness-Compulsiveness	0.65 ± 0.41	0.54 ± 0.77	0.8	NS	0.65 ± 0.41	0.48 ± 0.36	1.7	NS	0.65 ± 0.41	0.38 ± 0.39	3	<0.01
3. Interpersonal Sensitivity	0.44 ± 0.4	0.27 ± 0.28	2.3	<0.05	0.44 ± 0.4	0.22 ± 0.23	2.9	<0.01	0.44 ± 0.4	0.3 ± 0.38	1.9	NS
4. Depression	0.73 ± 0.56	0.43 ± 0.46	3.2	<0.005	0.73 ± 0.56	0.29 ± 0.24	4	<0.001	0.73 ± 0.56	0.3 ± 0.34	4.3	<0.0005
5. Anxiety	0.66 ± 0.38	0.48 ± 0.43	2.4	<0.05	0.66 ± 0.38	0.28 ± 0.28	5.9	<0.0005	0.66 ± 0.38	0.35 ± 0.27	4	<0.001
6. Hostility	0.51 ± 0.47	0.31 ± 0.39	1.8	NS	0.51 ± 0.47	0.29 ± 0.38	2.1	<0.05	0.51 ± 0.47	0.33 ± 0.37	1.9	NS
7. Phobic Anxiety	0.26 ± 0.33	0.18 ± 0.21	1.1	NS	0.26 ± 0.33	0.14 ± 0.22	1.7	NS	0.26 ± 0.33	0.14 ± 0.24	2.1	<0.05
8. Paranoid Ideation	0.39 ± 0.46	0.32 ± 0.33	0.9	NS	0.39 ± 0.46	0.21 ± 0.26	1.6	NS	0.39 ± 0.46	0.26 ± 0.45	1.8	NS
9. Psychoticism	0.42 ± 0.36	0.2 ± 0.32	3.6	<0.005	0.42 ± 0.36	0.14 ± 0.18	4.3	<0.0005	0.42 ± 0.36	0.28 ± 0.35	4.5	<0.0005
10. Sleep Disturbances	1.13 ± 1.06	0.95 ± 0.95	1.0	NS	1.13 ± 1.06	0.55 ± 0.66	2.9	<0.01	1.13 ± 1.06	0.4 ± 0.67	3.0	<0.01
11. Global	0.58 ± 0.33	0.41 ± 0.35	3.1	<0.005	0.58 ± 0.33	0.29 ± 0.22	5	<0.0005	0.58 ± 0.33	0.29 ± 0.27	5	<0.0005

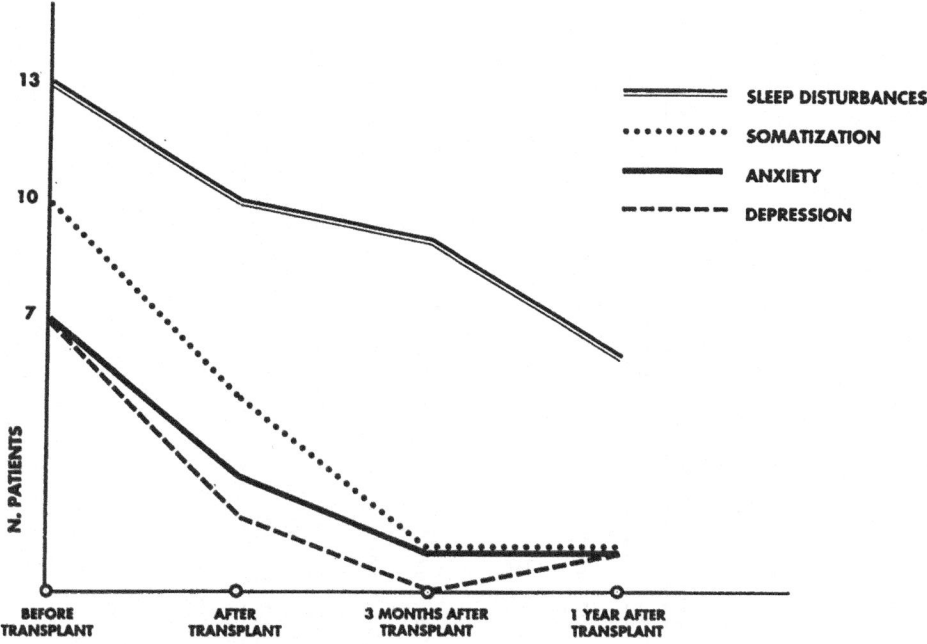

Figure 1. Scores of 1 or higher of four subscales of the SCL-90 before transplantation and at each assessment after transplantation. No. patients 26.

In our sample 80% of patients returned to full ot part-time work by the time of the 12 months' follow-up.

4. Discussion

We found in our transplant candidates a relatively high frequence of psycho-pathology (particulary affective and anxiety disorders), with slightly more than 40% of the sample presenting a psychiatric disturbance, and a relatively high level of psychological distress. The proportion of patients in this study who reported significant anxiety and depression before cardiac trans-plantation is similar to that reported by Mai et al. [1] and Jones et al. [2] in their prospective studies. With regard to the prevalence of panic disorder in transplant candidates, as previously reported [6], we definetely found lower percentage than Kahn et al. [7] who have proposed an association between idiophatic cardiomyopathy and panic disorder.

After transplant there was a general improvement of psychological distress which continued over time up to the twelve months assessment period. Only two patients still reported indices of moderate psychological distress one year after transplantation. The only exception to this respect is represented by sleep disorders which continue to be present in about one patient out of four

Table 2. Mean IBQ scores before transplantation and at each assessment after transplantation (No. Patients = 26).

	Pretransplant	Discharge	t	P	Pretransplant	3 Months	t	P	Pretransplant	1 year	t	P
1. General Hypochondriasis	2.85 ± 1.57	2.27 ± 1.48	1.4	NS	2.85 ± 1.57	2.65 ± 1.77	0.5	NS	2.85 ± 1.57	1.96 ± 1.54	2.8	<0.05
2. Disease Conviction	3.58 ± 1.58	2.62 ± 1.44	3.4	<0.005	3.58 ± 1.58	1.46 ± 1.27	7.6	<0.0005	3.58 ± 1.58	1.35 ± 1.35	6.4	<0.0005
3. Psycholoical vs somatic perception of illness	1.77 ± 0.82	2.04 ± 0.96	-1.3	NS	1.77 ± 0.82	1.65 ± 0.8	0.6	NS	1.77 ± 0.82	2.04 ± 0.6	-1.5	NS
4. Affective inhibition	2.81 ± 1.33	2.54 ± 1.39	0.8	NS	2.81 ± 1.33	2.0 ± 1.55	2.7	<0.05	2.81 ± 1.33	2 ± 1.5	3.4	<0.005
5. Affective disturbance	2.65 ± 1.5	2.15 ± 1.76	1.5	NS	2.65 ± 1.50	1.65 ± 1.74	2.6	<0.05	2.65 ± 1.5	1.08 ± 1.23	5.2	<0.0005
6. Denial	3.54 ± 1.5	3.27 ± 1.61	0.8	NS	3.54 ± 1.5	3.38 ± 1.1	0.5	NS	3.54 ± 1.5	4.12 ± 1.07	-1.9	<0.06
7. Irritability	2.08 ± 1.57	1.85 ± 1.74	0.7	NS	2.08 ± 1.57	1.58 ± 1.63	1.8	NS	2.08 ± 1.57	1.19 ± 1.23	2.6	<0.05

at the one year follow-up. The improvement of psychological distress may easily be explained by the dramatic improvement of the physical conditions after heart transplant. At the same time the presence of quite high levels of anxiety and depression before transplant could be correlated with the heavy symptomatology caused by the severe cardiological disease. However it is worthy here to mention that not all patients undergoing heart surgery show a similar pattern of virtually complete recovery in the great majority of the indices of psychological distress. In a previous study [8] we performed in subjects undergoing a cardiac valve replacement or an aortocoronary bypass, 25% of the sample did not show a significant improvement in psychological distress at the one year follow-up.

Illness behaviour measured with IBQ showed a general improvement, however apart from disease conviction which changed soon after surgery, the other indices took some time to change. Moreover we found an increase in denial one year after transplant. It may be conjectured that while the patients somewhat recognize themselves as being less ill, their attitudes toward the diseases and the emotional response to it do not undergo substantial modification before a certain lag of time. Moreover the presence and the increase over time of denial might suggest that it serves an important protective and adaptive function. An essential requirement for adaptation is the need to incorporate a new body image of a vital organ. Regarding this aspect Mai [9] reported 'that for some individuals a heart transplant is a traumatic event at a psychic level, and that denial serves a protective function during the period of adjustment.' Lastly, we wish to underline that the general improvement of IBQ scores found in this study appears to be in contrast with the findings of our previous prospective study on patients who received cardiac valve replacement or coronary artery bypass graft: except for the score for disease conviction, which had significantly decreased at the one-year follow-up evaluation there were no differences between scores before surgery and one year after surgery. This seems to indicate that though the changes in heart transplant patients are slow, they finally take place after some months. This was not the case for other cardiac surgery patients. As previously reported, it may well be true that some scales of the IBQ measure variables which are deeply rooted in the personality of the subject and therefore less likely to be influenced by the surgery. The change in heart transplant could be due to the high emotional content of the 'transplant' surgery.

It was extremely encouraging that 80% of patients returned to full or part-time work by the time of the 12 months follow-up. This finding was similar to the percentage obtained by Jones et al. [2] and better than those that have been published in other studies [10,11].

In conclusion this study has shown that heart transplant is accompanied by an overall improvement in several indices of psychosocial adjustment one year after surgery. Very few patients seem to be still 'symptomatic' from the psychological point of view, though sleep disturbances are still significantly present in about one patient out of four.

We are going to carefully reassess from the psychiatric point of view all the patients 2 and 3 years after the operation with the same psychiatric interview (SADS-L) used in the preoperative period.

5. Summary

Since 1987 we have been studying the emotional impact of cardiac transplantation on the recipients and their families.

This study presents the results for a group of recipients who have been assessed before transplantation, then followed-up at discharge from hospital and at three and 12 months after transplantation. We have evaluated the patients' psychological distress, illness behaviour, and psychiatric profile by means of the Symptom Distress Checklist (SCL-90), the Illness Behaviour Questionnaire (IBQ), and the Schedule for Affective Disorders and Schizophrenia Lifetime version (SADS-L). Before transplantation the most frequent psychiatric diagnoses were generalized anxiety disorder (35%) and major depression (19%). Only two patients developed a post-cardiotomy delirium after transplant. Immediately after transplantation psychological distress improved, in particular the depression, anxiety, psychoticism and interpersonal sensitivity subscales showed mean scores significantly lower than those before transplantation. This process continued through the follow-up period with all the relevant indices of psychological distress showing clear and significant improvement. Illness behaviours also improved, but this change required more time to take place. Eighty percent of the patients returned to full or part-time work by the time of the 12 months' follow-up.

References

1. Mai FM, McKenzie FN, Kostuk WJ: Psychiatric aspects of heart transplantation: preoperative evaluation and postoperative sequelae. Br Med J 1986;292:311–313.
2. Jones BM, Chang VP, Esmore D et al.: Psychological adjustment after cardiac transplantation. Med J Aust 1988;149:118–122.
3. Pilowski I, Spence ND: Manual for the Illness Behaviour Questionnaire (IBQ). Adelaide, Australia, University of Adelaide, 1981.
4. Derogatis LR, Rickels K. Rock AF: The SCL-90 and the MMPI: A step in the validation of a new self-report scale. Br J Psychiatry 1976;128:280–289.
5. Endicott J. Spitzer RL: Use of the Research Diagnostic Criteria and the Schedule for Affective Disorders and Schizophrenia to study affective disorders. Am J Psychiatry 1979;136:52–56.
6. Magni G, Borgherini G, Canton G: Idiopathic cardiomyopathy and panic disorder in cardiac transplant candidates (letter). Am J Psychiatry 1988;145:902–903.

7. Kahn JP, Drusin RE, Klein DF: Idiopathic cardiomyopathy and panic disorder: clinical association in cardiac transplant candidates. Am J Psychiatry 1987;144:1327–1330.
8. Magni G, Unger HP, Valfré C et al.: Psychosocial outcome one year after heart surgery: a prospective study. Arch Intern Med 1987;147:473–477.
9. Mai F, Burley J: Psychological aspects of heart transplantation. Transplantation Today 1985; 2: 52–56.
10. Lough ME, Lindsey AM, Shinn JA et al.: Life satisfaction following heart transplantation. J Heart Transplant 1985; 4: 446–449.
11. Meister ND, McAleer MJ, Meister IS: Returning to work after heart transplantation. J Heart Transplant 1986; 5: 154–161.

D: Performance of Social Roles

43. Psychosocial aspects of heart transplantation: a comparative analysis

ROGER W. EVANS

1. Introduction

Only recently has heart transplantation become considered as established therapy for end-stage cardiac disease. In the United States, completion of the National Heart Transplantation Study (NHTS), and the decision by the Health Care Financing Administration to extend Medicare benefits to eligible beneficiaries in need of a heart transplant, heralded a new era in cardiac replacement [1,2]. The experience was similar in the United Kingdom following completion of the U.K. Heart Transplant Study (UKHTS) [3–5]. Each of these studies evaluated both the costs and benefits of heart transplantation in an effort to respond to critics who were convinced that the costs associated with heart transplantation could hardly be justified based upon the benefits patients derived [6–15]. The generic underlying issue was essentially one of resource allocation, with critics maintaining that the resources expended on heart transplantation would be better allocated to other health care services intended to benefit a larger number of people at a substantially lower cost, an essentially utilitarian perspective [15–18].

In recent years, quality of life studies have become very popular in continuing efforts to provide a cost-benefit rationale for new and emerging health care technologies [19–21]. These technologies include drugs and devices, as well as medical and surgical procedures. Our earlier experience with heart transplantation has served as a worthy prototype for the analysis of a variety of new drugs (e.g., recombinant human erythropoietin, cyclosporine, antihypertensives) and transplant procedures (e.g., liver, heart-lung, pancreas) [22–39]. In each instance, these technologies are believed to offer considerable benefit, but at great expense to society [40,41]. Both the U.S. NHTS and the U.K. HTS demonstrated that it was possible to justify expensive procedures on the basis of cost-effectiveness. Now, in the United States, the Health Care Financing Administration plans to require, as one of its conditions for the payment of new technologies, that a cost-effectiveness analysis be performed [42,43]. Previously, coverage determinations were based upon

Paul J. Walter (ed.): Quality of Life after Open Heart Surgery, 469–482.
© 1992 Kluwer Academic Publishers.

affirmative answers to three questions: (1) was the technology safe? (2) was the technology effective? and (3) did the technology have widespread acceptance in the medical community [44,45].

Coupled with the foregoing concerns has been a greater appreciation of what is now referred to as 'outcomes' research [46–52]. While outcomes often refer to quality of care indicators, it is apparent that quality of life studies will also be captured under this same conceptual umbrella. Thus, what we have learned from quality of life studies in the field of cardiac transplantation has stimulated further inquiry and broader generalization across a number of health-related disciplines.

This paper focuses on three questions: (1) What is the quality of life of heart transplant recipients? (2) How does the quality of life of heart transplant recipients compare with that of kidney transplant recipients? and (3) What is the relationship between death, dying, and quality of life?

2. Conceptual framework

The concept of quality of life is multidimensional [30]. Of the many possible dimensions, two are foremost – the objective and the subjective. Several objective indicators have been systematically studied – ability to work, employment, functional ability, and health status [2,14,22,29–31]. Subjective indicators are often of a psychosocial or psychological orientation [30]. Several of these have also been empirically studied, including well-being, life satisfaction, psychological affect, and happiness. There are many other quality of life indicators that fall into either of these two categories, and most are deserving of study. However, in the course of developing a quality of life model, such as that proposed by Evans, the concept becomes very confusing [30]. Moreover, considering the existential basis of the quality of life concept, what qualifies as the 'purest' construct becomes more a matter of philosophy than of science.

Within the confines of this paper, it is impossible to either address or resolve all the conceptual and empirical issues underlying quality of life assessment. Several texts have been devoted to this subject, and most come up short on theory, are long methods, and steeped in philosophy [53–62]. To simplify matters, this analysis will be restricted to what we have found based upon a proven approach, an approach that has widespread acceptance.

3. Materials and methods

Data for this analysis have been obtained during the course of an ongoing series of quality of life studies at the Battelle-Seattle Research Center,

Seattle, Washington). These studies have been described at length elsewhere. We will only highlight here some of their more significant aspects.

During the course of the National Heart Transplantation Study, 152 heart transplant recipients from six transplant centers were interviewed regarding all aspects of their experience – quality of life, functional status, psychosocial adaptation, and social support [2,63]. The quality of life indicators used in the NHTS were identical to those previously used in the National Kidney Dialysis and Kidney Transplantation Study (NKDKTS) [22,30,64,65]. This study consisted of a survey of 859 patients from eleven dialysis and transplant centers located throughout the United States. These patients were on one of four end-stage renal disease treatment modalities – in-center hemodialysis, home hemodialysis, continuous peritoneal dialysis, and kidney transplantation. Finally, in a third study – the Kidney Transplant Immunosuppressive Protocols Study – the same quality of life indicators were used to survey 396 kidney transplant recipients associated with five renal transplant centers located throughout the United States [30,31].

Out of the many patients who participated in the foregoing studies, our attention will focus on four groups. These groups are as follows: (1) heart transplant recipients, (2) kidney transplant recipients transplanted under conventional immunosuppressive therapy (azathioprine and prednisone), and (3) kidney transplant recipients who received cyclosporine as their primary immunosuppressive agent. This latter group of patients is further divided into two groups – nondiabetics and diabetics.

The results presented here are descriptive. Our intent is to straightforwardly compare the quality of life of the patients in each of the foregoing groups. Often quality of life studies have been conducted in the abstract and, without comparison groups, it is difficult to interpret the meaning of the results.

4. Results

Studies have consistently shown that people who are chronically or terminally ill can be remarkably resilient in the face of extreme adversity [30]. Many patients even report a subjective quality of life which is on par with that of the general population [22,65]. The meaning of this is often difficult for health professionals to grasp. These studies have shown that there are many factors which enable an individual to adapt. Some patients have coping resources, both individual and social, that other people lack. These resources diminish the problems patients experience when facing their own mortality. This is remarkable, given that many patients in need of transplants are quite young – most have yet to live out half of their normal life expectancy.

Before presenting the results of this research, we will first provide a sociodemographic profile of the patient participants. We will then examine,

Table 1. Sociodemographic characteristics of patients.

Patient group	Age ($\bar{X}$)	Sex (%)		Race (%)			Education ($\bar{X}$)	Married (%)
		Male	Female	White	Black	Other		
Heart transplant	42.4	87.5	12.5	87.5	3.3	9.2	N/A	73.0
AZA kidney transplant[1]	37.2	56.3	43.8	84.7	11.8	3.5	12.2	64.6
CSA nondiabetic kidney transplant[2]	42.2	63.1	36.9	78.1	10.0	11.9	12.7	64.0
CSA diabetic kidney transplant[3]	39.8	65.3	34.7	96.4	0.0	3.6	13.0	65.2

N/A = not available as a statistical mean.
[1] Kidney transplant recipients on azathioprine and prednisone.
[2] Nondiabetic kidney transplant recipients on cyclosporine therapy.
[3] Diabetic kidney transplant recipients on cyclosporine therapy.

in detail, a variety of objective and subjective quality of life indicators. Finally, the paper concludes with the presentation of some data on the manner in which heart transplant recipients come to deal with the prospects of their mortality and their experience with dying.

4.1. *Sociodemographic characteristics*

As shown in Table 1, there are sociodemographic differences among the patients who have participated in our various studies. Age differences are rather insignificant, but over 87 percent of the heart transplant recipients are male. All patient groups are disproportionately white, consistent with several recent studies expressing concern over minority access to transplantation [66–69]. All patients are well-educated, according to today's standards. Although not shown, heart transplant recipients were, perhaps, the best-educated of the patients studied. Finally, about two-thirds to three-quarters of the patients were married. Social support has historically been a consideration in selecting transplant recipients [70,71].

Some of the sociodemographic differences identified in Table 1 could explain some of the variations we have observed in the quality of life variations among patients in our several studies. However, when we have statistically controlled for patient mix, quality of life differences have continued to persist between kidney dialysis and kidney transplant recipients [22].

Table 2. Sickness impact profile results.

Patient group	Score ($\bar{X}$)		
	Physical	Psychosocial	Total
Heart transplant	4.7	9.3	9.6
AZA kidney transplant[1]	3.3	4.1	5.5
CSA nondiabetic kidney transplant[2]	3.2	7.9	6.8
CSA diabetic kidney transplant[3]	11.9	12.8	15.0

[1] Kidney transplant recipients on azathioprine and prednisone.
[2] Nondiabetic kidney transplant recipients on cyclosporine therapy.
[3] Diabetic kidney transplant recipients on cyclosporine therapy.

4.2 *Objective quality of life indicators*

Health status and functional ability are critical aspects of the quality of life. In many respects, they determine quality of life and it could be argued, therefore, that rather than constituting quality of life indicators themselves, health status and functional ability act as independent predictors. Elsewhere we have debated the merits of this formulation and do not intend to extend it here [30].

4.2.1. *Health status*

The Sickness Impact Profile (SIP) is a health status measure we have used in each of our studies [2,30,31,65,73]. We have also used the Nottingham Health Profile, but will restrict our remarks to the SIP [31,72,74].

The SIP is a standardized questionnaire that measures sickness-related dysfunction. It consists of 136 questions that are grouped in 12 categories, each describing an area of activity in which dysfunctional behavior may occur. A score for each of the categories may be calculated, as well as a psychosocial dimension score, a physical dimension score, and an overall SIP score. Total SIP scores range from 0 to 100, where a high score indicates poor health status and a low score indicates good health. As the level of dysfunction experienced by the subject rises, so does the SIP score. In practice, the total mean score on the SIP ranges from 2 or 3 for a near typical control sample of the population to 35 or 37 for a homebound terminally ill or chronically ill sample [73].

Table 2 summarizes the mean physical, psychosocial, and total SIP scores for all four patient groups. In all respects, diabetic kidney transplant recipients are in the poorest health. Heart transplant recipients are considerably better, yet are not as well off as the remaining two groups of kidney transplant recipients.

The foregoing differences in objective health status are also reflected in the subjective assessments patients make of their health status, as is apparent

Table 3. Perceived health status.

Patient group	Health status (%)			
	Excellent	Good	Fair	Poor
Heart transplant	14.5	50.7	27.6	7.2
AZA kidney transplant[1]	29.4	43.4	22.4	4.9
CSA nondiabetic kidney transplant[2]	22.2	44.4	30.6	2.8
CSA diabetic kidney transplant[3]	4.1	44.9	36.7	14.3

[1] Kidney transplant recipients on azathioprine and prednisone.
[2] Nondiabetic kidney transplant recipients on cyclosporine therapy.
[3] Diabetic kidney transplant recipients on cyclosporine therapy.

from Table 3. Only 4.1 percent of the diabetic kidney transplant recipients felt they were in excellent health, compared with 14.5 percent of the heart transplant recipients, and between 22 and 29 percent of the other two patient groups. In the general population of the United States, 39 percent rate their health as excellent [75]. About 10 percent of the people rate their health as fair or poor.

4.2.2. *Functional limitations*

Compromised health status is usually reflected in the physical limitations people experience. This is very evident for the four groups of patients we studied using a standard set of questions taken from the Health Interview Survey (HIS) conducted by the National Center for Health Statistics. As shown in Table 4, diabetic kidney transplant recipients are the most debilitated of the patients we studied. Over 40 percent needed assistance in getting around the community. This compares with 8.6 percent of heart transplant recipients. The remaining two groups of kidney transplant recipients generally reported the lowest levels of functional impairment. However, regardless of patient group, over 50 percent of the patients we studied indicated that they were limited in doing something they would like to be able to do.

Despite the success of transplantation, it is clear that patients continue to have problems related to their activities of daily living. This is not always recognized by the clinicians involved in their care.

4.2.3. *Employment*

The goal of transplantation is to maximally rehabilitate the patient. The most direct indicator of rehabilitation is the productive capacity of the individual, usually represented by a return to the labor force. For many patients, return to work may be an unrealistic expectation. They may object to the harshness of judgments of social worth based upon employment.

As shown in Table 5, regardless of patient group, more people are able to work than do so. The gap between ability to work and employment is smallest for the diabetic kidney transplant recipients (8.1%). For the other

Table 4. Functional limitations.

Limitation	Patient group (%)			
	Heart transplant	AZA kidney transplant[1]	CSA nondiabetic kidney transplant[2]	CSA diabetic kindey transplant[3]
Need assistance traveling around community	8.6	7.7	4.9	40.8
Stay indoors most or all of the day because of health	6.6	9.0	3.5	18.4
Stay in bed most or all of the day because of health	6.6	9.0	2.1	18.4
Limited in vigorous activities	70.4	66.7	68.8	93.9
Trouble walking several blocks or climbing stairs because of health	34.2	39.9	32.3	63.3
Trouble bending, stooping, or lifting because of health	43.4	38.2	29.9	55.1
Trouble walking one block or climbing one flight of stairs because of health	16.4	17.4	15.9	38.8
Help in walking such as another person, cane, crutches, etc.	7.2	8.3	2.8	0.8
Unable to do certain amounts of work, housework, or schoolwork	52.6	38.9	38.9	71.4
Unable to work at job or do work around house	47.4	29.9	27.8	63.3
Need help eating, dressing, bathing, or using toilet	1.3	2.1	0.7	6.1
Limited in any way from doing anything he wants to	66.4	56.9	52.8	81.6

[1] Kidney transplant recipients on azathioprine and prednisone.
[2] Nondiabetic kidney transplant recipients on cyclosporine therapy.
[3] Diabetic kidney transplant recipients on cyclosporine therapy.

Table 5. Ability to work versus actually working.

Patient group	Work status (%)	
	Able to work	Working
Heart transplant	57.9	31.6
AZA kidney transplant[1]	74.1	45.9
CSA nondiabetic kidney transplant[2]	74.4	50.1
CSA diabetic kidney transplant[3]	34.7	26.6

[1] Kidney transplant recipients on azathioprine and prednisone.
[2] Nondiabetic kidney transplant recipients on cyclosporine therapy.
[3] Diabetic kidney transplant recipients on cyclosporine therapy.

Table 6. Patients receiving disability benefits.

Patient group	Percentage receiving disability benefits
Heart transplant	62.5
AZA kidney transplant[1]	41.0
CSA nondiabetic kidney transplant[2]	33.3
CSA diabetic kidney transplant[3]	59.2

[1] Kidney transplant recipients on azathioprine and prednisone.
[2] Nondiabetic kidney transplant recipients on cyclosporine therapy.
[3] Diabetic kidney transplant recipients on cyclosporine therapy.

three patient groups, the gap is very significant – between 24 and 26 percent of the patients who are able to work *are not doing so*.

It is often inappropriate to blame patients for their failure to return to the labor force. Many patients, because of physical and health-related limitations, may be unable to return to jobs they previously held. They may be unable to deal with physical demands. Employers may be reluctant to allow them to come back to work and, last but not least, the system by which disability benefits are administered in the United States may encourage people to retain their disability status. The financial rewards associated with disability may exceed the income earned through employment. Table 6 shows the percentage of patients receiving disability benefits, according to treatment modality, underscoring the tenuous relationship between income support and return to work.

4.3. *Subjective quality of life*

Numerous studies have shown that there may often be little association between objective and subjective quality of life [29]. In other words, severely debilitated patients may record a high level of life satisfaction, and a commendable level of happiness. Not every paraplegic prefers death to life. The same is true of transplant recipients.

In our many quality of life studies, we have used numerous standard subjective quality of life measures [30]. We have described these at length, and provided detailed reference material [31]. We prefer to use four indicators, as noted previously. These include the Index of Psychological Affect, the Index of Overall Life Satisfaction, and the Index of Well-Being. The Index of Psychological Affect, based on eight bipolar items, describes how patients feel about their present life, and responses are averaged for a mean score. The Index of Well-Being is calculated by combining the Index of Overall Life Satisfaction and the Index of Psychological Affect (giving slightly more weight to the former).

Both the Index of Psychological Affect and the Index of Life Satisfaction

Table 7. Subjective quality of life.

Patient group	Score		
	Well-being	Psychological affect	Life satisfaction
Heart Transplant			
Mean	11.11	5.49	5.11
Standard deviation	(2.53)	(1.32)	(1.28)
AZA Kidney Transplant[1]			
Mean	11.83	5.62	5.66
Standard deviation	(2.61)	(1.16)	(1.49)
CSA Nondiabetic Kidney Transplant[2]			
Mean	11.31	5.39	5.38
Standard deviation	(2.39)	(1.30)	(1.21)
CSA Diabetic Kidney Transplant[3]			
Mean	10.12	4.78	4.76
Standard deviation	(2.39)	(1.32)	(1.15)

[1] Kidney transplant recipients on azathioprine and prednisone.
[2] Nondiabetic kidney transplant recipients on cyclosporine therapy.
[3] Diabetic kidney transplant recipients on cyclosporine therapy.

range from a low of 1.0 (completely dissatisfied) to a high of 7.0 (completely satisfied). The Index of Well-Being ranges between 2.1 which indicates low well-being, and 14.7, which indicates high well-being.

The results of our analysis for the three measures just described are presented in Table 7. Once again, the general order of patient groups remains the same, with diabetic kidney transplant recipients having the poorest subjective quality of life. However, the equivalent scores for the general population on these indicators are also of interest. They are as follows: well-being ($\bar{X} = 11.77$, S.D. = 2.21); psychological affect ($\bar{X} = 5.68$, S.D. = 1.12) and life satisfaction ($\bar{X} = 5.54$, S.D. = 1.25) [22,53,65,76]. Although there is some variance between the transplant patient groups and the general population, these differences are not as substantial as might have been imagined.

Happiness can also be considered a quality of life indicator and, in general surveys of the U.S. public, a standard question is often used to ascertain the level of happiness of the population. We have incorporated this question in virtually all our quality of life studies. The question is as follows: 'Taking all things together, how would you say things are these days – would you say you're very happy, pretty happy, or not too happy?' The responses to this question are summarized in Table 8. As shown, diabetic kidney transplant recipients are least happy. However, on this measure, heart transplant recipients record a higher level of happiness than do the other two groups of kidney transplant recipients. It is noteworthy, that the general population reports a level of happiness far below that of patients in any of the four groups studied here. The general public responses are as follows: very happy, 22 percent; pretty happy, 68 percent; not too happy, 10 percent [2].

Table 8. Level of happiness.

Patient group	Level of happiness (%)		
	Very happy	Pretty happy	Not too happy
Heart transplant	50.0	37.5	11.8
AZA kidney transplant[1]	48.2	46.8	5.0
CSA nondiabetic kidney transplant[2]	34.7	53.5	11.8
CSA diabetic kidney transplant[3]	23.2	62.5	14.3

[1] Kidney transplant recipients on azathioprine and prednisone.
[2] Nondiabetic kidney transplant recipients on cyclosporine therapy.
[3] Diabetic kidney transplant recipients on cyclosporine therapy.

5. Discussion

The results presented here may, at first, appear to have little relationship to reality. People who have not yet confronted their own mortality may not, however, have the same appreciation of life as people who have been spared from death [77]. For most people, living is a preferred alternative to death, although it is yet unclear at precisely what point the quality of life becomes so compromised that death is a preferred alternative. Philosophically, we can assume that when the burdens of life outweigh the benefits of death, our own mortality becomes a desirable end. Perhaps people who commit suicide have grasped the very essence of what life should be yet, at the same time, cannot be. Death to the suicide victim is a preferred alternative, the ultimate act allowing one to escape an untenable reality. In this regard, it is unclear whether suicide is an act of the insane, or a release of creative energy (albeit self-destructive) that exceeds the boundaries of 'normal' human experience.

As these remarks suggest, the complex interplay between life and death must have as its common denominator some assessment of quality of life. A favorable assessment underscores our will to live, despite adversity, whereas a negative balance leads us to hasten, or at least envision, the consequences of premature death. We may grasp at every alternative to maintain our being but, at the same time, try to comprehend our nothingness. In isolation from the world around us, death becomes a more palatable event. However, if our own being is intricately intertwined with that of others around us, our own death is less acceptable, despite the level of our own quality of life experience. In effect, we view our life as a gift to be shared with others. Any act, overt or covert, by omission or commission, to suspend our existence, is considered selfish. Suicide is a selfish act, often intended to punish others.

Perhaps, therefore, the struggle to live is not so much for our own benefit, but for that of others upon whom we have come to depend or vice versa. The will to live is a powerful motivation. It surely allows many chronically and terminally ill people to go on living, despite enormous odds. Many a transplant surgeon will say that the most successful patient is a 'fighter' – a person who just does not give up. And, to aid in the fight for life, transplant teams frequently consider social and family support as critical in the patient selection process. Clearly, in the fight for life, we must enlist the support of others. Not only does this assure that the patient avoids isolation (and willingly embraces the terror of death) but, in addition, we create a social and emotional debt to others that can only be repaid by continuing our fight for life.

The existential dynamics of transplantation are generic to the experience of dying and the threat of death. Of the heart transplant survivors we have studied, over 85 percent consider their families to be close, supportive, and able to get along well. Families are close-knit and respond to the needs of their members. The transplant experience uniformly draws families together. Even still, most patients, despite what is clearly a complicated treatment regimen, do not feel they are excessively dependent upon others. Only 10 percent feel their dependence to be a great problem.

The majority of patients we have interviewed (79%) indicate that they have a very strong will to live but, even so, 64 percent do not find it difficult to accept the fact that they might die. Over 56 percent of the patients believe that there is life after death, and most (66%) have a religious or spiritual perspective on death. Only 15 percent of the patients acknowledge that the possibility of death makes them angry.

Dying makes us humble and death serves as the great equalizer. It appears, however, that some of us may be more capable of resetting the quality of life balance to sustain our own lives in an effort to repay what we may view as a debt we have inflicted upon our families and significant others. Dying is a social process, death an isolated event. Thus, it should come as no surprise that transplantation is a psychosocially demanding experience affecting patients and families alike. Nonetheless, the transplantation experience may increase family cohesion which, in turn, enables patients to cope with their life circumstances. No doubt this is why patients consistently say they are satisfied and happy with their lives, despite substantial physical limitations and enormous psychosocial trauma. At the same time, they are remarkably able to accept their own death as an inevitable event.

References

1. Evans RW, Manninen DL, Overcast TD, et al: The National Heart Transplantation Study: Final Report. Seattle, WA: Battelle Human Affairs Research Centers, 1984.
2. Roper WL: Medicare Program; Criteria for Medicare Coverage of Heart Transplants. Federal Register. 1987;52(65):10935–10951.
3. Buxton MJ, Acheson R, Caine N, Gibson S, O'Brien BJ: Costs and Benefits of the Heart Transplant Programmes at Harefield and Papworth Hospitals. DHHS Research Report No.12. London: HMSO, 1985.

4. Caine N, O'Brien V: Quality of life and psychological aspects of heart transplantation. In: Wallwork J. (ed.) Heart and Heart-Lung Transplantation. Philadelphia, PA: W.B. Saunders, 1989:389–422.

5. Caine N, Sharples LD, Smyth R, et al: Survival and quality of life of cystic fibrosis patients before and after heart-lung transplantation. Transplant Proc. 1991;23:1203–1204.

6. Knox RA: Heart transplants: to pay or not to pay. Science. 1980;209:570–575.

7. Centerwall BS: Cost-benefit analysis and heart transplantation – an editorial. N Engl J Med. 1981;304:901–903.

8. Evans DW: Cardiac transplantation (letter). Lancet. 1984;1(8376):567.

9. Evans RW: Heart transplants and priorities. Lancet. 1984;1(8381):852–853.

10. Evans RW: The socioeconomics of organ transplantation. Transplant Proc. 1985;17(6)Suppl 4:129–136.

11. Evans RW: Cost effectiveness analysis of transplantation. Surg Clin North Am. 1986;66:603–616.

12. Evans RW: The heart transplant dilemma. Iss in Sci Technol. 1986;2(3):91–101.

13. Evans RW: The economics of heart transplantation. Circulation. 1987;75:63–76.

14. Evans RW: A catastrophic disease perspective on organ transplantation. In: Ginzberg E. (ed.) Medicine and Society: Clinical Decisions and Societal Values. Boulder, CO: Westview Press 1987:61–95.

15. Dean M: Is your treatment economic, effective, efficient? Lancet. 1991;337(8739):480–481.

16. Welch HG, Larson EB: Dealing with limited resources: the Oregon decision to curtail funding for organ transplantation. N Engl J Med. 1988;319:171–173.

17. Drummond MF: Economic evaluation and the rational diffusion and use of health technology. Health Policy. 1987;7:309–324.

18. Drummond MF: Allocating resources. Int J Technol Assess Health Care. 1990;6:77–92.

19. Evans RW: Health care technology and the inevitability of resource allocation and rationing decisions. (First of two parts.) JAMA. 1983;249:2047–2053.

20. Evans RW: Health care technology and the inevitability of resource allocation and rationing decisions. (Second of two parts.) JAMA. 1983;249:2208–2219.

21. Mosteller F, Falotico-Taylor J (eds): Quality of Life and Technology Assessment. Washington, DC: National Academy Press 1989.

22. Evans RW, Manninen DL, Garrison LP, Jr., Hart LG, Blagg CR, Gutman RA, Hull AR, Lowrie EG: The quality of life of end-stage renal disease patients. N Engl J Med. 1985;312:553–559.

23. Croog SH, Levine S, Testa MA, et al: The effects of antihypertensive therapy on quality of life. N Engl J Med. 1986;314:1657–1664.

24. Fletcher A, McLoone P, Bulpitt C: Quality of life on angina therapy: a randomized controlled trail of transdermal glyceryl trinitrate against placebo. Lancet. 1988;2(8601):4–8.

25. Bankhead CD: EPO's cost stirs questions about rationing renal care. Medical World News. December 12 1988:48.

26. Eschbach JW, Abdulhadi MH, Browne JK, Delano BG, Downing MR, Egrie JC, Evans RW, Freedman RA, et al: Recombinant human erythropoietin in anemic patients with end-stage renal disease: results of a Phase III multicenter clinical trial. Ann Intern Med. 1989;111:992–1000.

27. Canadian Erythropoietin Study Group: Association between recombinant human erythropoietin and quality of life and exercise capacity of patients receiving dialysis. BMJ. 1990;300:573–578.

28. Evans RW: EPO: broader definitions of improved quality of life may be needed. Kidney '90. 1990;7(1):7–8.

29. Evans RW, Rader BL, Manninen DL, and the Cooperative Multicenter EPO Clinical Trial Group: The quality of life of hemodialysis recipients treated with recombinant human erythropoietin. JAMA. 1990;263:825–830.

30. Evans RW: Quality of life assessment and the treatment of end-stage renal disease. Transplantation Reviews. 1990;4(1):28–51.

31. Evans RW, Manninen DL, Thompson C: A Cost and Outcome Analysis of Kidney Transplantation: The Implications of Initial Immunosuppressive Protocol and Diabetes. Seattle, WA: Battelle Human Affairs Research Centers 1989.

32. Manninen DL, Evans RW: The costs and outcomes of kidney transplantation according to initial immunosuppressive drug protocol: In: Terasaki PI, (ed.) Clinical Transplants 1987. Los Angeles, CA: UCLA Tissue Typing Laboratory 1987:269–275.

33. Wall WJ, Grant DR, Ghent C, et al: Liver transplantation: the University Hospital-Children:s Hospital of Western Ontario experience. Terasaki PI: (ed.) Clinical Transplants 1988. Los Angeles, CA: UCLA Tissue Typing Laboratory 1988:45–51.

34. Zitelli BJ, Miller JW, Gartner JC, Jr. et al: Changes in life-style after liver transplantation. Pediatrics. 1988;82:173–180.

35. Tarter RE, Erb S, Biller PA, Switala JA, Van Thiel D: The quality of life following liver transplantation: a preliminary report. Gastroenterol Clin North Am. 1988;17:207–217.

36. Wolcott D, Norquist G, Busuttil K: Cognitive functions and quality of life in adult liver transplantation. Transplant Proc. 1989;21(3):3563.

37. Corry RJ, Zehr P: Quality of life in diabetic recipients of kidney transplants is better with the addition of the pancreas. Clin Transplant. 1990;4:238–241.

38. Nakache R, Tyden G, Groth CG: Quality of life in diabetic patients after combined pancreas-kidney or kidney transplantation. Diabetes. 1989;38(Suppl 1):40–42.

39. Voruganti LNP, Sells RA: Quality of life of diabetic patients after combined pancreatic renal transplantation. Clin Transplantation. 1989;3:78–82.

40. Erslev AJ: Erythropoietin. N Engl J Med. 1991;324:1339–1344.

41. Doolittle RF: Biotechnology – the enormous cost of success. N Engl J Med. 1991;324:1360–1362.

42. Roper WL: Medicare program;criteria and procedures for making medical services coverage decisions that relate to health care technology. Federal Register. 1989;54(18):4302–4318.

43. Leaf A: Cost effectiveness as a criterion for medicare coverage. N Engl J Med. 1989;321:898–900.

44. Office of Technology Assessment Medical Technology and Costs of the Medicare Program. Washington, DC: U.S. Congress, Office of Technology Assessment, OTA-H-227 1984.

45. National Advisory Council on Health Care Technology Assessment. The Medicare Coverage Process. Rockville, MD: National Center for Health Services Research and Health Care Technology Assessment 1988.

46. Ebbs SR, Fallowfield LJ, Fraser SCA, Baum XY: Treatment outcomes and quality of life. Int J Technol Assess Health Care. 1989;5:391–400.

47. Schroeder SA: Outcome assessment 70 years later: are we ready? N Engl J Med. 1987;316:160–162.

48. Ellwood PM: Outcomes management: a technology of patient experience. N Engl J Med. 1988;318:1549–1556.

49. Lohr KN: Outcome measurement: concepts and questions. Inquiry. 1988;25:37–50.

50. Bloom BS: Does it work? The outcomes of medical interventions. Int J Technol Assess Health Care. 1990;6:326–332.

51. Geigle R, Jones SB: Outcomes measurement: a report from the front. Inquiry. 1990;27:7–13.

52. Epstein AM: The outcomes movement – will it get us where we want to go? N Engl J Med. 1990;323:266–270.

53. Campbell A, Converse PE, Rodgers WL: The Quality of American Life: Perceptions, Evaluations, and Satisfactions. New York, NY: Russel Sage Foundation, 1976.

54. Campbell A: The Sense of Well-Being in America: Recent Patterns and Trends. New York: McGraw-Hill, 1980.

55. Bradburn, NM and Caplovitz D: Reports on Happiness. Chicago, IL: Aldine, 1965.
56. Wenger NK, Mattson ME, Finberg CD, Elinson (eds.): Assessment of Quality of Life in Clinical Trials of Cardiovascular Therapies. New York: Le Jacq Publishing, Inc., 1984.
57. McDowell I, Newell C: Measuring Health: A Guide to Rating Scales and Questionnaires. New York: Oxford University Press, 1987.
58. Walker SR, Rosser RM: Quality of Life: Assessment and Application. Boston, MA: MTP Press, 1988.
59. Smith G Teeling (ed.): Measuring Health: A Practical Approach. New York: Alan R. Liss, 1988.
60. Williams JI, Wood-Dauphinee S: Assessing quality of life: measures and utility. In: Mosteller F, Falotico-Taylor J, (eds.) Quality of Life and Technology Assessment. Washington, DC: National Academy Press, 1989.
61. Streiner DL, Norman GR: Health Measurement Scales: A Practical Guide to Their Development and Use. New York: Oxford University Press, 1989.
62. Spilker B (ed.): Quality of Life Assessments in Clinical Trials. New York: Raven Press, 1990.
63. Evans RW, Manninen DL, Maier A, Garrison LP, Jr., Hart LG: The quality of life of kidney and heart transplant recipients. Transplant Proc. 1985;17:1579–1582.
64. Evans RW, Hart LG, Manninen DL: A comparative assessment of the quality of life of successful kidney transplant patients according to source of graft. Transplant Proc. 1984;16:1353–1358.
65. Evans RW, Manninen DL, Garrison LP, Jr., Hart LG: Special Report: Findings from the National Kidney Dialysis and Kidney Transplantation Study. HCFA Pub. No. 03230. Baltimore, MD: Health Care Financing Administration, 1987.
66. Kjellstrand CM: Age, sex, and race inequality in renal transplantation. Arch Intern Med. 1988;148:135–139.
67. Hagle ME, Rosenberg JC, Lysz K, Kaplan MP, Sillix D, Jr: Racial perspectives on kidney transplant donors and recipients. Transplantation. 1989;48:421–424.
68. Office of Inspector General: Office of Evaluations and Inspections. The distribution of organs for transplantation: expectations and practices. Washington, DC: Government Printing Office 1990. (DHHS publication No (OEI) 01-89-0550.)
69. Kasiske BL, Neylan JF, III, Riggio RR, et al: The effect of race on access and outcome on transplantation. N Engl J Med. 1991;324:302–307.
70. Copeland J, Stinson EB: Human heart transplantation. Curr Probl Cardiol. 1979;4:1–51.
71. Baumgartner WA, Reitz BA, Oyer PE, Stinson EB, Shumway NE: Cardiac homotransplantation. Curr Probl Surg. 1979;16:2–61.
72. Bergner M: Development, testing, and use of the Sickness Impact Profile. In: Walker SR, Rosser RM: Quality of Life: Assessment and Application. Boston, MA: MTP Press Ltd. 1988:79–94.
73. Hart LG, Evans RW: The functional status of ESRD patients as measured by the Sickness Impact Profile. J Chron Disease. 1987;40(Suppl 1):117s–130s.
74. Hunt SM, McEwen J, McKenna SP: Measuring Health Status. Beckenham, Kent: Croom Helm, 1986.
75. Ries P: Americans assess their health: United States 1987. National Center for Health Statistics. Vital Health Stat. 1990;10(174).
76. Evans RW, Manninen DL, Livak C: The Kidney Transplant Health Insurance Study. Seattle, WA: Battelle Human Affairs Research Centers, 1990.
77. Becker E: The Denial of Death. New York, NY: The Free Press 1973.

44. Changes in partnership after cardiac transplantation

A. GRUNDBÖCK, B. BUNZEL and M.T. SCHUBERT

1. Introduction

Heart transplantation has become an acceptable therapeutic intervention for patients with end-stage heart disease. Coping with heart transplantation concerns not only one individual, but at least two. Although the disease threatens the life expectancy of only one partner, it does affect the life quality of both partners by forcing them to adapt to the new situation and cope with the problems.

Until recently, research involving the heart transplant patient's support systems and needs of family members has had low priority. Christopherson [1] reported changes in patterns of family interaction and role assignment during the *waiting period*. Patients have to leave pre-transplant functions to the spouses [2]. Usually they care for the welfare of the patient which is often very stressful for them. Possible conflicts in the marital relationship are blocked to ensure the patient's welfare [3]. These results were emphasized in a study by Rogers [4]: during the first 6 months to a year after heart transplantation, patients tend to become dependent on the spouse for material needs until they are capable of meeting their own needs. The waiting period is not only a stressful time, but even a time where partners are drawing closer together and a period of enrichment within their relationship [5,6].

In the *postoperative period* the couples realize that a new life-style must be structured, which is based on the patient's unpredictable future. Reversed roles adopted because of the patient's disease may no longer fit. Female partners must give up roles adopted preoperatively; the patients themselves have to change from the 'sick' to the 'well' role with all its pros and cons [7]. Furthermore the spouses are forced to modify their pattern of control and monitoring of the patient's welfare as this behaviour becomes unbearable for the patients, who are eager to regain self-control postoperatively. The success of this process depends on the degree of interpersonal conflict and on interpersonal resources for crisis management. Even one year after surgery

Paul J. Walter (ed.): Quality of Life after Open Heart Surgery, 483–490.
© 1992 Kluwer Academic Publishers.

Table 1. Patient data.

Number of patients		*N* = 43	
Age of patients	18–30	3	
	31–40	4	
	41–50	16	
	51–60	18	
	Older than 60	2	
Diagnosis	coronary heart disease	13	
	Cardiomyopathy	30	
Years married	up to 10	7	
	11–20	5	
	21–30	16	
	31–40	14	
	More than 40	1	
Number of children	0	7	
	1	11	
	2	15	
	3	4	
	4	4	
	More than 4	2	
Education	pre-high school	32	
	High school graduate	9	
	College	2	
Occupation	self-employed	3	
	Office worker	8	
	Manager	13	
	Farmer	3	
	Blue-collar worker	16	
Pre- and post-transplant employment		Preoperative	Postoperative
	Full-time	5	8
	Sick leave	15	0
	Retired early for		
	Health reasons	22	26
	Retired	1	9

patients and partners report that roles have not yet returned to their previous status [3].

It was the aim of our study to investigate (a) if and (b) in which areas changes in partnership could be found one year after surgery.

2. Methods

2.1. *Patients and study design*

We studied 43 transplant patients who had undergone surgery in 1988 and 1989 and their female partners. Table 1 shows the patient data and the indication for transplantation. Patients and partners were interviewed separately in a relaxed private setting. The data were collected by testing the subjects with the Dyadic Relationship Scale of the Family Assessment Measure (FAM) [8] and by using a short interview guide. Data were collected once more one year after heart transplantation.

2.2. *Instruments*

The Dyadic Relationship Scale of the Family Assessment Measure (FAM) was used in Cierpka's German version [9]. FAM is a self-report instrument that provides quantitative indices of family strengths and weaknesses. The Dyadic Relationship Scale, one component of FAM, examines the relationship between specific pairs. It consists of 42 items and 7 subscales called: task accomplishment (TA), role performance (RP), communication (COM), affective expression (AE), involvement (I), control (C), and values and norms (VN). Most scores for nonclinical families should be between 40 and 60. Scores below 40 indicate healthy functioning, scores of 60 and above considerable disturbance [10].

The theoretical dimensions of the scales were described by Steinhauer *et al.* [7] as follows: 'To accomplish these tasks requires that family members perform successfully a variety of roles (role performance). Effective role performance demands the communication of information essential to task accomplishment and ongoing role definition, including the communication of feeling that can either impede or facilitate task accomplishment and role performance (Affective Expression). Similarly, member's emotional involvement with each other (Affective Involvement) and their ways of influencing one another (Control), may either help or hinder the family task accomplishment.'

2.3. *Statistical methods*

There were two main questions we wanted to answer:

(1) Is there a significant difference between patients (men) and partners (women) in the pre- and postoperative period? Male/female profiles were compared by paired Student's *t*-tests.
(2) Is there a significant difference between the pre- and postoperative period if we consider the profiles of men and women separately?

The comparison of women's pre- and postoperative profiles was done by paired Student's *t*-tests. The same was done for men's profiles. The standard significance level was 0.05.

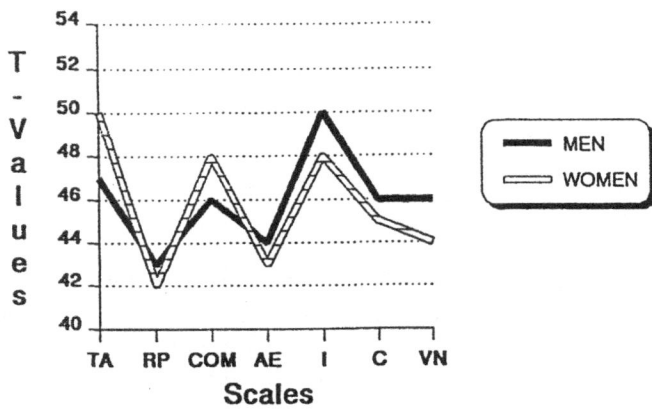

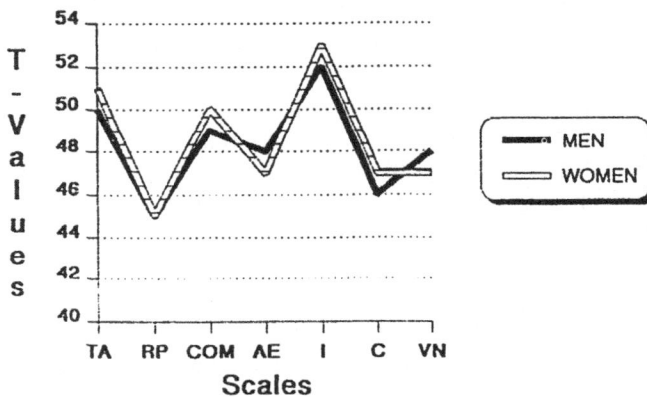

Figure 1. Dyadic relationship scale: Men–women profiles in the pre- and postoperative period.

3. Results

The assessment of partnership in the pre- and postoperative period is shown in Figure 1. The solid line shows the scores of men and the broken line indicates the scores of women. All profiles achieved are in the average range. No significant differences could be found. The same is true for the postoperative situation.

Figure 2 shows the profiles of the preoperative (solid line) and postoperative (broken line) situation, for both men and women. Although all scores achieved are in the average range, significant differences (marked with asterisks) could be found: postoperatively men showed significant differences in task accomplishment affective expression and involvement, whereas women

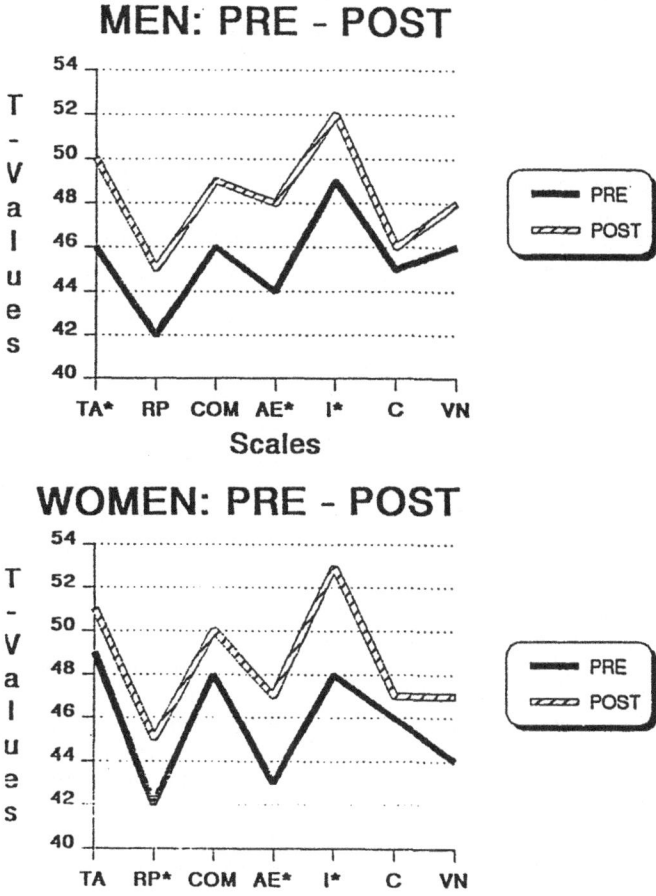

Figure 2. Dyadic relationship scale: pre- and postoperative profiles of women, pre- and postoperative profiles of men.

revealed significant differences in role performance and, in the same way as their partners in affective expression and involvement.

Table 2 lists the definitions of these scales [10].

4. Discussion

The most surprising aspect of the results was the fact that all values were in the normal range. On the basis of our experience with heart transplant patients and their female partners we would have expected results in the range of Family Problems of the FAM test. On the other hand, the scales where significant differences did occur confirm our clinical experience.

Clinical observation has shown that heart transplantation seems to have a

Table 2. The Family Assessment Measure (FAM) interpretation guide.

1. TASK ACCOMPLISHMENT

LOW SCORES (40 and below) STRENGTH	HIGH (60 and above) WEAKNESS
– basic tasks consistently met	– failure of some basic tasks
– flexibility and adaptability to change in developmental tasks	– inability to respond appropriately to changes in the family life cycle
– functional patterns of task accomplishment are maintained even under stress	– problems in task identification, generation of potential solutions, and implementation of change
– task identification shared by family members, alternative solutions are explored and attempted	– minor stress may precipitate a crisis

2. ROLE PERFORMANCE

LOW SCORES (40 and below) STRENGTH	HIGH SCORES (60 and above) WEAKNESS
– roles are well integrated: family members understand what is expected, agree to do their share and get things done	– insufficient role integration, lack of agreement regarding role definitions
– Members adapt to new roles required in the development of the family	– inability to adapt to new roles required in evolution of the family life cycle
– no idiosyncratic roles	– idiosyncratic roles

3. COMMUNICATION

LOW SCORES (40 and below) STRENGTH	HIGH SCORES (60 and above) WEAKNESS
– communications are characterized by sufficiency of information	– communications are insufficient, displaced or masked
– messages are direct and clear	– lack of mutual understanding among family members
– receiver is available and open to messages sent	– inability to seek clarification in case of confusion
– mutual understanding exists among family members	

4. AFFECTIVE EXPRESSION

LOW SCORES (40 and below) STRENGTH	HIGH SCORES (60 and above) WEAKNESS
– affective communication characterized by expression of a full range of affect, when appropriate and with correct intensity	– inadequate affective communication involving insufficient expression, inhibition of (or overly intense) emotions appropriate to a situation

5. AFFECTIVE INVOLVEMENT

LOW SCORES (40 and below) STRENGTH	HIGH SCORES (60 and above) WEAKNESS
– emphatic involvement	– absence of involvement among family members, or merely interest devoid of feelings
– family members' concern for each other leads to fulfillment of emotional need (security) and promotes autonomous function	– involvement may be narcissistic, or to an extreme degree, symbiotic
– quality of involvement is nurturant and supportive	– family members may exhibit insecurity and lack of autonomy

6. CONTROL

LOW SCORES (40 and below) STRENGTH	HIGH SCORES (60 and above) WEAKNESS
- patterns of influence permit family life to proceed in a consistent and generallly acceptable manner	- patterns of influence do not allow family to master the routines of ongoing family life
- able to shift habitual patterns of functioning in order to adapt to changing demands	- failure to perceive and adjust to changing life demands
- control style is predictable yet flexible enough to allow for some spontaneity	- may be extremely predictable (no spontaneity) or
- control attempts are constructive, educational and nurturant	- chaotic
	- control attempts are destructive or shaming
	- style of control may be too rigid or laissez-faire
	- characterized by overt or covert power struggles

7. VALUES AND NORMS

LOW SCORES (40 and below) STRENGTH	HIGH SCORES (60 and above) WEAKNESS
- consonance between various components of the family's value system	- components of the family's value system are dissonent resulting in confusion and tension
- family's values are consistent with their subgroup and the larger culture to which thefamily belongs	- conflict between the family's values and those of the culture as a whole
- explicit and implicit rules are consistent	- explicitly stated rules are subverted by implicit rules
- family members function comfortably with the existing latitude	- degree of latitude is inappropriate

great impact on partnership. Task accomplishment and role performance as well as affective expression and involvement have turned out to be the key problems of postoperative partnership. Coping with these difficulties may put a big strain on a partnership. Patients are forced to identify and meet their own needs (task accomplishment), whereas female partners are unwilling to give up all of the roles taken on in the preoperative period (role performance). Successful task accomplishment and role performance can be achieved only if the degree and quality of the partners' interest in and concern for one another are sufficient. But both involvement and affective expression are experienced as insufficient by the patient and his partner. This process seems to be gradual and is still going on one year after surgery. Patients and partners report that they are still in the process of redefining roles and redesigning a new life-style with an unpredictable future.

5. Summary

Terminal heart disease with all its somatic and psychological consequences does not only involve the patient; his family is also involved. It was the aim of our study to assess the dyadic relationship in couples before and after heart transplantation. Forty-three patients who had undergone heart transplantation in 1988 and 1989 and their female partners were tested preoperatively and one year postoperatively with the Dyadic Relationship Scale of the Family Assessment Measure (FAM; Skinner and Steinhauser, Cierpka). FAM is a self-report instrument that provides quantitative indices of family functioning and examines the relationship of couples. The basic concepts assessed by the scale include: task accomplishment, role performance, communication, affective expression, involvement, control and values and norms. Our results show that (1) all profiles achieved are within the average range and that (2) there are no significant differences between men and women in the way they view their relationship before and after heart transplantation, whereas (3) there are clear differences in intraindividual views: postoperatively men reveal significant changes in task accomplishment, affective expression and involvement, while women show problems in role performance, affective expression and involvement. Our results emphasize that after heart transplantation it is necessary to redefine roles, restore task accomplishment and redesign the relationship.

References

1. Christopherson LK: Cardiac transplantation: a psychological perspective. Circulation 1987;75:57–62.
2. Hyler BJ, Corley MC, McMahon D: The role of nursing in a support group for heart transplantation recipients and their families. J Heart Transplant 1985;4:453–456.
3. Mishel MH, Murdaugh CL: Family adjustment to heart transplantation: redesigning the dream. Nurs Res 1987;36:332–338.
4. Rogers K: Nature of spousal supportive behaviors that influence heart transplant patient compliance. J Heart Transplant 1987;6:90–95.
5. O'Brien VC: Psychological and social aspects of heart transplantation. J Heart Transplant 1985;4:229–231.
6. Jones BM, Chang VP, Esmore D, et al: Psychological adjustment after cardiac transplantation. Med J Aust 1988;149:118–122.
7. Gier MD, Levick MD, Blazina PJ: Stress Reduction with heart transplant patients and their families: a multi-disciplinary approach. J Heart Transplant 1988;7:342–347.
8. Steinhauer PD, Santa-Barbara J, Skinner H: The process model of family functioning. Can J Psychiatry 1984;29:77–88.
9. Cierpka M (ed.): Familiendiagnostik. Springer Verlag, Heidelberg Berlin, New York, Tokyo, 1987.
10. Skinner H, Steinhauer PD, Santa-Barbara J: The family assessment measure. Can J Community Mental Health 1983;2:91–105.

45. Quality of life before and after heart transplantation

N. CAINE, L. SHARPLES and J. WALLWORK

1. Introduction

It is now increasingly accepted that measurement of quality of life should form a part of any evaluation of the effectiveness of health care interventions. In the 1970s return to work was the main criterion because it was a simple and objective measurement. In the 1980s, however, subjective assessments of a wider range of quality of life criteria became accepted as being equally relevant to more objective measurements.

In measuring outcome of cardiac surgery at Papworth Hospital the same basic study design has been adopted: questionnaires are completed at intervals before and after surgery with follow-up to at least one year. One of the questionnaires used is a general health status measure used widely in the U.K., with other patient groups and the general population, thus enabling comparison of results. Other instruments are designed to address the issues relevant to the particular group of patients being studied. Quality of life studies of heart transplant patients began at Papworth Hospital with the DHSS sponsored project looking at the costs and benefits of heart transplantation in the U.K. during 1982–84 [1]. Work has continued since then, collecting additional data with the aims of confirming the changes in quality of life before and after heart transplantation and investigating longer term outcome.

2. Methods

Patients complete questionnaires immediately after acceptance to the waiting list for a heart transplant; at three monthly intervals prior to transplantation and at three months, six months, one year and thereafter at six monthly intervals after transplantation.

The Nottingham Health Profile (NHP) has been used throughout, it is in two parts; Part I contains 38 statements in six dimensions; physical mobility,

Paul J. Walter (ed.): Quality of Life after Open Heart Surgery, 491–498.

energy, pain, sleep, social isolation and emotional reactions. Patients are required to give yes or no responses to each of the statements and a score ranging from 0 to 100 is calculated for each dimension; the higher the score the more the problems being perceived by patients. In Part II of the NHP, patients are asked to indicate which of seven areas of daily life are being affected by their state of health; the seven areas being working life, ability to perform tasks in the home, social life, home relationships, sex life, hobbies and holidays.

Nonparametric methods are used to analyse the NHP results. In measuring changes in NHP scores over time the Kruskal–Wallis one-way ANOVA by ranks is used. To assess the significance of changes in the same individuals before and after transplantation, the Wilcoxon matched pairs signed rank test is used for Part I and the McNemar test for Part II.

The accompanying questionnaire was developed from the interviews carried out with patients during the DHSS study and work done at Stanford [2]. It comprises sections on working life; activity restrictions in home, leisure and social life; symptoms including breathlessness and chest pain, and problems like rejection and infection; and dependence on others because of health state.

More recently, in order to enhance the measurement of psychological factors, the Emotional Distress Subscale of the Psychological Adjustment to Illness Scale has been added to the second questionnaire.

This consists of questions covering anxiety, depression, irritability, guilt, worry, self-esteem and appearance. The patient's level of adjustment in each area is determined by answers on a scale from 0–3; the higher the score the greater the maladjustment.

3. Results

3.1. *General health status*

The mean scores from Part I of 492 Profiles completed by 276 patients at intervals while waiting for transplantation are shown in Figure 1. Deterioration was evident in three dimensions; pain ($p < 0.05$), social isolation ($p < 0.01$) and emotional reactions ($p < 0.001$). NHP scores from the questionnaires completed less than three months prior to transplantation and at three months following surgery, in the same 147 patients, showed improvements ($p < 0.001$) in all six dimensions (Figure 2).

In Part II of the NHP, the proportion of patients experiencing problems in their daily lives related to their state of health, was significantly fewer ($p < 0.001$) at three months after surgery when compared with less than three months before transplantation. Some 90% of patients were experiencing problems in home, social and sexual activities prior to transplantation,

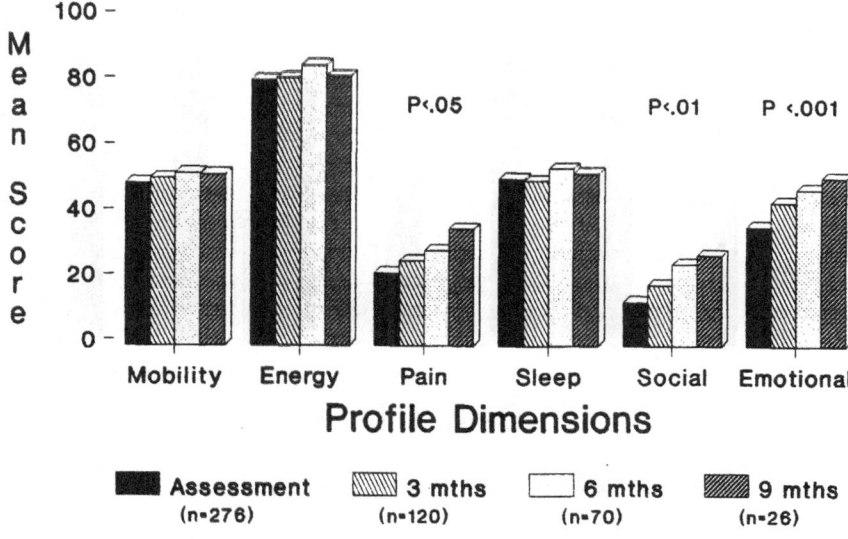

Figure 1. Nottingham Health Profile: Part I. Heart transplant patients – waiting list.

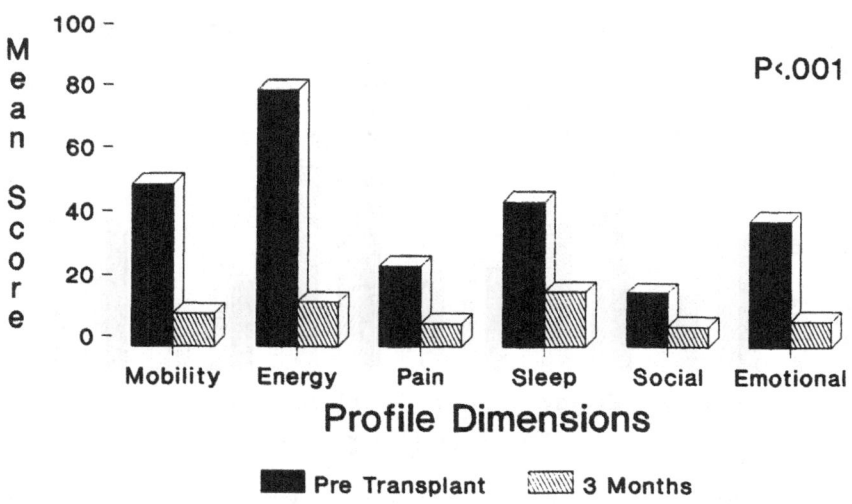

Figure 2. Nottingham Health Profile: Part I. Heart transplant patients ($n = 147$).

compared with a range of 20% to 40% at three months after. The smallest change was in working life, reducing from 69% to 42% (Figure 3).

Changes in the mean scores from Part I of 484 Profiles completed by 150 patients at intervals from one to five years after transplantation are shown in Figure 4. There was evidence of some improvement over time in the dimensions of social isolation and emotional reactions, and of deterioration

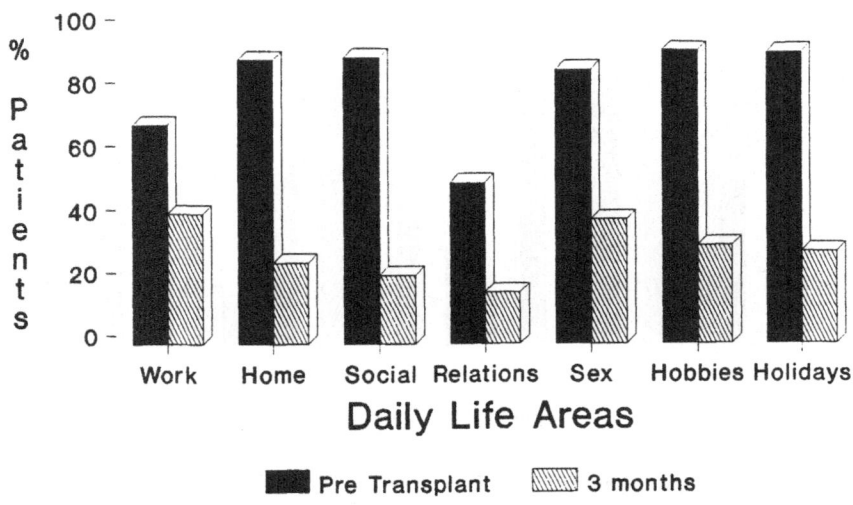

Figure 3. Nottingham Health Profile – Part II. Heart transplant patients (*n* = 147).

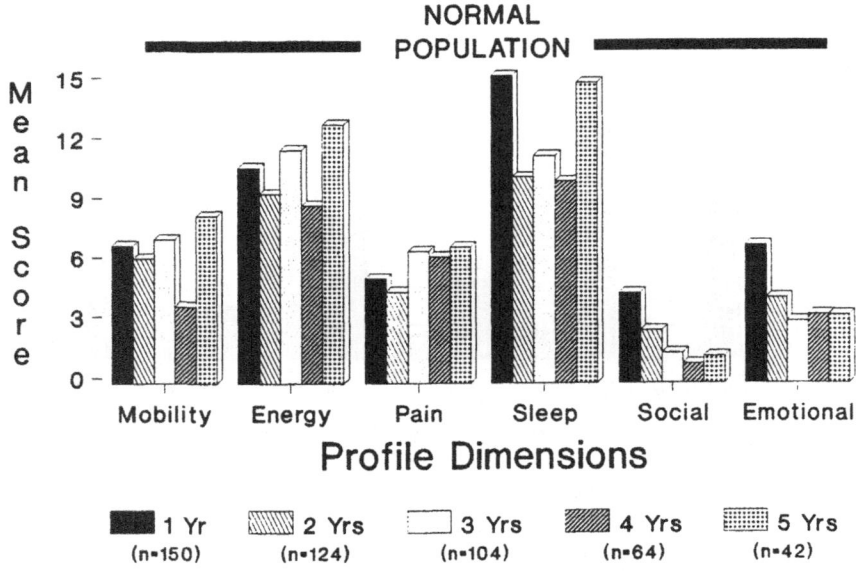

Figure 4. Nottingham Health Profile: Part I. Heart transplant patients – Post-op.

at five years in physical mobility, energy and sleep, but none of the differences were statistically significant. All these mean scores were in the 0 to 15 range which is comparable to the scores obtained from a general population sample [3].

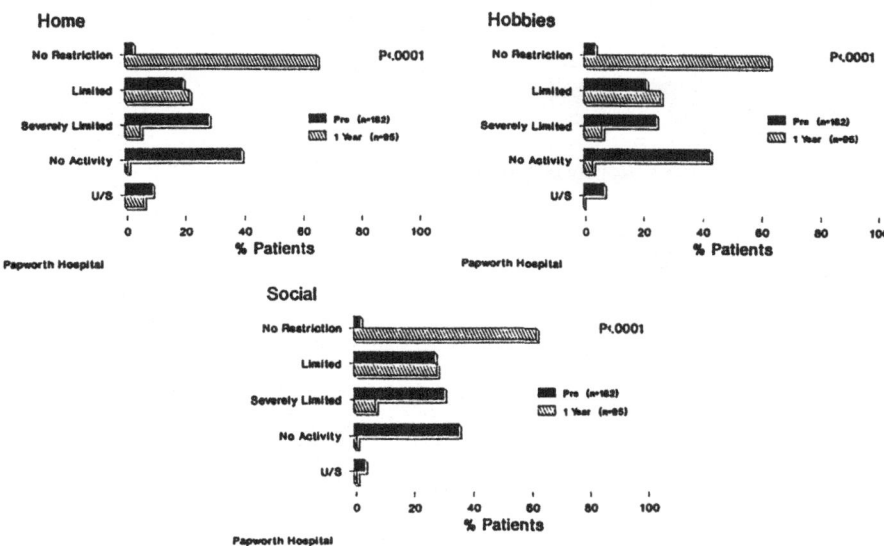

Figure 5. Heart transplant patients activity levels.

3.2 *Activity restrictions and dependence*

At the time of acceptance onto the waiting list for heart transplantation, 9 (4.9%) of patients were working. At one year after surgery 27 (28.4%) had returned to work. Restrictions in activity in the home, hobbies and social life were rated on a scale from 'no restriction', 'limited', 'severely limited' to 'no activity'. Patients' assessments of their activity at time of acceptance for transplantation and at one year after surgery are shown in Figure 5. Results are similar in the three groupings of activity; with 88–89% of patients indicating some level of restriction pre-transplant reducing to 29–36% at one year after transplant.

Dependence on others was rated from being no problem to being a slight, moderate or severe problem. Pre-transplant, 44.1% assessed their dependence on others to be a moderate problem and 47.1% a severe problem, reducing to 17.5% and 3.2% respectively at one year after transplantation.

3.3. *Symptoms*

As well as rating the frequency of symptoms, patients were asked to assess the level of exertion precipitating symptoms. Frequency of pain and breathlessness before and at three months and one year after transplantation are shown in Figure 6. The proportion of patients experiencing pain and breathlessness reduced from 76.2% and 100% pre transplant to 31.6% and 48.4%

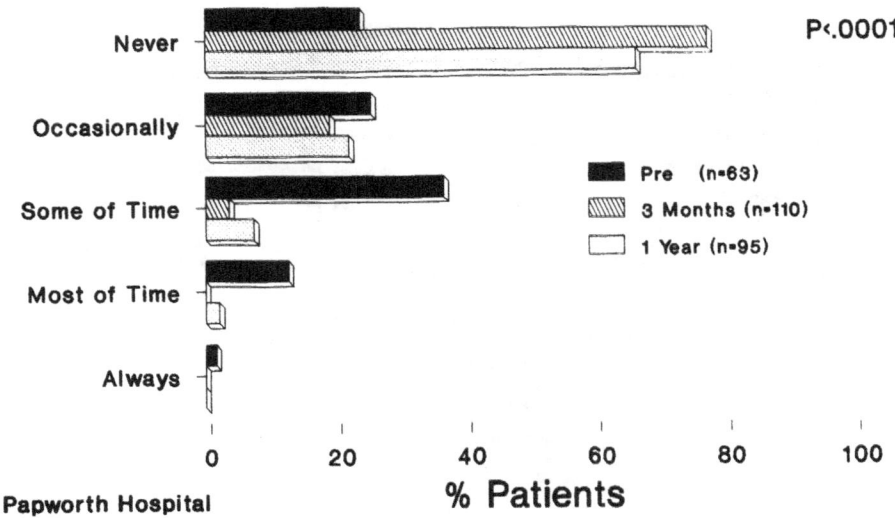

Figure 6a. Heart transplant patients, frequency of pain.

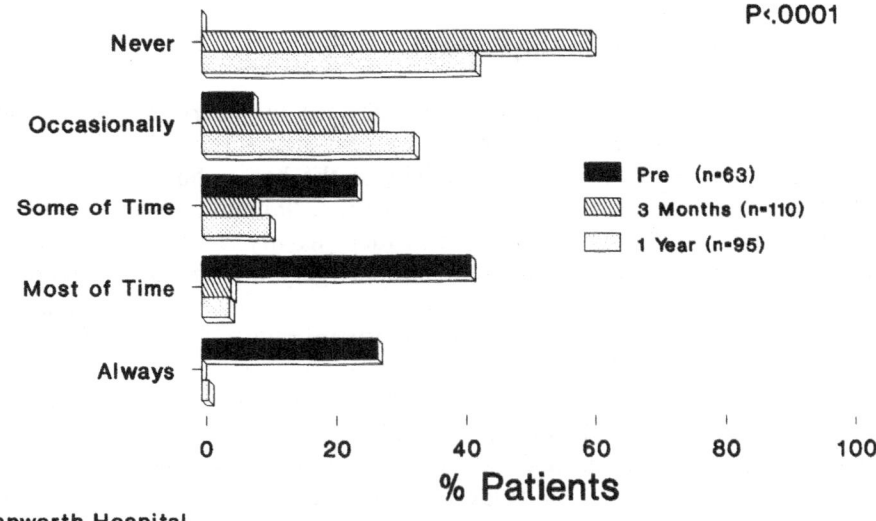

Figure 6b. Heart transplant patients, frequency of breathlessness.

at one year after surgery, when the frequency level was mostly 'occasionally' or 'some of the time'.

The level of exertion precipitating symptoms, is shown in Figure 7. The vast majority of patients were experiencing symptoms pre transplant at rest, walking slowly or normally, whereas at one year after transplantation the majority experienced symptoms after climbing stairs, running or heavy lifting.

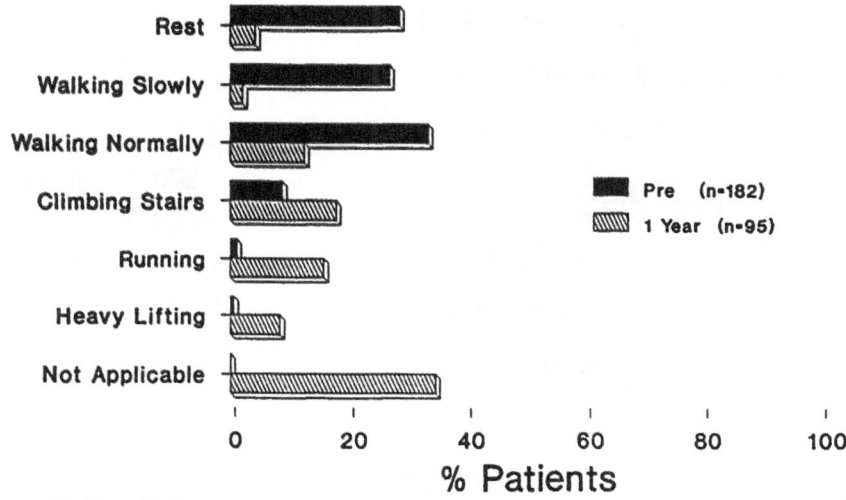

Papworth Hospital

Figure 7. Heart transplant patients. Level of exertion: symptoms.

3.4. *Patients assessment of outcome*

At one year after transplantation 42 (44%) of 95 patients said they were 'completely better' and 49 (52%) felt they were 'definitely improved' compared with their condition prior to surgery. On a quality of life scale from 1 'poor' to 10 'excellent'; 107 (59%) of 182 patients pre-transplant gave a rating between 1–3 with a further 63 (35%) in the 4–7 range. At one year after transplantation, 74 (78%) of 95 patients rated their quality of life in the 8–10 range.

3.5. *Psychological adjustment to illness scale (PAIS)*

The mean scores from the emotional distress subscale of the PAIS, for 34 patients pre-transplant and 63 patients at one year after surgery, are shown in Figure 8. The highest scores pre transplant were in anxiety, worry, depression and self-esteem and it was in these areas where there was greatest improvement when comparing scores at one year with those given at time of acceptance, pre-transplant.

4. Conclusion

Measurement of quality of life at intervals before and after transplantation provides insight to changes over time and comparisons before and after

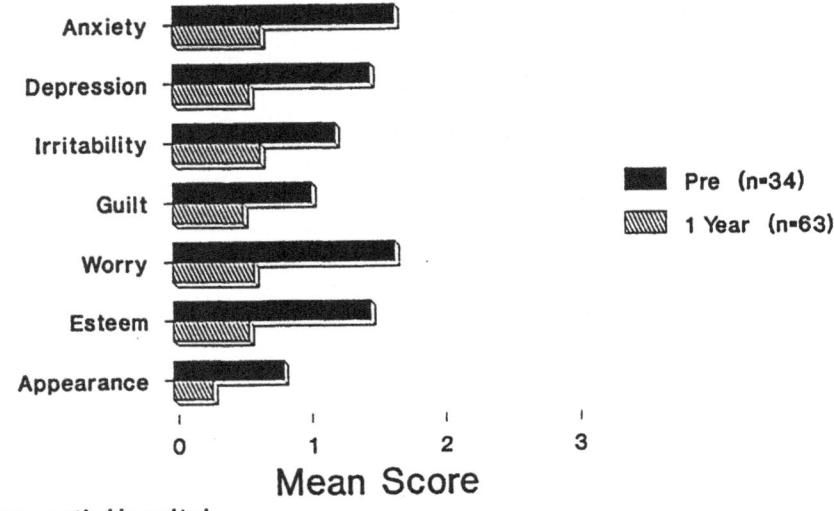

Papworth Hospital

Figure 8. Heart transplant patients. P.A.I.S mean score.

surgery. Results demonstrate patients return to a level of general health status comparable to the general population, soon after heart transplantation as measured by the NHP. From evidence so far available, this level is maintained in longer term survivors.

References

1. Buxton M, Acheson RM, Caine N, Gibson S, O'Brien B: Costs and Benefits of the Heart Transplant Programmes at Harefield and Papworth Hospitals: Final Report, London, HMSO, 1985.
2. Lough ME, Lindsey AM, Shinn JA et al: Life Satisfaction Following Heart Transplantation. Heart Transplant 1985;4:446–449.
3. Hunt SM, McEwen J, McKenna SP: Perceived health: age and sex comparisons in the community. J Epidemiol Comm Health 1984;38:156–160.

E: General Satisfaction

46. Quality of life and satisfaction after heart transplantation

B. BUNZEL, A. GRUNDBÖCK and G. WOLLENEK

1. Introduction

For persons with terminal heart disease heart transplantation has become the chosen method of therapy. The overall aim has been and remains to assess the long-term therapeutic.value-for patients, for whom neither standard forms of medication nor the usual surgical treatments are of any benefit. Improved suppression of graft rejection resulting from the discovery of cyclosporine in 1969 and its regular therapeutic application since 1980 triggered a sharp increase in heart transplantation worldwide [1].

At the beginning, survival rates were the focus of scientific interest [2–5]. The main question for many years was: *do* they survive? Later attention shifted from purely physical to psychosocial areas [6–10]. The question arose: *how* do they survive? In our investigation we have gone a step further: we concentrated on the question whether the transplant patients are *content* with their postoperative quality of life. Satisfaction with life is supposed to be a good, if not the best indicator for postoperative quality of life. If a person is satisfied with life, values for blood pressure and renal function, for example, although important for physical well-being, do not play a major role. Satisfaction expressed by the patients themselves is the best indicator of success of any operation. What the doctors want the patients to do after surgery (for instance, walk more than 3 miles) seems less important than what the patients themselves want to do and whether they are satisfied. Therefore primarily one should look at what is the aim of the patients and if they are content with the level of condition they have reached up to assessment [11].

2. Methods

By the end of the first postoperative year we mailed letters to 47 patients who had undergone heart transplantation in 1988 and 1989. Table 1 shows the patient data and the indication for transplantation.

Paul J. Walter (ed.): Quality of Life after Open Heart Surgery, 501–505.

Table 1. Patients data and indication for heart transplantation.

Number of patients		47
Age	up to 30	6
	31–40	4
	41–50	16
	51–60	19
	more than 60	2
Sex	male	46
	female	1
Family status	single	8
	married	37
	widowed	0
	divorced	2
	separated	0
Indication for HTx	coronary heart disease	14
	cardiomyopathy	27
	mitral vitium	6

We asked them to assess changes in condition as well as satisfaction with their present condition since admission to the waiting list as donor-organ recipient. This was to be done in eight areas of quality of life (physical, mental, emotional, vocational and financial status, sexual situation, leisure-time activities, family/partnership) as well as for overall quality of life [12]. Assessment was done by visual rating scales [13–17]: crosses drawn on 10 cm lines, with the extremes being maximal deterioration and maximal improvement or maximal and minimal satisfaction, represent the subjective assessment of the respective dimension. By measuring the distance of the marks to the reference line, numeric data were obtained and statistically evaluated (Wicoxon-, Kruskal–Wallis Test). Figure 1 shows this measurement method regarding, for instance, physical status.

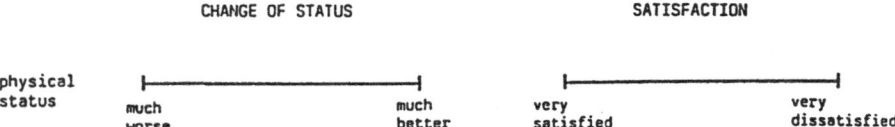

Figure 1. Visual rating scale: change of status and satisfaction.

3. Results

The results of our study are shown graphically in Figure 2.

The horizontal axis indicates the areas of quality of life, the vertical axis the arithmetic means of the data obtained. The basic level zero means no

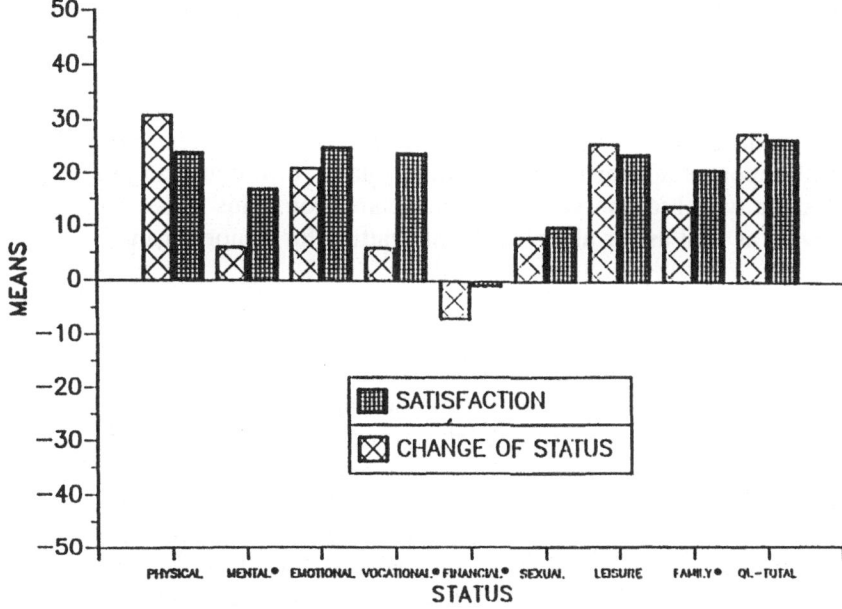

Figure 2. Results: Assessment of changes and satisfaction.

change at all. Values between 0 and 50 means improvement, whereas each value between 0 and −50 indicate deterioration. Apart from the financial situation, there are only improvements in the areas asked for. We may therefore talk about an absolute increase in quality of life as well as in satisfaction with life.

A few facts are worth mentioning: obviously, the best qualified dimensions are physical status, leisure-time activities and overall quality of life. Regarding physical condition it is interesting that, although no statistically significant difference could be detected, satisfaction is not as high as performance. This shows up a phenomenon which is typical for heart transplant patients: although performance is high, they are not content with it in the same way; they are never satisfied with the physical performance they have achieved. Statistically significant differences between change of status and satisfaction were obtained in the mental and financial situation as well as in partnership, where satisfaction was ranked even higher. In Figure 1 these dimensions are marked with points. This means that the patients are very satisfied with their skills, they have learned to appreciate partnership, and they are even content with a lower income.

The vocational situation is an exception, because only one third (*N* = 14) of the former patients work postoperatively. They are happy that they can work again; they appreciate being able to work more than ever before, when holding a job was something they took for granted.

Finally, statistical evaluation has shown that neither the age of the patients nor the indication for heart transplantation had any influence on the patient's assessment of quality and satisfaction of life.

Summing up, we may say that our brief survey shows that despite side effects of drugs and repeated invasive diagnostic procedures, our Austrian patients reported a clear improvement in quality of life and an even higher satisfaction with life one year after transplantation. This is assuring for the caregivers as well as for all patients still waiting for donor organs.

4. Summary

Over the last few years heart transplantation has become the chosen method to treat terminally ill patients suffering from severe cardiac disease. It was the aim of our retrospective study to give a survey on life quality of donor organ recipients who had undergone heart transplantation one year before. 47 patients were asked to evaluate their postoperative improvement/deterioration (change of status) and their satisfaction with the levels achieved on visual scales. Life quality was defined in 9 areas: physical, emotional, mental, vocational, sexual status, financial situation, leisure activities, partnership and overall quality of life. The following results were obtained: (1) the former patients reported a distinct improvement in almost all dimensions (except financial situation). We may therefore talk of an absolute increase in quality of life as well as in satisfaction with life after heart transplantation. (2) Although improvement was ranked highest for the physical status, there was also a good improvement in psychosocial areas. (3) Statistically significant differences between postoperative change of status and satisfaction with the level achieved were shown in the fields of mental, vocational, financial situation as well as in partnership, where satisfaction was ranked even higher than in the latter. (4) Neither the indication for transplantation (coronary heart disease, cardiomyopathy, mitral vitium) nor the age of the patients had any influence on the assessment of quality of life and life satisfaction.

Acknowledgement

This study was supported by the Austrian 'Fonds zur Förderung wissenschaftlicher Forschung' (FFwF).

References

1. Griffith B, Hardesby R, Thompson R, Drummer J. Bahnson H: Cardiac transplantation with cyclosporine: The Pittsburgh experience. Heart Transplant 1983;2:251–255.

2. British Cardiac Society: Report on cardiac transplantation in the United Kingdom. Br Heart J 1984;52:679–682.
3. Firth B: Southwestern internal medicine conference: replacement of the failing heart. Am J Med Science 1987;293(1):50–65.
4. Gail M: Does cardiac transplantation prolong life? Ann Intern Med 1982;76:815–817.
5. Pennock J, Oyer P, Reitz B, et al: Cardiac transplantation in perspective for the future. J Thorac Cardiovasc Surg 1982;83:168–177.
6. Christopherson, L: Cardiac transplantation: a psychological perspective. Circulation 1987;75(1): 57–62.
7. Harvison A, Jones B: Rehabilitation after heart transplantations: The Australian experience. J Heart Transplant 1988;7:337–341.
8. Jones B, Chang V, Esmore D, et al: Psychological adjustment after cardiac transplantation. Med J Australia 1988;149:118–122.
9. Mai F, Burley J: The psychosocial aspects of heart transplantation. Transplantation Today 1985;2:16–21.
10. McAleer M, Copeland J, Fuller J: Psychological aspects of heart transplantation.
11. Lough M, Lindsay A, Shinn J: Life satisfaction following heart transplantation. J. Heart Transplant 1985;4(4):446–449.
12. Levine S, Croog S: What constitutes quality of life? A conceptualization of the dimensions of life quality. In: Wenger NK, Mattson ME, Furberg CD (eds.) Assessment of quality of life. Le Jacq USA, 1989:46–59.
13. Bond A, Lader M: The use of visual analogue scales in rating subjective feelings. Br J Med Psychol 1974;47:211–218.
14. Bunzel B, Grundböck A, Laczkovics A, Teufeisbauer H: Quality of life after heart transplantation: a retrospective study of the first three years of transplantation in Vienna, Austria. J Heart Transplant 1991;10(3):455–459.
15. Guyatt GH, Townsend M, Berman LB, Keller JL: A comparison of Likert and visual analogue scales for measuring change in function. J Chron Dis 1987;40(1):1129–1133.
16. Huskisson EC, Jones J, Scott PJ: Application of visual analogue scales to the measurement of functional capacity. Rheu Rehabil 1976;15:185–187.
17. Scott PI, Huskisson EC: Measurement of functional capacity with visual analogue scales. Rheum Rehabil 1977;16:257–259.

47. Quality of life after open heart surgery: strategies to improve quality of life after heart transplantation

PETER A. SHAPIRO

1. Introduction

The astounding progress in the field of heart transplantation achieved over the past decade, the culmination of prior decades of intense effort to understand and modulate the immune response to the transplanted heart, has transformed this procedure from an experimental to a proven clinical therapy suitable for wide application, to the benefit of many thousands of patients. With the success of heart transplantation and the now commonplace expectation of long-term survival, our awareness of issues of quality of life after surgery has increased. In the past several years much has been learned about the quality of life of heart transplant recipients, and where the problems lie [1–3]. Much less is known about interventions to address these problems. I will attempt to summarize what I believe are key issues for the quality of life of heart transplant recipients, what we know about these issues, what has been described so far about attempts to improve the quality of life of heart transplant recipients, and what we do not know and might be able to study.

2. Health status

Without doubt, the most important determinant of a patient's perceived quality of life is his health [1,4]. Heart transplant recipients now enjoy five-year survival rates of 75–82% [5], but experience a variety of more or less debilitating medical problems, including benign but unpleasant side effects of medications such as acne and hirsutism, more serious side effects such as hypertension, osteoporosis and pain, and life-threatening problems such as infections, rejection graft atherosclerosis and malignancies. Outcome is worse for children thall for adults [6–8] and, in general, for patients in more debilitated condition or with relative medical contraindications. The more physical symptoms and disability, the worse the reported quality of life [9].

Paul J. Walter (ed.): Quality of Life after Open Heart Surgery, 507–515.
© 1992 Kluwer Academic Publishers.

In response to these problems, much attention has been devoted to improvement in immunosuppression protocols, and in particular, elimination of steroids from the medical regimen [10], which results in reduced medication side effects and weight gain. It appears that some patients can avoid rejection without use of steroids. Since it is not clear how to identify these patients prospectively, however, and since the morbidity of rejection may be substantial, universal treatment with steroids remains the general rule. New immunosuppressive agents such as FK 506 and protocols to induce tolerance of the graft without other immune suppression hold forth tantalizing promise but seem far from routine clinical application. In the meanwhile, trials of different combinations of antibiotics for prophylaxis of opportunistic infections continue. Little effort has been devoted to study of the long-term effects on graft atherosclerosis of improved nutritional status and lipid metabolism or enhanced exercise training.

It seems clear that quality of life of recipients would also be 'enhanced' by restrictive selection criteria and exclusion of patients at heightened risk of substantial morbidity after surgery [7]. Whether the greatest benefit for the greatest number of people would be obtained by tightening selection criteria, excluding some patients in endstage heart failure who might benefit from the procedure, in order to shorten waiting time for others, who might then undergo surgery in better condition, is a matter for ethical debate as well as empirical research. In any given case, it is extremely difficult to withhold treatment which has fairly good likelihood of benefit just because the risk of morbidity and mortality is somewhat greater than average.

3. Emploment and finances

Only a fraction of heart transplant recipients return to work, although physical capacity to return to work is achieved by most long-term survivors of heart transplantation [11,12]. Some do not because of medical problems after transplantation. It is noteworthy that Jones and colleagues [10] found that patients on a steroid-free regimen were more likely to be employed, presumably because they were as a group more fit than those on steroid maintenance. Many heart transplant candidates are not aware that they will be physically able to return to work after recovery: some look forward to maintaining the secondary gains of the disabled role. Many who would like to work have difficulty finding suitable employment [3,13,14]. Financial status is routinely noted to be impaired by transplantation one of the few areas of quality of life which patients report as worse after the procedure. In the United States, health insurance is provided by government programs for the disabled and the indigent, and by the employer for most workers. Insurance is a necessity for adequate medical care. Transplant recipients who have been insured through government programs may lose these benefits if they return to work, and may be unable to obtain other insurance through employment, due to the reluctance of employers to take on the anticipated burden of high health insurance costs for these workers. Consequently they are 'insurance-disabled'.

Ad hoc fund-raising and social work advocacy seem to be the methods of choice for dealing with financial problems of heart transplant recipients. Little has been written about interventions to improve this aspect of their quality of life. Informal support networks and formal patient organizations such as the United States group TRIO provide channels to organize monetary assistance for needy patients.

As work and finances remain a significant source of distress, however, further effort is required. At Columbia-Presbyterian Medical Center in New York, heightened attention has been paid recently to the expectations about return to work of newly evaluated patients. Patients are now informed that it is the program's expectation that they will be able to return to work and should not expect to continue to receive disability payment indefinitely. Pointed inquiry is made into their plans for return to work. The effects of this intervention are as yet unknown. Vocational counselling, pre- and postoperatively, could be of benefit to many patients who do not have a job waiting for them on recovery from surgery. So far as I know, there has been no study of the effect of vocational counselling on return to work after heart transplantation. Since society should have an interest in the return to productive contribution to society of transplant recipients, if for no other reason than to help defray the enormous cost of their care, organized lobbying to alter the system of eligibility for government-mandated insurance might be of considerable benefit; if prospective employers were relieved of the private burden of insuring these patients for transplant-related expenditures, transplant recipients vould be more likely to become employed, income-earning taxpayers instead of dependents of the welfare-disability system.

4. Psychiatric problems

Numerous studies have demonstrated a high prevalence of adjustment and affective disorders, organic mental syndromes and various other psychiatric problems in recipients of heart transplants [1,15–19]. The dramatic psychoses reported in up to one third of patients following heart transplantation in the late 1960s [20] are now rare, but distress and impairment in quality of life due to psychiatric problems remain significant. Episodes of major depressive disorder or steroid-induced depression may occur in up to 10–20% of heart transplant recipients: many of these are undiagnosed and untreated. Steroid-induced mood lability, irritability and grandiosity is a common problem of the early months after transplantation. Mild to moderate cognitive impairment is frequently overlooked [21]. Fortunately, it appears that for patients on the whole, ratings of mood, anxiety and overall adjustment to illness improve substantially over the first two years after transplantation [16].

Patient, social worker, nurse, or other staff-led support groups for transplant candidates, recipients, and families are commonly utilized to impart information, allay feelings of apprehension and anxiety, reduce social isolation, empower patients and families to deal more effectively with each other and with the 'system', and provide opportunity for ventilation and emotional support [22–25]. These groups are widely perceived as psychologically helpful, although little is reported about attempts to measure their effects. Models of group work apparently vary widely and have not been compared.

Anecdotal reports of individual psychotherapy of anxiety and depression of heart transplant recipients suggest that this treatment is widely utilized and of value for some patients. I have personally observed apparent significant benefit of brief courses of psychotherapy in selected patients with anxiety and depression problems after transplantation. Repeated explanation and clarification of distorted understanding of the medical course, help in communicating needs to family and staff, and exploration of dynamic issues may occur in psychotherapy. Significant themes include survivor guilt, mourning for the loss of the 'person I was before I got sick,' anger at persistent problems after the transplant, and conflicts about dependency and the sick role. Systematic study of the applicability of various forms of psychotherapy in the transplant population has not been conducted.

Somatic treatment of anxiety and depression in transplant recipients is important and described frequently in passing in the literature. Tricyclic antidepressants have been demonstrated to be safe and effective in treatment of depressed heart transplant recipients [26,27]: effects on cyclosporine blood levels require monitoring [26]. Elimination of steroids from the routine medication regimen of transplant recipients would undoubtedly reduce the prevalence of affective illnesses and post-operative delirium.

5. Body image

For many patients, heart transplantation creates a change in the sense of self which may be stressful. Fantasies of incorporation of personal aspects of the donor along with the heart are commonplace, and may be helpful or disturbing to the patient. For example, an adolescent boy with congenital heart disease and lifelong disability refused to accept a woman's heart out of fear of becoming feminine: one week after receiving a man's heart, he expressed his uncertainty about his identity in a drawing depicting himself as weak on one side of the body, powerful on the other (Figure 1). In a follow-up drawing a month later, he depicted himself as a brawny athlete. He was in fact developing Cushingoid features at that point.

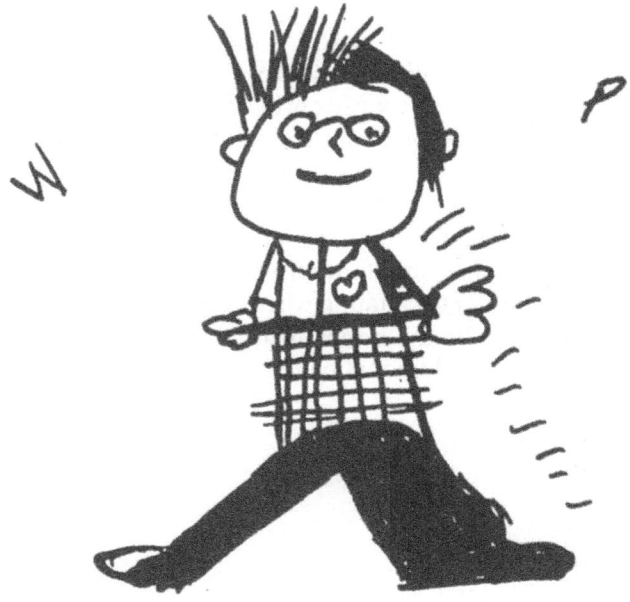

Figure 1. Drawing by a sixteen year old boy one week after undergoing heart transplantation. The patient was asked to draw a person, without further elaboration. W: 'weak', P: 'powerful'. The left side of the body, site of the transplanted heart, is hypertrophied and radiates force.

Distress about physical appearance affects quality of life for many patients, especially in the first year after transplantation, when hirsutism, acne, and Cushingoid habitus and facies may be most pronounced. In children especially, alterations in appearance may lead to severe social stigmatization with deleterious effects on role function such as school and peer avoidance [1,6]. The effects of consultation with a cosmetician, dietary counselling, and physical therapy, and the benefit of education about the transitory nature of these changes, should not be underestimated, but have not been evaluated. Peer support groups may provide a venue for feelings of acceptance by others and sharing of emotional support and practical suggestions. Again, no systematic research comparing effects of different forms of group counselling or other modes of support has been reported.

6. Marital and family relationships

Role strain and readjustment problems occur frequently in families of heart transplant recipients [1,28,29]. Chronically ill, often facing imminent death, patients awaiting transplants relinquish ordinary responsibilities and privileges to others in their families. who struggle with their need to be prepared for the patient's death while maintaining hope for his recovery, and with their anger at the patient for being ill while providing him with support. After transplantation the patient may provoke rage by being too slow to assume old responsibilities, or conversely by attempts to reclaim lost prerogatives in the family unit. Divorce and children's behavior problems may be precipitated during recovery.

Individual, group and family therapy have been used to treat these problems, which occur in all kinds of patients with chronic illnesses. Pre-operative teaching and support, and identification of couples at risk, with referral to marital therapy before transplantation when possible, are indicated interventions. The use of multi-family groups focused specifically on marriage and family issues might be of additional benefit.

7. Sexual function

American and British surveys of quality of life after heart transplantation differ markedly in their findings of sexual satisfaction in transplant recipients. Several British reports [11,30,31] utilizing the Nottingham Health Profile self-report instrument describe near-complete satisfaction with sexual adjustment. In contrast, sexual problems represent one of the main areas of dissatisfaction with quality of life in various American reports [4,32,33]. The reasons for this discrepancy are unknown. Sexual problems reported include poor libido, impotence, and anxiety. These conditions are generally treatable by psychotherapy, sex therapy techniques. psychoeducational counselling, and adjunctive use of medication for treatment of underlying depressive and anxiety disorders. Some sexual problems are due to medications, such as steroids, antihypertensive medication and possibly cyclosporine, and attention to elimination of organic etiologies of dysfunction requires coordinated attention by physician and therapist. Unfortunately, physicians frequently fail to inquire about sexual difficulties, or fail to realize that interventions are possible which may have significant benefits. Even cases of irreversible impotence may be helped through use of penile prostheses which have been reported to be well-tolerated in transplant recipients, and without infectious complications [34]. Contributions toward improving this aspect of quality of life of heart transplant recipients may include better sexual history-taking, peer support groups for patients and spouses, and referral for treatment. However, it must be noted that little is known of the premorbid sexual function of most patients complaining of difficulty after transplantation: how much of the problem is actually attributable to the transplantation process is unknown, and the likelihood of treatment benefit has not been established in any significant series.

8. Compliance

Noncompliance is closely associated with poor quality of life due to increased morbidity and mortality after heart transplantation. In attempting to improve quality of life for recipients of heart transplants, therefore, efforts to screen out the incorrigibly noncompliant patient and to enhance the compliance of selected patients have a kind of face validity. Considerable effort has been invested in psychosocial screening to identify traits predictive of poor compliance [1,35]. Severe personality disorders, particularly those with antisocial, narcissistic and borderline features, and active substance abuse up to the time of evaluation appear to be among the most powerful predictors of later compliance problems, along with behavior management problems during the preoperative evaluation period. In contrast, preoperative depression, anxiety and transient organic brain syndromes appear to have little predictive power [16,18,36]. Since it is difficult to deny a patient a life-saving procedure on the grounds of past behavior, application of this information for exclusionary purposes is problematic. It does provide a guide, however, for closer supervision of selected patients, and if a consensus can be achieved among program staff, the patient may be motivated to enter psychotherapy to help anticipate future problems and to deal with them in less maladaptive fashion than through noncompliance. The use of extended waiting periods, with enrollment in a heart failure management program and opportunity to observe and confront compliance problems in the here and now, rather than through the history, gives questionable candidates an opportunity to demonstrate their ability to comply with a treatment regimen [37]. While support groups and classes appear to be useful to patients, the actual effectiveness of transplant recipient educational classes, support groups, family member support groups and other psychosocial interventions in improving compliance has never been rigorously investigated with a randomized prospective study.

9. Coping skills

The instrumental relationship of coping ability to quality of life seems intuitively obvious. Efforts to operationalize coping skills and teach them to transplant patients and their families, including programs of relaxation, assertiveness, and social skills training, have been reported to lead to improved psychological wellbeing and greater feelings of satisfaction with life and family adjustment [28,38]. Their effects on other aspects of quality of life have not been described. Preoperative teaching about procedures and complications commonly encountered after surgery may have a prophylactic effect against subsequent anxiety [39].

10. Summary

There is little dispute that heart transplantation itself provides a remarkable improvement in survival and quality of life for patients in endstage heart failure, but many problems in quality of life remain. Now that we have achieved longterm survival and documented the quality of life issues, more attention must be turned to evaluating secondary interventions in order to establish which strategies may be most effective in improving quality of life after heart transplantation. Increasing availability of transplants so that patients' waiting time is reduced and transplantation is undertaken on a healthier patient, improvements in immunosuppression to reduce side effects and health problems, and social policy changes regarding insurance and employment are longterm 'strategies' likely to have significant beneficial effects on the quality of life of transplant recipients. Psychosocial treatments such as support groups and classes aimed at stress and strain for patients and families have not yet been adequately evaluated to demonstrate what works best and for whom, though preliminary evidence strongly suggests that they do some good for some patients. Treatment of depression, other psychiatric problems and sexual dysfunction can be expected to have positive effects if more widely applied. Finally, the development of coherent strategies to address problems of noncompliance related to character disorders will remain a challenge for transplantation programs.

References

1. Shapiro PA: Life after heart transplantation. Prog Cardiovasv Dis 1990;32:105–418.
2. Packa DR: Quality of life of adults after a heart transplant. J Cardiovasc Nurs 1989;3:12–22.
3. Gutkind L: Life after transplantation Transplant Proc 1988;20(Suppl 1):1092–1099.
4. Lough ME, Lindsey AM, Shinn JA, et al: Life satisfaction following heart transplantation. J Heart Transplant 1985;4:446–449.
5. Kaye MP: The long-term effects of cyclosporine in heart transplant patients. Transplant Proc 1990;22(3 Suppl 1):12–14.
6. Lawrence KS, Fricker FJ: Pediatric heart transplantation: quality of life. J Heart Transplant 1987;6:329–333.
7. Bailey LL: Pediatric heart transplantation (editorial). Ann Thorac Surg 1989;48:612.
8. Trento A, Griffith BP, Fricker FJ, Kormos RL, Armitage J, Hardesty RL: Lessons learned in pediatric heart transplantation. Ann Thorac Surg 1989;48:617–623.
9. Lough ME, Lindsey AM, Shinn JA, Stotts NA: Impact of symptom frequency and symptom distress on self-reported quality of life in heart transplant recipients. Heart Lung 1987;16:193–200.
10. Jones BM, Taylor FJ, Wright OM, et al: Quality of life after heart transplantation in patients assigned to double or triple-drug therapy. J Heart Transplant 1990;9:392–396.
11. Wallwork J, Caine N: A comparison of the quality of life of cardiac transplant recipients and CABG patients before and after surgery. Quality of Life in Cardiovascular Care 1985;1:317–331.

12. Niset G, Coustry-Degre C, Degre S: Psychosocial and physical rehabilitation after heart transplantation: 1-year follow-up. Cardiology 1988;75:311–317.
13. Meister ND, McAleer MJ, leister JS, Riley JE, Copeland JG: Returning to work after heart transplantation. J Heart Transplant 1986;5:154–161.
14. Harvison A, Jones BM, McBride M, Taylor F, Wright O, Chang VP: Rehabilitation after heart transplantation: the Australian experience. J Heart Transplant 1988;7:337–341.
15. Shapiro PA, Kornfeld DS: Psychiatric outcome of heart transplantation. Gen Hosp Psychiatry 1989;11:352–357.
16. Freeman AM, Folks DG, Sokol RS, et al: Cardiac transplantation: clinical correlates of psychiatric outcome. Psychosomatics 1988;29:47–54.
17. Kuhn WF, Myers B, Brennan AF, et al: Psychopathology in heart transplant candidates. J Heart Transplant 1988;7:223–226.
18. Mai FM, McKenzie FN, Kostuk WJ: Psychiatric aspects of heart transplantation: preoperative evaluation and postoperative sequelae. Br Med J 1986;292:311–317.
19. Brennan AF, Davis MH, Buchholz DJ, Kuhn WF, Gray LA Jr: Predictors of quality of life following cardiac transplantation. Psychosomatics 1987;28:566–571.
20. Lunde DT: Psychiatric complications of heart transplants. Am J Psychiatry 1969;126:369–373.
21. Schall RR, Petrucci RJ, Brozena SC, Cavarocchi NC, Jessup M: Cognitive function in patients with symptomatic dilated cardiomyopathy before and after cardiac transplantation. J Am Coll Cardiol 1989;14:166–172.
22. McAleer MJ, Copeland J, Fuller J, Copeland JG: Psychological aspects of heart transplantation. J Heart Transplant 1985;4:232–233.
23. Suszycki LH: Psychosocial aspects of heart transplantation. Social Work 1988;33:205–209.
24. Hyler BJ, Corley MC, McMahon D: The role of nursing in a support group for heart transplantation recipients and their families. J Heart Transplant 1985;4:453–456.
25. Suszycki LH, Midelfort J, Gibson J, Lysandrou S: Social workers' responsibilities in heart transplantation programs. Prog Cardiovasc Dis 1990;33:35–48.
26. Shapiro PA: Nortriptyline treatment of depressed cardiac transplant recipients. Am J Psychiatry 1991;148:371–373.
27. Kay J, Bienenfeld D, Slomowitz M, et al: Use of tricyclic antidepressants in recipients of heart transplants. Psychosomatics 1991;32:165–170.
28. Suszycki LH: Social work groups on a heart transplant program. J Heart Transplant 1986;5:166–170.
29. Uzark K, Crowley D: Family stress after pediatric heart transplantation. Prog Cardiovasc Nurs 1989;4:23–27.
30. Yacoub MH, Reid CJ, Al-Khadimi RH, et al: Cardiac transplantation – the London experience. Z Kardiol 1985;6(Suppl 74):45–50.
31. Hunt SM: Quality of life considerations in cardiac transplantation. Quality of Life in Cardiovascular Care 1985;1:308–316.
32. Tabler JB, Frierson RL: Sexual concerns after heart transplantation. J Heart Transplant 1990;9:397–403.
33. Mulligan T, Sheehan H, Hanrahan J: Sexual function after heart transplantation. J Heart Lung Transplant 1991;10:125–128.
31. Kabalin JM, Kessler R: Successful implantation of penile prostheses in organ transplant patients. Urology 1989;33:282–284.
35. Mai FM, McKenzie FN, Kostuk WJ: Psychosocial adjustment and quality of life following heart transplantation. Can J Psychiatry 1990;35:223–227.
36. Maricle RA, Hosenpud JD, Norman DJ, et al: Depression in patients being evaluated for heart transplantation. Gen Hosp Psychiatry 1989;11:418–424.
37. Herrick CM, Mealey PC, Tischner LL, Holland CS: Combined heart failure-transplant program: advantages in assessing patient compliance. J Heart Transplant 1987;6:141–146.
38. Gier MD, Levick MD, Blazina PJ: Stress reduction with heart transplant recipients and their families: a multidisciplinary approach. J Heart Transplant 1988;7:342–347.
39. Berron K: Transplant patients' perceptions about effective preoperative teaching. J Heart Transplant 1986;5:162–165.

F: Summary

Quality of life after heart transplantation

PETER A. SHAPIRO

It is exciting and revealing to read chapters ranging from a single case study to the broadest possible overview of survival after heart transplantation. These studies bring out both the great success and the remaining problems affecting quality of life of heart transplant recipients, and point out some of the tasks ahead of us.

It is abundantly clear that heart transplantation has moved from the realm of experiment to that of proven therapy [1]. Approximately 16 100 heart transplant operations have been performed worldwide. The rate of long-term survival afforded by modern surgical technique, immunosuppression protocols, and infection management now approaches 75% for five years. Their surgeons have described the survivors as 'virtually normal' with respect to social and family life [1]. Survivors have had children, competed in sports and returned to work. Many problems are associated with cyclosporine immunosuppression, including hypertension, renal dysfunction, hirsutism, tremor, hepatic dysfunction and malignancies. However, its introduction has permitted reduced use of steroid medications, with reduced steroid side effects. Graft atherosclerosis remains a major issue, with a diffuse form of coronary artery occlusive disease believed to result from chronic immunological injury representing the major cause of late morbidity and mortality of heart transplant recipients. Advances in the non-invasive assessment of rejection, for example by Doppler echocardiography techniques, may reduce its morbidity.

Nevertheless, questions about the quality of life of heart transplant recipients remain. Systematic and detailed attempts to measure life satisfaction and functioning of transplant recipients are in a very early stage, and our knowledge of the effects of interventions to further improve patients' quality of life remains rudimentary.

Every surgeon knows that patient selection bears a relation to patient outcome. Healthier patients respond better than sicker ones to surgical intervention, as is illustrated by the data presented by Caine, Sharples and Wallwork [2]. Abou-Awdi and Frazier [3]. reported that for patients in severe

Paul J. Walter (ed.): Quality of Life after Open Heart Surgery, 519–522.
© 1992 Kluwer Academic Publishers.

congestive heart failure, the left ventricular assist device (LVAD) can restore cardiac output, restore circulation to vital organs, improve nutritional status, and ultimately help patients recover more quickly after transplantation and with improved survival. Other factors measurable at preoperative assessment may have a bearing on outcome. Mai [4] and Shapiro [5] have noted that preoperative psychiatric assessment can identify patients at substantial risk of life-threatening non-compliance; I have raised the question whether selection criteria should be more stringent in an attempt to increase the utility of the procedure; a decision on this question is necessarily political rather than medical.

After surgery, although many patients experience difficulty in the recovery process, most patients end up fairly well. Bullinger, Angermann and Kemkes [6], Bunzel, Wollenek and Grundböck [7] and Caine, Sharples and Wallwork [2] report generally high ratings of quality of life and psychological wellbeing. In the National Heart Transplant Study, as reported by Evans [8], most patients experience a high level of satisfaction. The most universal difficulties encountered have to do with employment, finances and sexual function.

Cabrol and colleagues [1] noted 45% employment and 35% 'retirement' in survivors. Jones [9]. noted 65% return to employment. Mai [4] also noted a substantial percentage unemployed. Health insurance, welfare benefits and employment status are tied together in ways which may create obstacles to reemployment or disincentives to work. The effects of structured programmatic interventions designed to promote post-recovery employment are unknown.

Evans [8] noted that only 45% of patients in the National Heart Transplant Study were satisfied with their sexual relationships. Grundböck, Bunzel and Schubert [10] also noted that relationships change under the stress of the chronic illness preceding tranplantation and during the course of recovery, and that sexual aspects of relationships often continue to deteriorate after transplantation. Sexual dysfunction, especially impotence, has been noted in a substantial number of patients by Mai [4] and in my own work [5]. Impotence may affect up to 50% of men after heart transplantation, particularly those on antihypertensive medications. Little systematic effort has been undertaken to evaluate and optimize sexual function after transplantation.

Most investigators, among them Mai [4], Bunzel, Wollenek and Grundböck [7] and myself, have found that heart transplantation tends to lead to worsened financial status. The financial burden of missed workdays for family members, relocation and travel expenses, and a variety of out-of-pocket costs is superimposed on the cost of medical care itself, which may vary according to the health insurance system involved. As was pointed out by Lawrence and colleagues [11], in some cases financial ruin is the cost of survival, and may lead to the destruction of the family unit, and to guilt and depression. The employment problems tied to discrimination in health insurance and eligibility for insurance, welfare and disability benefits for transplant recipients are closely linked to the financial difficulties of recipient families, and social policy changes more than intervention at the level of the individual case may be necessary to change this situation.

Aspects of psychological and psychiatric status of patients after transplantation have been described by Mai [4]; Jones and colleagues [9], Bullinger and colleagues [6], Bornstein and Starling [12], and Kavanaugh and Yacoub [13]. In general, patients improve in mood state and global psychological wellbeing as they recover from illness. Exercise training was reported to have a positive effect on mood. Improved cardiac output following transplantation was associated with improved neuropsychological test performance. I have noted that mood disorders are common, underdiagnosed and undertreated in the heart transplant population. Steroid medications appear to be a frequent contributor to psychiatric problems, both directly through their central nervous system effects and indirectly through their tendency to cause unpleasant somatic side effects which may provoke emotional reactions.

The psychological adjustment of children may be particularly difficult as they struggle with changes in body image and the effects on their families of the experience of transplantation. Kachaner and colleagues [14] described normal growth, school attendance and socialization for many pediatric heart recipients, but also frequent problems of compliance, and noted that for up to half of their patients, the course was stormy and left a 'bitter taste'. Lawrence and colleagues [11] cited difficulties in peer relationships and dating, family troubles, discrimination encountered at school and at work, financial hardship, uninsurability, and lack of control over life as sources of significant distress for preadolescent and teenaged heart recipients, and illustrated in a harrowing case study the contributing role of these factors in a patient's eventual depression and suicide.

This case underscores the importance of looking not only at heart transplantation's successes but also at its limits and failures [5]. If quality of life is to improve further for heart transplant recipients, the change will likely occur through shortening waiting time, better screening and optimization of patient status in the preoperative period, less toxic and more effective immune suppression, more aggressive management of psychosocial problems, including educational and group support interventions, and advocacy for changes in social systems of insurance and disability benefits which interfere with recovery and the sense of wellbeing of heart transplant recipients. We may hope for continuing advances in the already dramatic improvement in quality of life afforded to patients with severe heart disease by heart transplantation.

References

1. Cabrol C, Gandjbakhch I, Pavie A, et al: Long-term results: morbidity and mortality of

patients after heart transplantation. In: Walter PJ editor. Quality of life after open heart surgery. Dordrecht: Kluwer Acad Publ, 1992: 389–395 (this volume).

2. Caine N, Sharples L, Wallwork J: Quality of life before and after heart transplantation. In: Walter PJ editor. Quality of life after open heart surgery. Dordrecht: Kluwer Acad Publ, 1992: 491–498 (this volume).

3. Abou-Awdi N, Frazier OH: Quality of life of patients on LVAD support. In: Walter PJ editor. Quality of life after open heart surgery. Dordrecht: Kluwer Acad Publ, 1992: 397–401 (this volume).

4. Mai FM, McKenzie FN: The emotional state of the individual after heart transplantation. In: Walter PJ editor. Quality of life after open heart surgery. Dordrecht: Kluwer Acad Publ, 1992: 439–444 (this volume).

5 Shapiro PA: Quality of life after open-heart surgery: strategies to improve quality of life after heart transplantation. In: Walter PJ editor. Quality of life after open heart surgery. Dordrecht: Kluwer Acad Publ, 1992: 507–515 (this volume).

6. Bullinger M, Angermann CE, Kemkes BM: Psychological well-being of heart transplant patients – cross-sectional and longitudinal results. In: Walter PJ editor. Quality of life after open heart surgery. Dordrecht: Kluwer Acad Publ, 1992: 445–455 (this volume).

7. Bunzel B, Grundböck A, Wollenek G: Quality of life and satisfaction after heart transplantation. In: Walter PJ editor. Quality of life after open heart surgery. Dordrecht: Kluwer Acad Publ, 1992: 501–505 (this volume).

8. Evans RW: Psychosocial aspects of heart transplantation: a comparative analysis. In: Walter PJ editor. Quality of life after open heart surgery. Dordrecht: Kluwer Acad Publ, 1992: 469–482 (this volume).

9. Jones B, Taylor F, Downs K, Spratt P: Long-term follow-up of the emotional adjustment of patients after heart transplantation. In: Walter PJ editor. Quality of life after open heart surgery. Dordrecht: Kluwer Acad Publ, 1992: 427–437 (this volume).

10. Grundböck A, Bunzel B, Schubert MT: Changes in partnership after heart transplantation. In: Walter PJ editor. Quality of life after open heart surgery. Dordrecht: Kluwer Acad Publ, 1992: 483–489 (this volume).

11. Lawrence KS, Fricker FJ, Cardillo S: Pediatric heart transplantation: the recipient's perspective. In: Walter PJ editor. Quality of life after open heart surgery. Dordrecht: Kluwer Acad Publ, 1992: 363–370 (this volume).

12. Bornstein RA, Starling RC, Myerowitz PD: Neuropsychological function before and after cardiac transplantation. In: Walter PJ editor. Quality of life after open heart surgery. Dordrecht: Kluwer Acad. Publ, 1992: 419–424 (this volume).

13. Kavanagh T: Physiological and psychological benefits of exercise rehabilitation after cardiac transplantation. In: Walter PJ editor. Quality of life after open heart surgery. Dordrecht: Kluwer Acad Publ, 1992: 403–416 (this volume).

14. Kachaner J, Le Bidois J, Sidi D, Piéchaud JF, Vouhé P: Quality of life of children having undergone heart transplantation. In: Walter PJ editor. Quality of life after open heart surgery. Dordrecht: Kluwer Acad Publ, 1992: 371–379 (this volume).

Index

ability index 385
abnormal vs. normal left ventricular
    function 451
accelerated coronary atherosclerosis 377
'acting out' 326
activity restrictions and dependence 495
adherence 3
adolescent transplant 363
adolescents 325
    achievement-oriented 330
    ambitious 330
adults 325
affective disorders 509
age 453
aging 278, 282
airway patency 304
allocation of resources 4
AMDP 74
    apathy 74
    depression 74
    hostility 74
    mania 75
    paranoid-hallucinatory syndromes 75
    psycho-organic syndromes 75
    system 73
Anamnestic Comparative Self Assessment
    Scale (ACSA) 446
anger 510
anticoagulant therapy 33
anticoagulation 93
(anti) conception 326
antithymocyte polyclonal globulines 375
anxiety 177, 198, 329, 449
arrhythmias 256, 280, 283
assessing quality of life 398
association between psychological well-

being and global quality of life 453
atrial septal defects 278, 329
atypical complaints 330
azathioprine 374

bacterial endocarditis 257
Beck Depression Inventory 428, 430
behavioural problems 330
biological valve 9
biological vs. artificial valves 78
bioprosthesis 10, 13
body concept 326
body image 510, 521
bypass surgery 193

Campbell Well-Being Scale 431, 452
Canadian Cardiovascular Society
    Classification 2
cardiac complications 189
cardiac transplantation 397, 419
cardiac valve surgery 39, 63
cardiomyopathies 371
cardiovascular surgery 71
Carpentier valvuloplasty 14
CASS studies 71
central nervous system (CNS) complica-
    tion 47
changes in partnership 483
character disorders 514
childish behaviour 326
children 325, 335, 347, 371, 521
    psychological adjustment of 521
chronic illness 1, 3
circulatory support 391
clinical data 74
clinical improvement 24

clinical neurological disorders 143
clinical trials 115
clinical variables 453
CMV infection 376
cognition 155, 158
cognitive aspects 326
cognitive dysfunction 141
cognitive function 39, 247
cognitive impairment 509
complex congenital heart defects 315
compliance 521
complications 451
comprehensive cardiac care 133
comprehensive rehabilitation programme
    179
conceptual level analogy test (CLAT) 39
congenital cardiac malformation 303
congenital heart defects 277, 281, 293
congenital heart disease (CHD) 335, 347,
    355
  impact of, on brothers and sisters 352
  impact of, on the child 351
  perception of parents 349
  physical aspects 325
  surgical correction of 383
congenital heart malformations 371
coping ability 513
coronary aortic bypass grafting (CABG)
    133, 141, 156, 169, 177, 227
coronary artery bypass surgery 39, 107,
    155, 185, 203, 215, 235, 245, 419
coronary artery disease (CAD) 133, 447
coronary disease vs. no disease 451
coronary risk factors 235
corrective open heart surgery 293
cost-effectiveness 4
courtship/marriage 326
crisis management 483
cyclosporine 374, 375
cytomegalovirus (CMV) 374

deficient knowledge 331
denial 326
dependency 510
depression 177, 326, 449, 450, 514
diabetes 122
dilated cardiomyopathy (CMP) 447
disability 283
discrimination 521
Doppler echocardiography 283
Dyadic Relationship Scale of Family
    Assessment Measure (FAM) 485

dysfunction 285
dysfunctional families 282
dyspnea 65

EBV infection 376
education 326
  counselling 2
  programmes 181
Eisenmengers' Syndrome 294
elderly patients 122, 248
emboli 160
emotional adjustment of patients 427
emotional aspects 326
emotional changes 206
emotional problems 342
emotional reactions 177
emotional state 64, 177
employment 203, 247, 470, 508, 514,
    520
  status 453
endomyocardial biopsy 373–376
enlightened consumerism 3
Epstein-Barr virus (EBV) 374
exercise 283, 377, 521
  programme 405
  rehabilitation 403
  training 508
extracardiac anomalies 280
extracardiac factors 281
extracorporal circulation (ECC) 253

factorial studies 84
family 282, 286
  needs of 179
  perspective 76
  ratings 83
  relationships 326, 511
  therapy 512
fatigue 450
FEKB 81
  acceptance 81
  coping styles 73, 81
  religiosity 81
  social support seeking 81
  social withdrawal 81
female patients 74
finances 508, 520
follow-up period 385
FPI 80
  achievement orientation 80
  extraversion 80
  low inhibition 80

personality 73, 74
  satisfaction 81
friends 330
functional capacity 2
functional deterioration 375

gancyclovir 376
gender 123
general health questionnaire (GHQ) 457
genetic risk 286
great arteries, transposition of 329, 335
growth 376, 521

Hamburg Rating Scale for Psychic
    Disturbances (HRPD) 194
Hamilton Anxiety Scale (HAM-A) 194
Hamilton Psychiatric Rating Scale for
    Depression (HAM-D) 194
health 449
  insurance 508
  problems 514
  -related policy 4
  status 470
healthy comparison group 446
healthy reference group 83
heart surgery 303
heart transplantation 363, 403, 427, 439,
    457, 469, 483, 491, 501, 507
  emotional state after 439
  long-term results after 389
  psychological responses to exercise
    after 403
  psychosocial outcome after 457
heart valve replacement 19, 21, 47, 101
heart valve surgery 91
Heartmate 397
Hemopum 397
herpes viruses 374, 376
Holter 24-hour ambulatory ECG 298, 315
homesickness 330
homograft 9
Hospital Anxiety and Depression Scale
    180

identification of problems 187
immunosuppression 375, 508, 514, 521
  complications due to 392
immunosuppressive regimen 391
immunosuppressive therapy 372
impotence 512, 520
impulsive 330
infections 372, 374

in-patient psychopathology 84
insurance 509, 514, 520
intellectual dysfunction 141, 149
intelligence 327, 337
intercourse 326
intraaortic balloon pump (IABP) 397
intracardiac correction 253
irritability 450

job hunting 326
Joint Study on the Natural History of
    Congenital Heart Defects 296

Kuglers' criteria 299

late postoperative mortality 21
late survival 267
learning difficulties 330
left main stenosis 117
left ventricular assist device (LVAD)
    397, 520
left ventricular function 122
life 453
  -satisfaction 4
long-term follow-up 427
long term mortality 15
long-term outcome and psychological
    variables 457
lung compliance 304
lung function in children 303
lung volumes 304
lymphoproliferative process 376

malformations 383
  additional non-cardiac 384
malignancies 374, 376
marital relationship 483
marital therapy 512
maternal anxiety 326
mechanical prostheses 91
mechanical valve 10
medical rehabilitation 216
Medical Outcomes Study 4
mental function 71
methodological weaknesses 328
methylprednisolone 375
mitral valve insufficiency 14
mitral valve repair 13
mitral vs. aortic valve replacement 78
monoclonal antibodies 373
mood 158, 160
morbidity and mortality 389

mourning 510
Mustard repair 295
myocardial infarction 235
myocardial revascularization 107

National Heart Transplant Study 452, 520
Natural History Study 278
neuropsychologic complications 50, 189
neuropsychological assessment 155
neuropsychological deficits 156, 419
  prediction of 146
neuropsychological deterioration 143,
  144
neuropsychological dysfunction 49,
  147
neuropsychological performance 81
neuropsychological tests 41 , 155
neuropsychology 419
New York Heart Association (NYHA)
  398
  criteria 259
  Functional Classification 2
Newcastle CABG study 146, 151
nightmares 330
noncompliance 513, 514, 520
nonpharmacologic interventions 3
Nottingham Health Profile (NHP) 2, 428,
  432, 491, 512
nutritional status 508

occlusive coronary lesions 390
occupational rehabilitation 215
open heart surgery 419
operative mortality 21
operative techniques 72
organic mental syndromes 509
overcompensation 326
overprotection 326

pampering 326
Papworth Hospital 491
parental attitude towards the child 350
parents' organization 355
patient assessment 497
patient motivation 453
patient profiles 108
patient selection 519
pediatric heart transplantation 363, 371
perceived health status 2
personality disorders 513
PGWB 78
  anxiety 78

depression 78
health 78
self-control 78
vitality 78
well-being 78
physical retardation 325
pneumocystis 376
polyclonal antibodies 373, 376
possibility to speak with doctors 349
postoperative complications 446
postoperative employment, strategies for
  improving 209
postoperative neurologic complications
  48
postoperative psychosocial problems 441
postoperative recovery 187
postoperative treatment 103
pre-adolescent transplant 363
prediction 173
preoperative diagnosis 451
preoperative treatment 101, 103
presurgical psychological data 171
preventive care 2
professional education 342
Profile of Mood States (POMS) 73, 76,
  446
  depression 76
  fatigue 76
  irritability 76
  vigor 76
prostheses 19
prosthetic valve-related morbidity 22
psychiatric assessment 520
psychiatric problems 439, 509
psychiatric ratings 72
psychiatry 185
psychointellectual performance 315
psychological adjustment 71
  to illness scale (PAIS) 497
psychological evolution 172
psychological examination 335, 337
psychological factors 233
psychological status of patients 169
Psychological General Well-Being Index
  (PGWB) 73, 446, 449
psychology 160, 185
psychoneurological function 64
psychopathology 71, 193, 445
psychosocial aspects 28, 278, 325, 336,
  470, 471
psychosocial background measures 72
psychosocial development 335

psychosocial endpoints 71
psychosocial problems 335
psychosocial support 453
psychotherapeutic support 85
psychotherapy 510
pulmonary insufficiency 285
pulmonary stenosis 329
PW-CW-Color-Doppler study 315
pyschological adjustment 445

quality of life 1, 2, 4, 9, 133, 185, 227,
    363, 389, 442, 470, 501
  after heart transplantation 519
  after open heart surgery 507
  assessment 398
  before and after heart transplantation
    491
  global rating 79, 446
  multifactorial approach to 72
  social aspects of 206
  strategies to improve 507
  studies 297, 469
Quality of Well-Being Index 2, 278, 287
questionnaires 170

rage 326
recovery process 68
recurrent disease 123
rehabilitation 403
rehabilitation programmes, psychological
    benefits of 180
rehabilitative aspects 445
rehabilitative efforts 85
rejection episodes 372, 374, 376, 389
renal damage 374, 377
renal dysfunction 375
reoperation 15, 126, 269
retired vs. employed patients 451
retransplantation 391
return to work 2, 67, 71, 133, 203, 508
Rose Chest Pain Questionnaire 2
Rotterdam Follow-Up Study on Quality of
    Life 297, 299, 328

sample size 452
satisfaction with life 501
school 330
  attendance 377, 521
screening 521
selection criteria 508
self-assessment questionnaires 457
self-control 449

self-esteem 325
self reports 157, 159
semi-standardized interviews 194
Senning-type repair 295
separation anxieties 330
sexual dysfunction 514
sexual function 512, 520
sexual problems 512
sexuality 445
siblings 327
sick role 510
Sickness Impact Profile 2
side effects 514
  of medication 507
single vessel disease 119
SKF 81
  health locus of control 73, 81
sleeping difficulties 330
social activities 326
social aspects 327
social integration 270
social isolation 325
social problems 439
social support (SSF) 73
socialization 521
sociodemographic information 74
socioeconomic 282
Somerville's Ability Index 298
special education 329
Specific Activity Scale 2
Spielberger State-Trait Anxiety Scale
    194, 428, 432, 430
Stark's criteria 295
steroid medications 521
steroids 373, 374, 376, 508
stroke 93
subgroup analyses 453
subjective cognitive function, effect of
    205
subjective improvement 24
substance abuse 513
sudden death, fear of 326
support groups 510, 514
supportive psychotherapy 198
surgical intervention 101, 102
survival 117
survivor guilt 510
symptoms 116
syndromes 281
systemic hypertension 374, 375

teased children 330

technolgoy assessment 299
ten-item Affect-Balance Scale (ABS) 446
tetralogy of Fallot 277, 279, 294, 296,
    315, 329
thromboembolism 15
time-dependent changes 195
time span since transplantation 451
toxoplasm 376
transplantation
    healthiest candidates for 397
    long-term outcome after 457
transposition 279
    of great vessels (TGA) 267
treatment of specific problems 188
tricyclic antidepressants 510
triple vessel disease 121
two vessel disease 119

University of Minnesota Hosptial 253,
    254

valve and bypass patients, differences
    between 83
valve failure 91
valve sound 91
ventricular assist devices 397
ventricular function 279
ventricular septal defects (VSD) 253,
    278, 294, 296, 329
vigor 450
viral infections 374, 376
viruses 376
vitality 449
vocational counselling 509
vocational studies 285

waiting time 514, 521
Wechsler adult intelligence-scale 434
well-being 449, 470
withdrawal 326
women, surgical morality in 246

Developments in Cardiovascular Medicine

1. Ch.T. Lancée (ed.): *Echocardiology*. 1979 ISBN 90-247-2209-8
2. J. Baan, A.C. Arntzenius and E.L. Yellin (eds.): *Cardiac Dynamics*. 1980
   ISBN 90-247-2212-8
3. H.J.Th. Thalen and C.C. Meere (eds.): *Fundamentals of Cardiac Pacing*. 1979
   ISBN 90-247-2245-4
4. H.E. Kulbertus and H.J.J. Wellens (eds.): *Sudden Death*. 1980 ISBN 90-247-2290-X
5. L.S. Dreifus and A.N. Brest (eds.): *Clinical Applications of Cardiovascular Drugs*.
   1980 ISBN 90-247-2295-0
6. M.P. Spencer and J.M. Reid: *Cerebrovascular Evaluation with Doppler Ultrasound*.
   With contributions by E.C. Brockenbrough, R.S. Reneman, G.I. Thomas and D.L.
   Davis. 1981 ISBN 90-247-2384-1
7. D.P. Zipes, J.C. Bailey and V. Elharrar (eds.): *The Slow Inward Current and Cardiac
   Arrhythmias*. 1980 ISBN 90-247-2380-9
8. H. Kesteloot and J.V. Joossens (eds.): *Epidemiology of Arterial Blood Pressure*. 1980
   ISBN 90-247-2386-8
9. F.J.Th. Wackers (ed.): *Thallium-201 and Technetium-99m-Pyrophosphate. Myocardial Imaging in the Coronary Care Unit*. 1980 ISBN 90-247-2396-5
10. A. Maseri, C. Marchesi, S. Chierchia and M.G. Trivella (eds.): *Coronary Care Units*.
    Proceedings of a European Seminar, held in Pisa, Italy (1978). 1981
    ISBN 90-247-2456-2
11. J. Morganroth, E.N. Moore, L.S. Dreifus and E.L. Michelson (eds.): *The Evaluation of
    New Antiarrhythmic Drugs*. Proceedings of the First Symposium on New Drugs and
    Devices, held in Philadelphia, Pa., U.S.A. (1980). 1981 ISBN 90-247-2474-0
12. P. Alboni: *Intraventricular Conduction Disturbances*. 1981 ISBN 90-247-2483-X
13. H. Rijsterborgh (ed.): *Echocardiology*. 1981 ISBN 90-247-2491-0
14. G.S. Wagner (ed.): *Myocardial Infarction*. Measurement and Intervention. 1982
    ISBN 90-247-2513-5
15. R.S. Meltzer and J. Roelandt (eds.): *Contrast Echocardiography*. 1982
    ISBN 90-247-2531-3
16. A. Amery, R. Fagard, P. Lijnen and J. Staessen (eds.): *Hypertensive Cardiovascular
    Disease*. Pathophysiology and Treatment. 1982 IBSN 90-247-2534-8
17. L.N. Bouman and H.J. Jongsma (eds.): *Cardiac Rate and Rhythm*. Physiological,
    Morphological and Developmental Aspects. 1982 ISBN 90-247-2626-3
18. J. Morganroth and E.N. Moore (eds.): *The Evaluation of Beta Blocker and Calcium
    Antagonist Drugs*. Proceedings of the 2nd Symposium on New Drugs and Devices,
    held in Philadelphia, Pa., U.S.A. (1981). 1982 ISBN 90-247-2642-5
19. M.B. Rosenbaum and M.V. Elizari (eds.): *Frontiers of Cardiac Electrophysiology*.
    1983 ISBN 90-247-2663-8
20. J. Roelandt and P.G. Hugenholtz (eds.): *Long-term Ambulatory Electrocardiography*.
    1982 ISBN 90-247-2664-6
21. A.A.J. Adgey (ed.): *Acute Phase of Ischemic Heart Disease and Myocardial
    Infarction*. 1982 ISBN 90-247-2675-1
22. P. Hanrath, W. Bleifeld and J. Souquet (eds.): *Cardiovascular Diagnosis by
    Ultrasound*. Transesophageal, Computerized, Contrast, Doppler Echocardiography.
    1982 ISBN 90-247-2692-1

Developments in Cardiovascular Medicine

23. J. Roelandt (ed.): *The Practice of M-Mode and Two-dimensional Echocardiography.*
    1983   ISBN 90-247-2745-6
24. J. Meyer, P. Schweizer and R. Erbel (eds.): *Advances in Noninvasive Cardiology.*
    Ultrasound, Computed Tomography, Radioisotopes, Digital Angiography. 1983
                                                                     ISBN 0-89838-576-8
25. J. Morganroth and E.N. Moore (eds.): *Sudden Cardiac Death and Congestive Heart
    Failure.* Diagnosis and Treatment. Proceedings of the 3rd Symposium on New Drugs
    and Devices, held in Philadelphia, Pa., U.S.A. (1982). 1983   ISBN 0-89838-580-6
26. H.M. Perry Jr. (ed.): *Lifelong Management of Hypertension.* 1983
                                                                     ISBN 0-89838-582-2
27. E.A. Jaffe (ed.): *Biology of Endothelial Cells.* 1984   ISBN 0-89838-587-3
28. B. Surawicz, C.P. Reddy and E.N. Prystowsky (eds.): *Tachycardias.* 1984
                                                                     ISBN 0-89838-588-1
29. M.P. Spencer (ed.): *Cardiac Doppler Diagnosis.* Proceedings of a Symposium, held in
    Clearwater, Fla., U.S.A. (1983). 1983   ISBN 0-89838-591-1
30. H. Villarreal and M.P. Sambhi (eds.): *Topics in Pathophysiology of Hypertension.*
    1984   ISBN 0-89838-595-4
31. F.H. Messerli (ed.): *Cardiovascular Disease in the Elderly.* 1984
                                           Revised edition, 1988: see below under Volume 76
32. M.L. Simoons and J.H.C. Reiber (eds.): *Nuclear Imaging in Clinical Cardiology.*
    1984   ISBN 0-89838-599-7
33. H.E.D.J. ter Keurs and J.J. Schipperheyn (eds.): *Cardiac Left Ventricular Hyper-
    trophy.* 1983   ISBN 0-89838-612-8
34. N. Sperelakis (ed.): *Physiology and Pathology of the Heart.* 1984
                                           Revised edition, 1988: see below under Volume 90
35. F.H. Messerli (ed.): *Kidney in Essential Hypertension.* Proceedings of a Course, held
    in New Orleans, La., U.S.A. (1983). 1984   ISBN 0-89838-616-0
36. M.P. Sambhi (ed.): *Fundamental Fault in Hypertension.* 1984   ISBN 0-89838-638-1
37. C. Marchesi (ed.): *Ambulatory Monitoring.* Cardiovascular System and Allied
    Applications. Proceedings of a Workshop, held in Pisa, Italy (1983). 1984
                                                                     ISBN 0-89838-642-X
38. W. Kupper, R.N. MacAlpin and W. Bleifeld (eds.): *Coronary Tone in Ischemic Heart
    Disease.* 1984   ISBN 0-89838-646-2
39. N. Sperelakis and J.B. Caulfield (eds.): *Calcium Antagonists.* Mechanism of Action
    on Cardiac Muscle and Vascular Smooth Muscle. Proceedings of the 5th Annual
    Meeting of the American Section of the I.S.H.R., held in Hilton Head, S.C., U.S.A.
    (1983). 1984   ISBN 0-89838-655-1
40. Th. Godfraind, A.G. Herman and D. Wellens (eds.): *Calcium Entry Blockers in
    Cardiovascular and Cerebral Dysfunctions.* 1984   ISBN 0-89838-658-6
41. J. Morganroth and E.N. Moore (eds.): *Interventions in the Acute Phase of Myocardial
    Infarction.* Proceedings of the 4th Symposium on New Drugs and Devices, held in
    Philadelphia, Pa., U.S.A. (1983). 1984   ISBN 0-89838-659-4
42. F.L. Abel and W.H. Newman (eds.): *Functional Aspects of the Normal, Hyper-
    trophied and Failing Heart.* Proceedings of the 5th Annual Meeting of the American
    Section of the I.S.H.R., held in Hilton Head, S.C., U.S.A. (1983). 1984
                                                                     ISBN 0-89838-665-9

Developments in Cardiovascular Medicine

43. S. Sideman and R. Beyar (eds.): [3-D] *Simulation and Imaging of the Cardiac System.* State of the Heart. Proceedings of the International Henry Goldberg Workshop, held in Haifa, Israel (1984). 1985   ISBN 0-89838-687-X

44. E. van der Wall and K.I. Lie (eds.): *Recent Views on Hypertrophic Cardiomyopathy.* Proceedings of a Symposium, held in Groningen, The Netherlands (1984). 1985

     ISBN 0-89838-694-2

45. R.E. Beamish, P.K. Singal and N.S. Dhalla (eds.), *Stress and Heart Disease.* Proceedings of a International Symposium, held in Winnipeg, Canada, 1984 (Vol. 1). 1985   ISBN 0-89838-709-4

46. R.E. Beamish, V. Panagia and N.S. Dhalla (eds.): *Pathogenesis of Stress-induced Heart Disease.* Proceedings of a International Symposium, held in Winnipeg, Canada, 1984 (Vol. 2). 1985   ISBN 0-89838-710-8

47. J. Morganroth and E.N. Moore (eds.): *Cardiac Arrhythmias.* New Therapeutic Drugs and Devices. Proceedings of the 5th Symposium on New Drugs and Devices, held in Philadelphia, Pa., U.S.A. (1984). 1985   ISBN 0-89838-716-7

48. P. Mathes (ed.): *Secondary Prevention in Coronary Artery Disease and Myocardial Infarction.* 1985   ISBN 0-89838-736-1

49. H.L. Stone and W.B. Weglicki (eds.): *Pathobiology of Cardiovascular Injury.* Proceedings of the 6th Annual Meeting of the American Section of the I.S.H.R., held in Oklahoma City, Okla., U.S.A. (1984). 1985   ISBN 0-89838-743-4

50. J. Meyer, R. Erbel and H.J. Rupprecht (eds.): *Improvement of Myocardial Perfusion.* Thrombolysis, Angioplasty, Bypass Surgery. Proceedings of a Symposium, held in Mainz, F.R.G. (1984). 1985   ISBN 0-89838-748-5

51. J.H.C. Reiber, P.W. Serruys and C.J. Slager (eds.): *Quantitative Coronary and Left Ventricular Cineangiography.* Methodology and Clinical Applications. 1986

     ISBN 0-89838-760-4

52. R.H. Fagard and I.E. Bekaert (eds.): *Sports Cardiology.* Exercise in Health and Cardiovascular Disease. Proceedings from an International Conference, held in Knokke, Belgium (1985). 1986   ISBN 0-89838-782-5

53. J.H.C. Reiber and P.W. Serruys (eds.): *State of the Art in Quantitative Cornary Arteriography.* 1986   ISBN 0-89838-804-X

54. J. Roelandt (ed.): *Color Doppler Flow Imaging and Other Advances in Doppler Echocardiography.* 1986   ISBN 0-89838-806-6

55. E.E. van der Wall (ed.): *Noninvasive Imaging of Cardiac Metabolism.* Single Photon Scintigraphy, Positron Emission Tomography and Nuclear Magnetic Resonance. 1987   ISBN 0-89838-812-0

56. J. Liebman, R. Plonsey and Y. Rudy (eds.): *Pediatric and Fundamental Electrocardiography.* 1987   ISBN 0-89838-815-5

57. H.H. Hilger, V. Hombach and W.J. Rashkind (eds.), *Invasive Cardiovascular Therapy.* Proceedings of an International Symposium, held in Cologne, F.R.G. (1985). 1987   ISBN 0-89838-818-X

58. P.W. Serruys and G.T. Meester (eds.): *Coronary Angioplasty.* A Controlled Model for Ischemia. 1986   ISBN 0-89838-819-8

59. J.E. Tooke and L.H. Smaje (eds.): *Clinical Investigation of the Microcirculation.* Proceedings of an International Meeting, held in London, U.K. (1985). 1987

     ISBN 0-89838-833-3

Developments in Cardiovascular Medicine

60. R.Th. van Dam and A. van Oosterom (eds.): *Electrocardiographic Body Surface Mapping*. Proceedings of the 3rd International Symposium on B.S.M., held in Nijmegen, The Netherlands (1985). 1986   ISBN 0-89838-834-1

61. M.P. Spencer (ed.): *Ultrasonic Diagnosis of Cerebrovascular Disease*. Doppler Techniques and Pulse Echo Imaging. 1987   ISBN 0-89838-836-8

62. M.J. Legato (ed.): *The Stressed Heart*. 1987   ISBN 0-89838-849-X

63. M.E. Safar (ed.): *Arterial and Venous Systems in Essential Hypertension*. With Assistance of G.M. London, A.Ch. Simon and Y.A. Weiss. 1987

     ISBN 0-89838-857-0

64. J. Roelandt (ed.): *Digital Techniques in Echocardiography*. 1987

     ISBN 0-89838-861-9

65. N.S. Dhalla, P.K. Singal and R.E. Beamish (eds.): *Pathology of Heart Disease*. Proceedings of the 8th Annual Meeting of the American Section of the I.S.H.R., held in Winnipeg, Canada, 1986 (Vol. 1). 1987   ISBN 0-89838-864-3

66. N.S. Dhalla, G.N. Pierce and R.E. Beamish (eds.): *Heart Function and Metabolism*. Proceedings of the 8th Annual Meeting of the American Section of the I.S.H.R., held in Winnipeg, Canada, 1986 (Vol. 2). 1987   ISBN 0-89838-865-1

67. N.S. Dhalla, I.R. Innes and R.E. Beamish (eds.): *Myocardial Ischemia*. Proceedings of a Satellite Symposium of the 30th International Physiological Congress, held in Winnipeg, Canada (1986). 1987   ISBN 0-89838-866-X

68. R.E. Beamish, V. Panagia and N.S. Dhalla (eds.): *Pharmacological Aspects of Heart Disease*. Proceedings of an International Symposium, held in Winnipeg, Canada (1986). 1987   ISBN 0-89838-867-8

69. H.E.D.J. ter Keurs and J.V. Tyberg (eds.): *Mechanics of the Circulation*. Proceedings of a Satellite Symposium of the 30th International Physiological Congress, held in Banff, Alberta, Canada (1986). 1987   ISBN 0-89838-870-8

70. S. Sideman and R. Beyar (eds.): *Activation, Metabolism and Perfusion of the Heart*. Simulation and Experimental Models. Proceedings of the 3rd Henry Goldberg Workshop, held in Piscataway, N.J., U.S.A. (1986). 1987   ISBN 0-89838-871-6

71. E. Aliot and R. Lazzara (eds.): *Ventricular Tachycardias*. From Mechanism to Therapy. 1987   ISBN 0-89838-881-3

72. A. Schneeweiss and G. Schettler: *Cardiovascular Drug Therapoy in the Elderly*. 1988   ISBN 0-89838-883-X

73. J.V. Chapman and A. Sgalambro (eds.): *Basic Concepts in Doppler Echocardiography*. Methods of Clinical Applications based on a Multi-modality Doppler Approach. 1987   ISBN 0-89838-888-0

74. S. Chien, J. Dormandy, E. Ernst and A. Matrai (eds.): *Clinical Hemorheology*. Applications in Cardiovascular and Hematological Disease, Diabetes, Surgery and Gynecology. 1987   ISBN 0-89838-807-4

75. J. Morganroth and E.N. Moore (eds.): *Congestive Heart Failure*. Proceedings of the 7th Annual Symposium on New Drugs and Devices, held in Philadelphia, Pa., U.S.A. (1986). 1987   ISBN 0-89838-955-0

76. F.H. Messerli (ed.): *Cardiovascular Disease in the Elderly*. 2nd ed. 1988

     ISBN 0-89838-962-3

77. P.H. Heintzen and J.H. Bürsch (eds.): *Progress in Digital Angiocardiography*. 1988

     ISBN 0-89838-965-8

Developments in Cardiovascular Medicine

78. M.M. Scheinman (ed.): *Catheter Ablation of Cardiac Arrhythmias.* Basic Bioelectrical Effects and Clinical Indications. 1988   ISBN 0-89838-967-4

79. J.A.E. Spaan, A.V.G. Bruschke and A.C. Gittenberger-De Groot (eds.): *Coronary Circulation.* From Basic Mechanisms to Clinical Implications. 1987   ISBN 0-89838-978-X

80. C. Visser, G. Kan and R.S. Meltzer (eds.): *Echocardiography in Coronary Artery Disease.* 1988   ISBN 0-89838-979-8

81. A. Bayés de Luna, A. Betriu and G. Permanyer (eds.): *Therapeutics in Cardiology.* 1988   ISBN 0-89838-981-X

82. D.M. Mirvis (ed.): *Body Surface Electrocardiographic Mapping.* 1988   ISBN 0-89838-983-6

83. M.A. Konstam and J.M. Isner (eds.): *The Right Ventricle.* 1988   ISBN 0-89838-987-9

84. C.T. Kappagoda and P.V. Greenwood (eds.): *Long-term Management of Patients after Myocardial Infarction.* 1988   ISBN 0-89838-352-8

85. W.H. Gaasch and H.J. Levine (eds.): *Chronic Aortic Regurgitation.* 1988   ISBN 0-89838-364-1

86. P.K. Singal (ed.): *Oxygen Radicals in the Pathophysiology of Heart Disease.* 1988   ISBN 0-89838-375-7

87. J.H.C. Reiber and P.W. Serruys (eds.): *New Developments in Quantitative Coronary Arteriography.* 1988   ISBN 0-89838-377-3

88. J. Morganroth and E.N. Moore (eds.): *Silent Myocardial Ischemia.* Proceedings of the 8th Annual Symposium on New Drugs and Devices (1987). 1988   ISBN 0-89838-380-3

89. H.E.D.J. ter Keurs and M.I.M. Noble (eds.): *Starling's Law of the Heart Revisited.* 1988   ISBN 0-89838-382-X

90. N. Sperelakis (ed.): *Physiology and Pathophysiology of the Heart.* (Rev. ed.) 1988   ISBN 0-89838-388-9

91. J.W. de Jong (ed.): *Myocardial Energy Metabolism.* 1988   ISBN 0-89838-394-3

92. V. Hombach, H.H. Hilger and H.L. Kennedy (eds.): *Electrocardiography and Cardiac Drug Therapy.* Proceedings of an International Symposium, held in Cologne, F.R.G. (1987). 1988   ISBN 0-89838-395-1

93. H. Iwata, J.B. Lombardini and T. Segawa (eds.): *Taurine and the Heart.* 1988   ISBN 0-89838-396-X

94. M.R. Rosen and Y. Palti (eds.): *Lethal Arrhythmias Resulting from Myocardial Ischemia and Infarction.* Proceedings of the 2nd Rappaport Symposium, held in Haifa, Israel (1988). 1988   ISBN 0-89838-401-X

95. M. Iwase and I. Sotobata: *Clinical Echocardiography.* With a Foreword by M.P. Spencer. 1989   ISBN 0-7923-0004-1

96. I. Cikes (ed.): *Echocardiography in Cardiac Interventions.* 1989   ISBN 0-7923-0088-2

97. E. Rapaport (ed.): *Early Interventions in Acute Myocardial Infarction.* 1989   ISBN 0-7923-0175-7

98. M.E. Safar and F. Fouad-Tarazi (eds.): *The Heart in Hypertension.* A Tribute to Robert C. Tarazi (1925-1986). 1989   ISBN 0-7923-0197-8

99. S. Meerbaum and R. Meltzer (eds.): *Myocardial Contrast Two-dimensional Echocardiography.* 1989   ISBN 0-7923-0205-2

Developments in Cardiovascular Medicine

100. J. Morganroth and E.N. Moore (eds.): *Risk/Benefit Analysis for the Use and Approval of Thrombolytic, Antiarrhythmic, and Hypolipidemic Agents*. Proceedings of the 9th Annual Symposium on New Drugs and Devices (1988). 1989   ISBN 0-7923-0294-X

101. P.W. Serruys, R. Simon and K.J. Beatt (eds.): *PTCA - An Investigational Tool and a Non-operative Treatment of Acute Ischemia*. 1990   ISBN 0-7923-0346-6

102. I.S. Anand, P.I. Wahi and N.S. Dhalla (eds.): *Pathophysiology and Pharmacology of Heart Disease*. 1989   ISBN 0-7923-0367-9

103. G.S. Abela (ed.): *Lasers in Cardiovascular Medicine and Surgery*. Fundamentals and Technique. 1990   ISBN 0-7923-0440-3

104. H.M. Piper (ed.): *Pathophysiology of Severe Ischemic Myocardial Injury*. 1990
    ISBN 0-7923-0459-4

105. S.M. Teague (ed.): *Stress Doppler Echocardiography*. 1990   ISBN 0-7923-0499-3

106. P.R. Saxena, D.I. Wallis, W. Wouters and P. Bevan (eds.): *Cardiovascular Pharmacology of 5-Hydroxytryptamine*. Prospective Therapeutic Applications. 1990
    ISBN 0-7923-0502-7

107. A.P. Shepherd and P.A. Öberg (eds.): *Laser-Doppler Blood Flowmetry*. 1990
    ISBN 0-7923-0508-6

108. J. Soler-Soler, G. Permanyer-Miralda and J. Sagristà-Sauleda (eds.): *Pericardial Disease*. New Insights and Old Dilemmas. Preface by Ralph Shabetai. 1990
    ISBN 0-7923-0510-8

109. J.P.M. Hamer: *Practical Echocardiography in the Adult*. With Doppler and Color-Doppler Flow Imaging. 1990   ISBN 0-7923-0670-8

110. A. Bayés de Luna, P. Brugada, J. Cosin Aguilar and F. Navarro Lopez (eds.): *Sudden Cardiac Death*. 1991   ISBN 0-7923-0716-X

111. E. Andries and R. Stroobandt (eds.): *Hemodynamics in Daily Practice*. 1991
    ISBN 0-7923-0725-9

112. J. Morganroth and E.N. Moore (eds.): *Use and Approval of Antihypertensive Agents and Surrogate Endpoints for the Approval of Drugs affecting Antiarrhythmic Heart Failure and Hypolipidemia*. Proceedings of the 10th Annual Symposium on New Drugs and Devices (1989). 1990   ISBN 0-7923-0756-9

113. S. Iliceto, P. Rizzon and J.R.T.C. Roelandt (eds.): *Ultrasound in Coronary Artery Disease*. Present Role and Future Perspectives. 1990   ISBN 0-7923-0784-4

114. J.V. Chapman and G.R. Sutherland (eds.): *The Noninvasive Evaluation of Hemodynamics in Congenital Heart Disease*. Doppler Ultrasound Applications in the Adult and Pediatric Patient with Congenital Heart Disease. 1990
    ISBN 0-7923-0836-0

115. G.T. Meester and F. Pinciroli (eds.): *Databases for Cardiology*. 1991
    ISBN 0-7923-0886-7

116. B. Korecky and N.S. Dhalla (eds.): *Subcellular Basis of Contractile Failure*. 1990
    ISBN 0-7923-0890-5

117. J.H.C. Reiber and P.W. Serruys (eds.): *Quantitative Coronary Arteriography*. 1991
    ISBN 0-7923-0913-8

118. E. van der Wall and A. de Roos (eds.): *Magnetic Resonance Imaging in Coronary Artery Disease*. 1991   ISBN 0-7923-0940-5

119. V. Hombach, M. Kochs and A.J. Camm (eds.): *Interventional Techniques in Cardiovascular Medicine*. 1991   ISBN 0-7923-0956-1

Developments in Cardiovascular Medicine

120. R. Vos: *Drugs Looking for Diseases*. Innovative Drug Research and the Development of the Beta Blockers and the Calcium Antagonists. 1991   ISBN 0-7923-0968-5

121. S. Sideman, R. Beyar and A. G. Kleber (eds.): *Cardiac Electrophysiology, Circulation, and Transport*. Proceedings of the 7th Henry Goldberg Workshop (Berne, Switzerland, 1990). 1991   ISBN 0-7923-1145-0

122. D.M. Bers: *Excitation-Contraction Coupling and Cardiac Contractile Force*. 1991   ISBN 0-7923-1186-8

123. A.-M. Salmasi and A.N. Nicolaides (eds.): *Occult Atherosclerotic Disease*. Diagnosis, Assessment and Management. 1991   ISBN 0-7923-1188-4

124. J.A.E. Spaan: *Coronary Blood Flow*. Mechanics, Distribution, and Control. 1991   ISBN 0-7923-1210-4

125. R.W. Stout (ed.): *Diabetes and Atherosclerosis*. 1991   ISBN 0-7923-1310-0

126. A.G. Herman (ed.): *Antithrombotics*. Pathophysiological Rationale for Pharmacological Interventions. 1991   ISBN 0-7923-1413-1

127. N.H.J. Pijls: *Maximal Myocardial Perfusion as a Measure of the Functional Significance of Coronary Arteriogram*. From a Pathoanatomic to a Pathophysiologic Interpretation of the Coronary Arteriogram. 1991   ISBN 0-7923-1430-1

128. J.H.C. Reiber and E.E. v.d. Wall (eds.): *Cardiovascular Nuclear Medicine and MRI*. Quantitation and Clinical Applications. 1992   ISBN 0-7923-1467-0

129. E. Andries, P. Brugada and R. Stroobrandt (eds.): *How to Face 'the Faces' of Cardiac Pacing*. 1992   ISBN 0-7923-1528-6

130. M. Nagano, S. Mochizuki and N.S. Dhalla (eds.): *Cardiovascular Disease in Diabetes*. 1992   ISBN 0-7923-1554-5

131. P.W. Serruys, B.H. Strauss and S.B. King III (eds.): *Restenosis after Intervention with New Mechanical Devices*. 1992   ISBN 0-7923-1555-3

132. P.J. Walter (ed.): *Quality of Life after Open Heart Surgery*. 1992   ISBN 0-7923-1580-4

133. E.E. van der Wall, H. Sochor, A. Righetti and M.G. Niemeyer (eds.): *What is new in Cardiac Imaging?* SPECT, PET and MRI. 1992   ISBN 0-7923-1615-0

134. P. Hanrath, R. Uebis and W. Krebs (eds.): *Cardiovascular Imaging by Ultrasound*. 1992   ISBN 0-7923-1755-6

135. F.H. Messerli (ed.): *Cardiovascular Disease in the Elderly*. 3rd ed. 1992   ISBN 0-7923-1859-5

136. J. Hess and G.R. Sutherland (eds.): *Congenital Heart Disease in Adolescents and Adults*. 1992   ISBN 0-7923-1862-5

137. J.H.C. Reiber and P.W. Serruys (eds.): *Advances in Quantitative Coronary Arteriography*. 1992   ISBN 0-7923-1863-3

Previous volumes are still available

KLUWER ACADEMIC PUBLISHERS – DORDRECHT / BOSTON / LONDON

The manufacturer's authorised representative in the EU is Springer
Nature Customer Service Centre GmbH, Europaplatz 3, 69115 Heidelberg,
Germany. If you have any concerns regarding our products, please
contact ProductSafety@springernature.com

Printed and bound by CPI Group (UK) Ltd, Croydon, CR0 4YY

23/04/2026

02095625-0014